Dermatology

FOURTH EDITION

AN ILLUSTRATED COLOUR TEXT

Commissioning Editor: Timothy Horne
Development Editor: Ailsa Laing
Project Manager: Susan Stuart
Designer: Erik Bigland
Illustrator: David Graham
Illustration Manager: Gillian Richards

Dermatology

FOURTH EDITION

AN ILLUSTRATED COLOUR TEXT

David J. Gawkrodger MD FRCP FRCPE
Consultant Dermatologist and Honorary Professor of Dermatology
University of Sheffield
Royal Hallamshire Hospital
Sheffield
UK

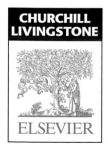

CHURCHILL LIVINGSTONE

ELSEVIER

EDINBURGH   LONDON   NEW YORK   OXFORD   PHILADELPHIA   ST LOUIS   SYDNEY   TORONTO   2008

CHURCHILL
LIVINGSTONE
ELSEVIER

© Longman Group UK 1992
© Pearson Professional 1997
© Elsevier Science Limited 2002. Reprinted 2003
© 2008, Elsevier Limited. All rights reserved

First edition 1992
Second edition 1997
Third edition 2002
Fourth edition 2008

ISBN: 978-0-443-10421-3

British Library Cataloguing in Publication Data
A catalogue record for this book is available from the British Library

Library of Congress Cataloging in Publication Data
A catalog record for this book is available from the Library of Congress

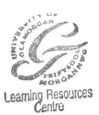

Printed in China

Preface to the fourth edition

Advances in medicine occur all the time and often in an unprecedented way. The manner in which clinicians practise changes almost on a day-to-day basis, and often we do not notice that we are doing things differently until we take stock of how we work. In the case of the common diseases, the philosophy of our practice can alter quite radically. One example is the higher degree of involvement of patients in deciding on their treatment (and taking some responsibility for it). Another is the detail given to patients regarding their diagnosis and prognosis. Yet another is the decline in the use of inpatient treatments for skin disease, resulting from economic pressures and patient expectation. What may seem quite normal to us these days in terms of medical practice would have been seen as strange or even incorrect 25 years ago. This is why a systematic and disciplined approach is needed when revising a textbook. To take account of such changes in the fourth edition has sometimes required the philosophical approach to the clinical problem to be altered and the text to be rewritten in a different light.

The use of technology increases all the time, not only in its accessibility and the amount of information available to physicians and patients through the Internet but also in the technological advances that allow clinicians to do more for patients. Traditionally, dermatology has been regarded as rather low-tech and has been seen by those who do not understand what it involves as merely the application of creams to conditions that do not get better. However, treatments in dermatology are moving ahead apace, with the increased use of biological agents in psoriasis and other diseases. The use of biological agents is likely to become more widespread over the coming years, and mention of this has been made in the text. The diagnostic skills of the dermatologist have been enhanced by the now widespread availability of dermoscopy, which is especially useful in differentiating pigmented lesions that are benign from those that may be malignant. The use of the dermoscope is included in a new section on practical clinical procedures.

Over the last decade, the range of surgical treatments undertaken by dermatologists, who have traditionally been regarded as physicians, has increased. This is partly an expansion of the role of the dermatologist as an 'organ specialist', but is also a response to the remarkable increase in skin cancer seen in western countries and the better definition of the correct surgical management of skin cancer. It is vital for all those who see patients with skin cancer to know what sort of surgical procedures are available. A new section outlines the advanced techniques practised by dermatological surgeons.

I hope that medical students, family practitioners, residents or specialist registrars in dermatology or general internal medicine and specialist nurses will find that the revisions made in this fourth edition keep them well informed on the current state of play in skin disease. I trust that the knowledge base is sufficiently up to date and detailed for them to practise clinically at the high level that all patients deserve.

Sheffield
2007

David J. Gawkrodger

Preface to the first edition

Recent advances in publishing technology and book presentation demand that a modern text be attractively and concisely presented, in colour and at an affordable price. This is essential for success in a very competitive market. In writing this book, I have attempted to present an introductory dermatology text for the 1990s, using a format of individually designed double-page spreads, generously illustrated with colour photographs, line drawings, tables, bulleted items and 'key point' summaries. This unique approach, which deals with each topic as an educational unit, allows the reader better accessibility to the facts and greater ease in revision than is possible with a conventional textbook.

The book is aimed at medical students but contains sufficient detail to be of use to family practitioners, physicians in internal medicine, registrars or residents in dermatology, and dermatological nurses. The contents are divided into three sections. The first presents a scientific basis for the understanding of and clinical approach to skin disease. The second details the major dermatological conditions, and the third outlines special topics, such as photoageing and dermatological surgery, that are of current importance or that are poorly dealt with in other textbooks.

Sheffield
1992

David J. Gawkrodger

Acknowledgements

In the production of the fourth edition of this book, it is a pleasure to acknowledge the contribution of the publishing staff at Elsevier Science, particularly Timothy Horne, commissioning editor, and Ailsa Laing, development editor. I am grateful to colleagues who have advised me on various aspects of the book, including Dr M.D. Talbot, of the Royal Hallamshire Hospital, Sheffield, and Dr S.M. Morley of the University of Dundee. Dr M. Liovic and colleagues from the Universities of Ljubljana, Wales, Uppsala and Dundee kindly permitted the use of the diagram of the keratin molecule (p. 8: published in *J Invest Dermatol* 2001: 116; 964–969, and reproduced with permission of Blackwell Publishing).

I thank colleagues who have generously provided figures for this and previous editions, including Dr E.C. Benton of Edinburgh, Dr J.E. Bothwell of Barnsley, Dr J.S.C. English of Nottingham, Dr J. Bowling of Oxford (for dermoscopy images), Dr F.M. Lewis of Slough, Dr S.M. Morley of Dundee, Dr M. Shah of Dewsbury, and Dr A.J.G. McDonagh, Dr H.S. Ghura, Dr A.G. Messenger, Dr C. Yeoman, Mr D. Dobbs, Professor S.S. Bleehen and Dr C.I. Harrington of Sheffield. Figure 2 (p. 28) is reproduced by permission of the British Medical Association (originally used in *ABC of Dermatology* by P.K. Buxton, 1988) and Figure 2 (p. 16) is reproduced by permission of Blackwell Publishing (originally used in *Clinical Dermatology* by J.A.A. Hunter, J.A. Savin and M.V. Dahl, 1989). Figure 4 (p. 117) is reproduced courtesy of the editor of the *British Journal of Dermatology* and previous editions, including and Dr E.F. Bernstein of Jefferson Medical College, Philadelphia, PA, USA. Figures 2 and 4 (pp. 134 and 135) are reproduced courtesy of Blackwell Publishing (having originally appeared in the *Textbook of Dermatology*, fifth edition, edited by R.H. Champion, J.L. Burton and F.J.G. Ebling, 1982).

I am grateful to the following for advice or for the provision of illustrations: Professor R.StC. Barnetson, Dr G.W. Beveridge, Dr P.K. Buxton, Dr G.B. Colver, the late Professor F.J.G. Ebling, Dr M.E. Kesseler, Dr C. McGibbon, Dr A. McMillan, Mrs E. McVittie, Dr C.StJ. O'Doherty, Miss M.J. Spencer and Dr A.E. Walker. I also thank those patients who gave permission for their faces to be shown without eyebars.

Contents

Basic Principles

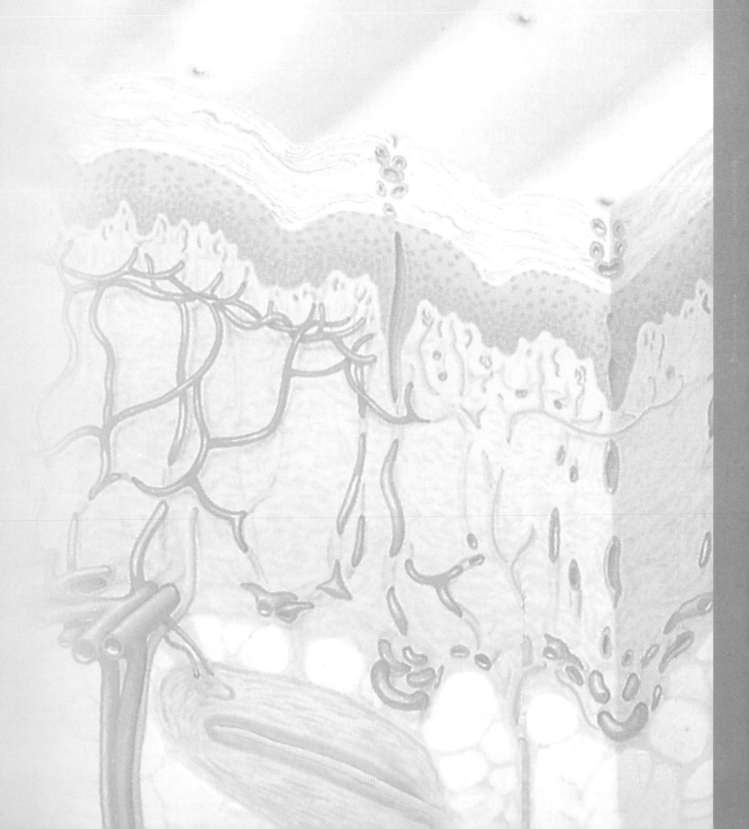

Microanatomy of the skin

Introduction

The skin is one of the largest organs in the body, having a surface area of 1.8 m² and making up about 16% of body weight. It has many functions, the most important of which is as a barrier to protect the body from noxious external factors and to keep the internal systems intact.

Skin is composed of three layers: the epidermis, the dermis and the subcutis (Fig. 1).

Epidermis

The epidermis is defined as a stratified squamous epithelium that is about 0.1 mm thick, although the thickness is greater (0.8–1.4 mm) on the palms and soles. Its prime function is to act as a protective barrier. The main cells of the epidermis are *keratinocytes*, which produce the protein keratin. The four layers of the epidermis (Fig. 2) represent the stages of maturation of keratin by keratinocytes (p. 6).

Basal cell layer (stratum basale)

The basal cell layer of the epidermis is composed mostly of keratinocytes, which are either dividing or non-dividing. The cells contain keratin tonofibrils (p. 6) and are secured to the basement membrane (Fig. 2) by hemidesmosomes. *Melanocytes* make up 5–10% of the basal cell population. These cells synthesize melanin (p. 8) and transfer it via dendritic processes to neighbouring keratinocytes. Melanocytes are most numerous on the face and other exposed sites, and are of neural crest origin. *Merkel cells* are also found, albeit infrequently, in the basal cell layer. These cells are closely associated with terminal filaments of cutaneous nerves and seem to have a role in sensation. Their cytoplasm contains neuropeptide granules, as well as neurofilaments and keratin. Basal keratinocytes synthesize antimicrobial peptides, important in defence against bacteria.

Prickle cell layer (stratum spinosum)

Daughter basal cells migrate upwards to form this layer of polyhedral cells, which are interconnected by desmosomes (the 'prickles' seen at light microscope level). Keratin tonofibrils form a supportive mesh in the cytoplasm of these cells. *Langerhans* cells are mostly found in this layer; these dendritic, immunologically active cells are described fully on page 10.

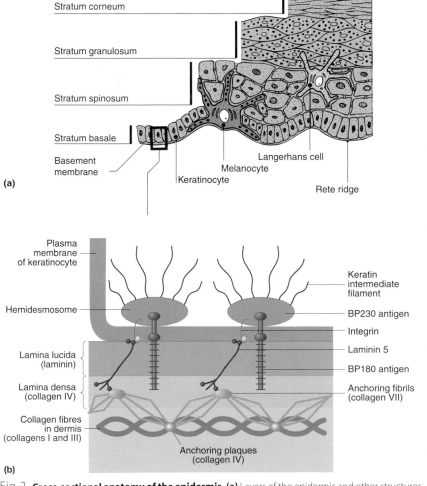

(a)

Stratum corneum
Stratum granulosum
Stratum spinosum
Stratum basale
Basement membrane

Langerhans cell
Melanocyte
Keratinocyte
Rete ridge

(b)

Plasma membrane of keratinocyte
Hemidesmosome
Lamina lucida (laminin)
Lamina densa (collagen IV)
Collagen fibres in dermis (collagens I and III)

Keratin intermediate filament
BP230 antigen
Integrin
Laminin 5
BP180 antigen
Anchoring fibrils (collagen VII)

Anchoring plaques (collagen IV)

Fig. 2 **Cross-sectional anatomy of the epidermis. (a)** Layers of the epidermis and other structures. **(b)** Detailed view of the basement membrane zone at the dermoepidermal junction. Components are arranged in three layers. The lamina lucida is traversed by filaments connecting the basal cells with the lamina densa, from which anchoring fibrils extend into the papillary dermis. These laminae are the sites of cleavage in certain bullous disorders (p. 82).

Fig. 1 **Structure of the skin.** The diagram shows a comparison between thick, hairless skin (plantar and planar) and thinner, hirsute skin.

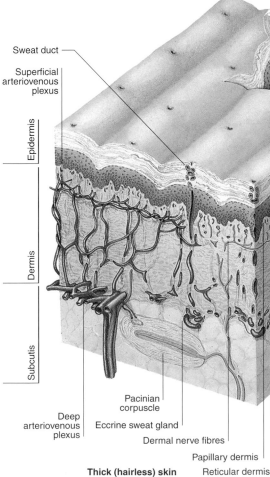

Sweat duct
Superficial arteriovenous plexus
Epidermis
Dermis
Subcutis

Deep arteriovenous plexus
Pacinian corpuscle
Eccrine sweat gland
Dermal nerve fibres
Papillary dermis
Thick (hairless) skin Reticular dermis

Embryology of the skin

The epidermis (ectoderm) begins to develop at 4 weeks of life, and, by 7 weeks, flat cells overlying the basal layer form the periderm (which is eventually cast off). Nails start to take shape at 10 weeks. The dermis (mesoderm) develops at 11 weeks, and, by 12 weeks, indented basal buds of the epidermis form the hair bulbs, with dermal papillae supplying vessels and nerves. Fingerprint ridges are determined by 17 weeks' gestation.

Granular cell layer (stratum granulosum)

Cells become flattened and lose their nuclei in the granular cell layer. Keratohyalin granules are seen in the cytoplasm together with membrane-coating granules (which expel their lipid contents into the intercellular spaces).

Horny layer (stratum corneum)

The end-result of keratinocyte maturation can be found in the horny layer, which is composed of sheets of overlapping polyhedral cornified cells with no nuclei (corneocytes). The layer is several cells thick on the palms and soles, but less thick elsewhere. The corneocyte cell envelope is broadened, and the cytoplasm is replaced by keratin tonofibrils in a matrix formed from the keratohyalin granules. Cells are stuck together by lipid glue that is partly derived from membrane-coating granules.

Dermis

The dermis is defined as a tough supportive connective tissue matrix, containing specialized structures, found immediately below and intimately connected with the epidermis. It varies in thickness, being thin (0.6 mm) on the eyelids and thicker (3 mm or more) on the back, palms and soles. The *papillary dermis* – the thin upper layer of the dermis – lies below and interdigitates with the epidermal rete ridges. It is composed of loosely interwoven collagen. Coarser and horizontally running bundles of collagen are found in the deeper and thicker *reticular dermis*.

Collagen fibres make up 70% of the dermis and impart a toughness and strength to the structure. *Elastin* fibres are loosely arranged in all directions in the dermis and provide elasticity to the skin. They are numerous near hair follicles and sweat glands, and less so in the papillary dermis. The *ground substance* of the dermis is a semisolid matrix of glycosaminoglycans (GAGs), which allows dermal structures some movement (p. 9).

The dermis contains fibroblasts (which synthesize collagen, elastin, other connective tissue and GAGs), dermal dendrocytes (dendritic cells with a probable immune function), mast cells, macrophages and lymphocytes.

Subcutaneous layer

The subcutis consists of loose connective tissue and fat (up to 3 cm thick on the abdomen).

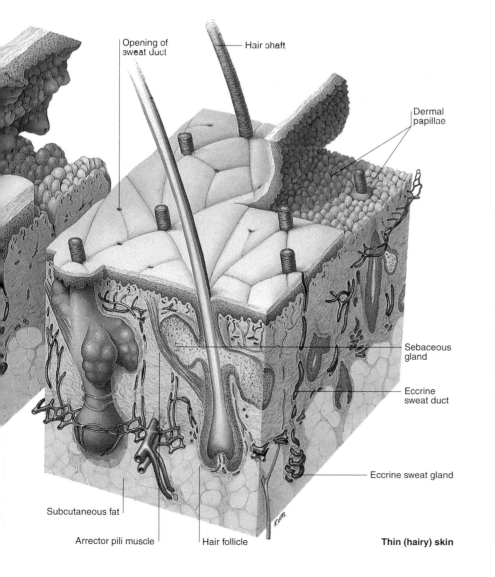

Opening of sweat duct — Hair shaft — Dermal papillae — Sebaceous gland — Eccrine sweat duct — Eccrine sweat gland — Subcutaneous fat — Arrector pili muscle — Hair follicle — **Thin (hairy) skin**

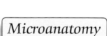

Microanatomy

- The skin constitutes 16% of body weight, with a surface area of 1.8 m².
- Structure and thickness vary with site.
- The epidermis is the outer covering, mainly composed of keratinocytes arranged in four layers, namely stratum corneum, stratum granulosum, stratum spinosum and stratum basale.
- The epidermis also contains melanocytes and Langerhans cells.
- The thickness of the epidermis varies from 0.1 mm to, on the palms and soles, 0.8–1.4 mm.
- The dermis is supportive connective tissue, mainly collagen, elastin and glycosaminoglycans. The thickness varies between 0.6 mm (e.g. eyelids) and 3 mm (e.g. back and soles).
- The dermis contains fibroblasts that synthesize the collagen, elastic fibres and glycosaminoglycans. Dermal dendritic cells are also found together with other immunocompetent cells.

Derivatives of the skin

Hair

Hairs are found over the entire surface of the skin, with the exception of the glabrous skin of the palms, soles, glans penis and vulval introitus. The density of follicles is greatest on the face. Embryologically, the hair follicle has an input from the epidermis, which is responsible for the matrix cells and the hair shaft, and the dermis, which contributes the papilla, with its blood vessels, and nerves.

There are three types of hair:

- *Lanugo* hairs are fine and long, and are formed in the fetus at 20 weeks' gestation. They are normally shed before birth, but may be seen in premature babies.
- *Vellus* hairs are the short, fine, light-coloured hairs that cover most body surfaces.
- *Terminal* hairs are longer, thicker and darker and are found on the scalp, eyebrows, eyelashes and also on the pubic, axillary and beard areas. They originate as vellus hair; differentiation is stimulated at puberty by androgens.

Structure

The hair follicle is an invagination of the epidermis containing a hair. The portion above the site of entry of the sebaceous duct is the infundibulum. The hair shaft consists of an *outer cuticle* that encloses a cortex of packed keratinocytes with (in terminal hairs) an *inner medulla* (Fig. 1). The germinative cells are in the hair bulb; associated with these cells are melanocytes, which synthesize pigment. The *arrector pili* muscle is vestigial in man; it contracts with cold, fear and emotion to erect the hair, producing 'goose pimples'.

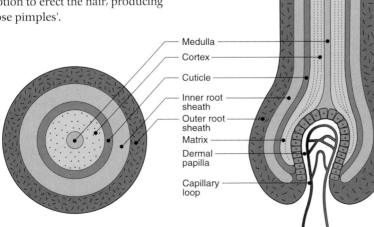

Medulla
Cortex
Cuticle
Inner root sheath
Outer root sheath
Matrix
Dermal papilla
Capillary loop

Fig. 1 **Structure of the hair follicle.**

Nails

The nail is a phylogenetic remnant of the mammalian claw and consists of a plate of hardened and densely packed keratin. It protects the finger tip and facilitates grasping and tactile sensitivity in the finger pulp.

Structure

The *nail matrix* contains dividing cells which mature, keratinize and move forward to form the *nail plate* (Fig. 2). The nail plate has a thickness of 0.3–0.5 mm and grows at a rate of 0.1 mm/24 h for the fingernail. Toenails grow more slowly. The *nail bed*, which produces small amounts of keratin, is adherent to the nail plate. The adjacent dermal capillaries produce the pink colour of the nail; the white lunula is the visible distal part of the matrix. The *hyponychium* is the thickened epidermis, which underlies the free margin of the nail.

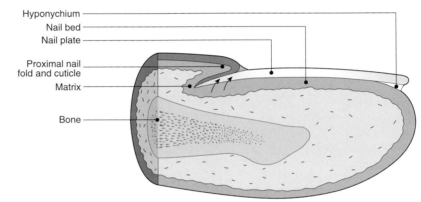

Hyponychium
Nail bed
Nail plate
Proximal nail fold and cuticle
Matrix
Bone

Fig. 2 **Structure of the fingernail.**

Sebaceous glands

Sebaceous glands are found associated with hair follicles (Fig. 3), especially those of the scalp, face, chest and back, and are not found on non-hairy skin. They are formed from epidermis-derived cells and produce an oily sebum, the function of which is uncertain. The glands are small in the child, but become large and active at puberty, being sensitive to androgens. Sebum is produced by holocrine secretion in which the cells disintegrate to release their lipid cytoplasm.

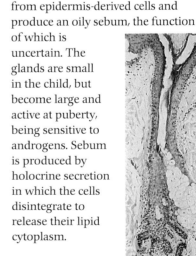
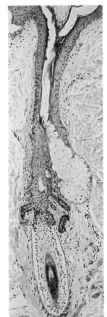
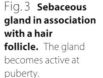

Fig. 3 **Sebaceous gland in association with a hair follicle.** The gland becomes active at puberty.

Sweat glands

Sweat glands (Fig. 4) are tube-like and coiled glands, located within the dermis, which produce a watery secretion. There are two separate types: eccrine and apocrine.

Eccrine

Eccrine sweat glands develop from downbudding of the epidermis. The secretory portion is a coiled structure in the deep reticular dermis; the excretory duct spirals upwards to open onto the skin surface. An estimated 2.5 million sweat ducts are present on the skin surface. They are universally distributed, but are most profuse on the palms, soles, axillae and forehead where the glands are under both psychological and thermal control (those elsewhere being under thermal control only). Eccrine sweat glands are innervated by sympathetic (cholinergic) nerve fibres.

Apocrine

Also derived from the epidermis, apocrine sweat glands open into hair follicles and are larger than eccrine glands. They are most numerous around the axillae, perineum and areolae. Their sweat is generated by 'decapitation' secretion of the gland's cells and is odourless when produced; an odour develops after skin bacteria have acted upon it. Sweating is controlled by sympathetic (adrenergic) innervation. The apocrine glands represent a phylogenetic remnant of the mammalian sexual scent gland.

Other structures in skin

Nerve supply

The skin is richly innervated (Fig. 5), with the highest density of nerves being found in areas such as the hands, face and genitalia. All nerves supplying the skin have their cell bodies in the dorsal root ganglia. Both myelinated and non-myelinated fibres are found. The nerves contain neuropeptides, e.g. substance P.

Free sensory nerve endings are seen in the dermis and also encroaching into the epidermis where they may abut onto *Merkel cells*. These nerve endings detect pain, itch and temperature. Specialized corpuscular receptors are distributed in the dermis, such as the *Pacinian corpuscle* (detecting pressure and vibration) and the touch-sensitive *Meissner's corpuscles*, which are mainly seen in the dermal papillae of the feet and hands.

Autonomic nerves supply the blood vessels, sweat glands and arrector pili muscles. The nerve supply is dermatomal with some overlap.

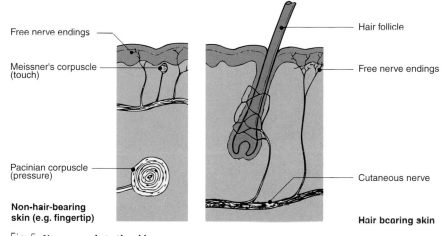

Free nerve endings
Meissner's corpuscle (touch)
Pacinian corpuscle (pressure)
Non-hair-bearing skin (e.g. fingertip)

Hair follicle
Free nerve endings
Cutaneous nerve
Hair bearing skin

Fig. 5 **Nerve supply to the skin.**

Blood and lymphatic vessels

The skin also has a rich and adaptive blood supply. Arteries in the subcutis branch upwards, forming a superficial plexus at the papillary/reticular dermal boundary. Branches extend to the dermal papillae (Fig. 6), each of which has a single loop of capillary vessels, one arterial and one venous. Veins drain from the venous side of this loop to form the mid-dermal and subcutaneous venous networks. In the reticular and papillary dermis, there are arteriovenous anastomoses that are well innervated and concerned with thermoregulation (see p. 7).

The lymphatic drainage of the skin is important, and abundant meshes of lymphatics originate in the papillae and assemble into larger vessels which ultimately drain into the regional lymph nodes.

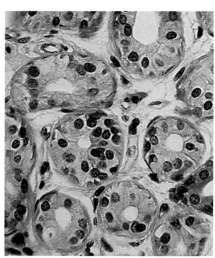

Fig. 4 **Sweat gland.** A cross-section through the coiled secretory portion of an eccrine sweat gland, situated deep in the dermis.

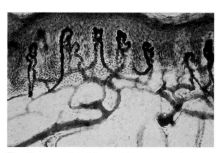

Fig. 6 **Superficial dermal blood vessels.** Capillary loops branch off the superficial vascular plexus and extend into each dermal papilla.

Derivatives

- Sebaceous glands, associated with hair follicles, are androgen sensitive.
- Vellus hairs cover most body surfaces; terminal hairs occur on the scalp, beard, axillary and pubic areas.
- Skin has extensive nerve networks with specialized nerve endings.
- Skin has a rich and adaptive blood supply; lymphatics drain to regional lymph nodes.
- Eccrine sweat glands, with sympathetic innervation, are under thermal/ psychological control; apocrine glands are largely vestigial in humans.

Physiology of the skin

The skin is a metabolically active organ with vital functions (Table 1), including the protection and homeostasis of the body.

Table 1 **Functions of skin**
Presents barrier to physical agents
Protects against mechanical injury
Antimicrobial peptides have a bactericidal effect
Prevents loss of body fluids
Reduces penetration of UV radiation
Helps to regulate body temperature
Acts as a sensory organ
Affords a surface for grip
Plays a role in vitamin D production
Acts as an outpost for immune surveillance
Cosmetic association

Keratinocyte maturation

The differentiation of basal cells into dead, but functionally important, corneocytes is a unique feature of the skin. The horny layer is important in preventing all manner of agents from entering the skin, including microorganisms, water and particulate matter. Antimicrobial peptides of the defensin and cathelicidin classes, present on the epidermal surface, have bactericidal activity. The epidermis also prevents the body's fluids from getting out.

Epidermal cells undergo the following sequence during keratinocyte maturation (Fig. 1).

1 Undifferentiated cells in the *basal layer* and the layer immediately above divide continuously. Half of these cells remain in place, and half progress upwards and differentiate.

2 In the *prickle cell layer*, cells change from being columnar to polygonal. Differentiating keratinocytes synthesize keratins, which aggregate to form tonofilaments. The *desmosomes* connecting keratinocytes are composed of the structural molecules cadherins, desmogleins and desmocollins. Desmosomes distribute structural stresses throughout the epidermis and maintain a distance of 20 nm between adjacent cells.

3 In the *granular layer*, enzymes induce degradation of nuclei and organelles. Keratohyalin granules containing filaggrin mature the keratin and provide an amorphous protein matrix for the tonofilaments. Membrane-coating granules attach to the cell membrane and release an impervious lipid containing cement, which contributes to cell adhesion and to the *horny layer* barrier.

4 In the *horny layer*, the dead, flattened corneocytes have developed thickened cornified envelopes containing involucrin, which encase a matrix of keratin macrofibres aligned by filaggrin. The strong disulphide bonds of the keratin provide strength to the stratum corneum, but the layer is also flexible and can absorb up to three times its own weight in water. However, if it dries out (i.e. water content falls below 10%), pliability fails.

5 The corneocytes are eventually shed from the skin surface after degradation of the lamellated lipid and loss of desmosomal intercellular connections.

Rate of maturation

Kinetic studies show that, on average, the dividing basal cells replicate every 200–400 h. The resultant differentiating cells in normal skin take 52–75 days to be shed from the stratum corneum. The epidermal transit time is considerably reduced in keratinization disorders such as psoriasis.

Hair growth

In most mammals, hair or fur plays an essential role in survival, especially in the conservation of heat; this is not the case in 'nude' humans. Scalp hair in humans does function as a protection against the cancer-inducing effects of ultraviolet (UV) radiation; it also protects against minor injury. However, the main role of hair in human society is as an organ of sexual attraction, and therein lies its importance to the cosmetics industry.

The rate of hair growth differs depending on the site. For example, eyebrow hair grows faster and has a shorter anagen (see below) than scalp hair. On average, there are about 100 000 hairs on the scalp, and the normal rate of growth is 0.4 mm/24 h. Hair growth is cyclical, with three phases, and is randomized for individual hairs, although synchronization does occur during pregnancy. The three phases of hair development (Fig. 2) are anagen, catagen and telogen.

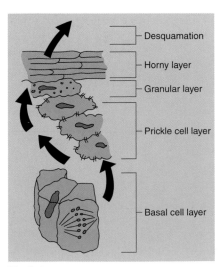

Fig. 1 **Keratinocyte maturation.**

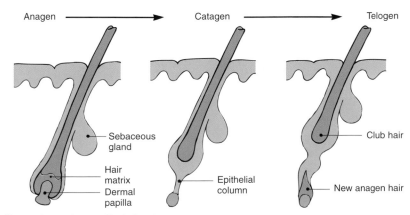

Fig. 2 **The three phases of hair development.**

1 *Anagen* is the growing phase. For scalp hair, this lasts from 3 to 7 years but, for eyebrow hair, it lasts only 4 months. At any one time, 80–90% of scalp hairs are in anagen, and about 50–100 scalp follicles switch to catagen per day.

2 *Catagen* is the resting phase and lasts 3–4 weeks. Hair protein synthesis stops, and the follicle retreats towards the surface. At any one time, 10–20% of scalp hairs are in catagen.

3 *Telogen* is the shedding phase, distinguished by the presence of hairs with a short club root. Each day 50–100 scalp hairs are shed, with less than 1% of hairs being in telogen at any one time.

Melanocyte function

Melanocytes (located in the basal layer) produce the pigment melanin in elongated, membrane-bound organelles known as melanosomes (Fig. 3). These are packaged into granules, which are moved down dendritic processes and transferred by phagocytosis to adjacent keratinocytes. Melanin granules form a protective cap over the outer part of keratinocyte nuclei in the inner layers of the epidermis. In the stratum corneum, they are uniformly distributed to form a UV-absorbing blanket, which reduces the amount of radiation penetrating the skin. Thickening of the epidermis also blocks UV.

UV radiation – mainly the wavelengths of 290–320 nm (UVB) – darkens the skin firstly by immediate photo-oxidation of preformed melanin and secondly over a period of days by stimulating melanocytes to produce more melanin. UV radiation also induces keratinocyte proliferation, resulting in thickening of the epidermis.

Variations in racial pigmentation result not from differences in melanocyte numbers, but in the number and size of melanosomes produced. Red-haired people have phaeomelanin, not the more usual eumelanin (p. 8), and their melanosomes are spherical rather than oblong.

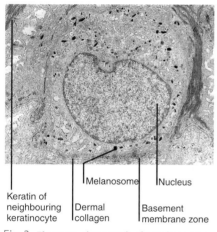

Fig. 3 **Electron micrograph of a melanocyte.**

Labels: Melanosome — Nucleus — Keratin of neighbouring keratinocyte — Dermal collagen — Basement membrane zone

Thermoregulation

The maintenance of a near-constant body core temperature of 37°C is a great advantage to humans, allowing a constancy to many biochemical reactions that would otherwise fluctuate widely with temperature changes. Thermoregulation depends on several factors, including metabolism and exercise, but the skin plays an important part in control through the evaporation of sweat and by direct heat loss from the surface.

Blood flow
Skin temperature is highly responsive to skin blood flow. Dilatation or contraction of the dermal blood vessels results in vast changes in blood flow, which can vary from 1 to 100 mL/min per 100 g of skin for the fingers and forearms. Arteriovenous anastomoses under the control of the sympathetic nervous system shunt blood to the superficial venous plexuses (Fig. 4), affecting skin temperature. Local factors, both chemical and physical, can also have an effect.

Sweat
The production of sweat cools the skin through evaporation. The minimum insensible perspiration per day is 0.5 L. Maximum daily secretion is 10 L, with a maximum output of about 2 L/h. Men sweat more than women.

Watery isotonic sweat, produced in the sweat gland, is modified in the excretory portion of the duct so that the fluid delivered to the skin surface has:

■ a pH of between 4 and 6.8
■ a low concentration of Na^+ (30–70 mEq/L) and Cl^- (30–70 mEq/L)
■ a high concentration of K^+ (up to 5 mEq/L), lactate (4–40 mEq/l), urea, ammonia and some amino acids.

Only small quantities of toxic substances are lost.

Sweating may also occur in response to emotion and after eating spicy food. In addition to thermoregulation, sweat also helps to maintain the hydration of the horny layer and improves grip on the palms and soles.

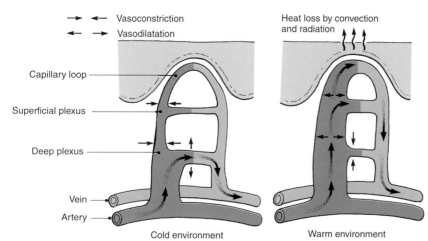

Fig. 4 **Variations in blood supply to the skin under cold and warm conditions.**

Labels: Vasoconstriction — Vasodilatation — Heat loss by convection and radiation — Capillary loop — Superficial plexus — Deep plexus — Vein — Artery — Cold environment — Warm environment

Physiology

■ Basal cell replication rate: once every 200–400 h.
■ Transepidermal cycle time: 52–75 days.
■ Growth rate for scalp hair: 0.4 mm/24 h.
■ Normal hair fall (scalp): 50–100/24 h.
■ Fingernail growth: 0.1 mm/24 h (toenail is less).
■ Skin blood flow is controlled by shunting at arteriovenous anastomoses.
■ Minimum insensitive perspiration: 0.5 L/24 h.

http://www.siumed.edu/~dking2/intro/skin.htm#regions

Biochemistry of the skin

The important molecules synthesized by the skin include keratin, melanin, collagen and glycosaminoglycans.

Keratins

Keratins are high-molecular-weight polypeptide chains produced by keratinocytes (Fig. 1). They are the major constituent of the stratum corneum, hair and nails. The stratum corneum comprises 65% keratin (along with 10% soluble protein, 10% amino acid, 10% lipid and 5% cell membrane).

Keratin proteins are of varying molecular weight (between 40 kDa and 67 kDa). Different keratins are found at each level of the epidermis, depending on the stage of differentiation. Epidermal keratin contains less cystine and more glycine than the harder hair keratin.

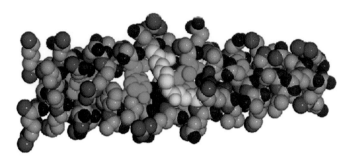

Fig. 1 **Molecular structure of alpha-keratin.** The molecule forms a helical coil which, if stretched, unwinds irreversibly to produce the beta form. The covalent bonds linking the cystine molecules provide extra strength.

Melanins

Melanin is produced from tyrosine (Fig. 2) in melanocytes and takes two forms:

- *eumelanin*, which is more common and gives a brown–black colour
- *phaeomelanin*, which is less common and produces a yellow or red colour.

Most natural melanins are mixtures of eumelanin and phaeomelanin. Melanins act as an energy sink and as free radical scavengers, and absorb the energy of ultraviolet (UV) radiation.

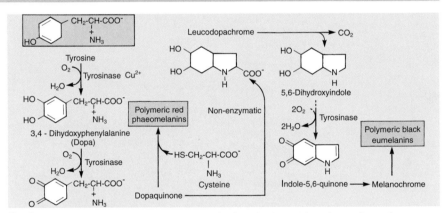

Fig. 2 **Biosynthesis of melanin.** Eumelanin is a high-molecular-weight polymer of complex structure formed by oxidative polymerization. The phaeomelanin polymer is synthesized from dopaquinone and cysteine (via cysteinyl dopa).

Collagens

Collagens are synthesized by fibroblasts (Fig. 3) and are the major structural proteins of the dermis, forming 70–80% of its dry weight. The main amino acids in collagens are glycine, proline and hydroxyproline. Collagens are broken down, e.g. in wound healing, by collagenases, of which the matrix metalloproteinases are important. There are over 22 types of collagen; at least five are found in skin:

- *type I* – found in the reticular dermis
- *type III* – found in the papillary dermis
- *types IV* and *VII* – found in the basement membrane structures
- *type VIII* – found in endothelial cells.

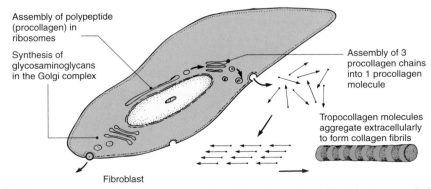

Fig. 3 **Collagen production.** Tropocollagen is formed from three polypeptide chains that are coiled around each other in a triple helix. Assembled collagen fibrils are 100 nm wide, with cross-striations visible with electron microscopy every 64 nm.

Glycosaminoglycans (GAG)

The 'ground substance' of skin is largely made up of GAGs, providing viscosity and hydration. In the dermis, chondroitin sulphate is the main GAG, along with dermatan sulphate and hyaluronan.

GAGs often exist as high-molecular-weight polymers with a protein core. These structures are known as *proteoglycans* (Fig. 4).

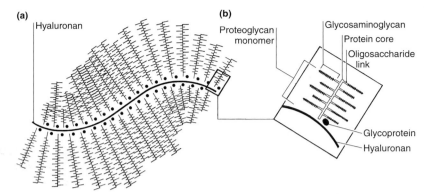

Fig. 4 **Proteoglycan. (a)** Proteoglycan aggregate with central filament of hyaluronan. **(b)** Detailed view of proteoglycan monomer with protein core.

Skin surface secretions

The skin surface has a slightly acidic pH (between 6 and 7). Sebum (Table 1), sweat and the horny layer (including intercellular lipid) contribute to the surface conditions, which generally discourage microbial proliferation.

Table 1 Sebum and epidermal lipid composition

Component	Sebum (%)	Epidermal lipid (%)
Glyceride/free fatty acid	58	65
Wax esters	26	0
Squalene	12	0
Cholesterol esters	3	15
Cholesterol	1	20

Subcutaneous fat

Triglyceride is synthesized from α-glycerophosphate and acyl coenzyme A (CoA). Triglyceride is broken down by lipase to give free fatty acid (FFA) – an energy source – and glycerol (Fig. 5).

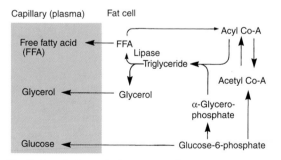

Fig. 5 **Metabolism of subcutaneous fat.**

HORMONES AND THE SKIN

The skin is the site of production of one hormone (vitamin D), but it is often a target organ for other hormones and is frequently affected in endocrine diseases.

Hormone	Site of production	Effects
Vitamin D	Produced in the dermis from precursors though the action of UV radiation	Important for the absorption of calcium and for calcification
Corticosteroids	Adrenal cortex	Receptors on several cells in both epidermis and dermis Produce vasoconstriction Reduce mitosis by basal cells Generate anti-inflammatory effects on leucocytes Inhibit phospholipase A
Androgens	Adrenal cortex Gonads	Receptors on hair follicles and sebaceous glands Stimulate terminal hair growth and increased output of sebum
Melanocyte-stimulating hormone (MSH) Adrenocorticotrophic hormone (ACTH)	Pituitary gland	Stimulates melanogenesis
Oestrogens	Adrenal cortex Ovaries	Stimulates melanogenesis
Epidermal growth factor (EGF)	Skin (probably produced at several sites in, as well as outside, the skin)	Receptors found on keratinocytes, hair follicles, sebaceous glands and sweat duct cells Stimulates differentiation Alters calcium metabolism
Cytokines and eicosanoids	Cell membrane (may be produced by several skin cells, including keratinocytes and lymphocytes)	Effects on immune function, inflammation and cell proliferation

Biochemistry

- **Keratins** are made up of polypeptide helical coils linked by covalent bonds. They form the horny layer, nails and hair.
- **Melanin** is a complex polymer synthesized from tyrosine. There are eu- and phaeo- types. Melanins absorb free radicals and energy including UV.
- **Collagens** are polypeptide polymers that constitute 75% of the dry weight of the dermis. They are synthesized by fibroblasts.
- **Glycosaminoglycans** make up the ground substance of skin. They provide viscosity and hydration, and can exist as high-molecular-weight polymers.
- **Vitamin D:** cutaneous UV activation produces the active form vitamin D3 from the inactive 7-dehydrocholesterol via the precursor previtamin D3.
- **Androgen receptors** in hair/sebaceous glands make these structures sensitive to the androgen surge of puberty.

Immunology of the skin

The skin is an important immunological organ and normally contains nearly all the elements of cellular immunity, with the exception of B cells. Much of the original research into immunology was done using the skin as a model.

Immunological components of skin

The immunological components of skin can be separated into structures, cells, functional systems and immunogenetics.

Structures

The epidermal barrier is an important example of innate immunity, as most microorganisms that have contact with the skin do not penetrate it. Equally, the generous blood and lymphatic supplies to the dermis are important channels through which immune cells can pass to or from their sites of action.

Cells

Langerhans cell

The Langerhans cells of the epidermis are the outermost sentinels of the cellular immune system (Fig. 1). They are dendritic, bone marrow-derived cells characterized ultrastructurally by a unique cytoplasmic organelle known as the *Birbeck granule*. Langerhans cells play an important role in antigen presentation. Dendritic cells are also seen in the dermis; these lack the Birbeck granule, but their other characteristics suggest that they too can present antigen.

T lymphocyte

T lymphocytes circulate through normal skin. Different types of T cell with differing functions are recognized, for example:

- *helper* (Th: facilitate immune reactions)
- *delayed hypersensitivity* (Th: specifically sensitized)
- *cytotoxic* (Tc: kill other cells)
- *suppressor* (Ts: regulate other lymphocytes).

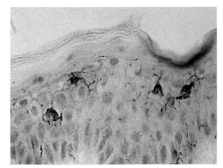

Fig. 1 **Langerhans cell.** The dendritic Langerhans cells form a network in the epidermis. In this section, the Langerhans cells have been stained with a monoclonal antibody to HLA-DR.

Surface receptors, detectable using monoclonal antibodies, help to categorize subgroups. Th cells are CD4 positive and may be divided into Th1 (promote inflammation, secrete interleukin (IL)-3, interferon-γ and tumour necrosis factor-β) and Th2 (stimulate B cells to produce antibodies, secrete IL-4, IL-6 and IL-10). Ts cells can probably be CD4 or CD8 positive. B lymphocytes are not found in normal skin, but are seen in some disease states.

Mast cell

Mast cells (which release histamine and other vasoactive molecules) are normal residents of the dermis, as are macrophages. Both may be recruited to the site during inflammatory reactions.

Keratinocyte

Keratinocytes may have an immunological function. They synthesize antimicrobial peptides, produce proinflammatory cytokines (especially IL-1) and express on their surface immune reactive molecules such as major histocompatibility complex (MHC) class II antigens (e.g. human leucocyte antigen (HLA)-DR) and intercellular adhesion molecules (notably ICAM-1).

Functional systems

Skin-associated lymphoid tissue

The skin, with its afferent blood supply, lymphatic drainage, regional lymph nodes, circulating lymphocytes and resident immune cells, can be viewed as forming a regulatory immunological unit.

Cytokines and eicosanoids

Cytokines are soluble molecules that mediate actions between cells. They are produced by T lymphocytes and sometimes by other skin cells, including Langerhans cells, keratinocytes, fibroblasts, endothelial cells and macrophages (Table 1). Certain cytokines activate the nuclear factor (NF)-κB cell signalling pathway, which regulates genes involved in inflammation. Eicosanoids are non-specific inflammatory mediators (e.g. prostaglandins, thromboxanes and leukotrienes), and are produced from

Table 1 **Some cytokines**		
Cytokine	**Source**	**Actions**
Interleukin (IL)-1	Langerhans cells, T cells, macrophages, keratinocytes	Enhances T-helper (Th) and B-cell proliferation, induces intercellular adhesion molecule (ICAM)-1, stimulates natural killer (NK) cells
IL-2	CD4 and CD8 T cells	Potentiates B cells, activates T cells
IL-10	T cells	Favours Th2 cells, inhibits Th1 cells
Interferon (IFN)-γ	T cells, NK cells	Inhibits Th2 cells, favours Th1 cell development

arachidonic acid by mast cells, macrophages and keratinocytes.

Complement

Activation of the complement cascade down either the classical or the alternative pathways results in molecules that have powerful effects. These include opsonization, lysis, mast cell degranulation, smooth muscle contraction and chemotaxis for neutrophils and macrophages.

Adhesion molecules

The adhesion molecules, particularly ICAM-1, are cell surface molecules found on lymphocytes and sometimes on endothelial cells and keratinocytes. By interacting with leucocyte functional antigens, they help to bind T cells and increase cell trafficking to the area.

Immunogenetics

The tissue type antigens of an individual are found in the MHC, located in man on the *HLA* gene cluster on chromosome 6. The MHC class II antigens, of which the commonest is HLA-DR, are expressed on B lymphocytes, Langerhans cells, some T cells, macrophages, endothelial cells and keratinocytes (in certain situations). They are vital for immunological recognition, but are also involved in transplant rejection.

In addition, the appearance of specific *HLA* genes is associated with an increased likelihood of certain diseases, some of which are 'autoimmune' in nature (Table 2).

Table 2	**Skin disease associations of HLA antigens**	
Disease	**HLA antigen**	**Relative risk**
Behçet's disease	B5	10
Dermatitis herpetiformis	B8	15
	DRw3	> 15
Pemphigus	DRw4	10
Psoriasis	B13	4
	Dw7	10
	Cw6	12
Psoriatic arthropathy	B27	10
	Bw38	9
Reiter's disease	B27	35

Hypersensitivity reactions and the skin

Hypersensitivity is the term applied when an adaptive immune response is inappropriate or exaggerated to the degree that tissue damage results. The skin can exhibit all the main types of hypersensitivity response.

Type I (immediate)

Allergen-specific immunoglobulin (Ig)E is bound to the surface of mast cells by Fc receptors. On encountering antigen (e.g. house dust mite, latex or pollen), the IgE molecules become cross-linked, producing degranulation and the release of inflammatory mediators. These include preformed mediators (such as histamine) and newly formed ones (e.g. prostaglandins or leukotrienes). The result in the skin is urticaria, although massive histamine release can cause anaphylaxis. The response occurs within minutes, although a delayed component is recognized. Factors other than IgE can cause mast cell degranulation.

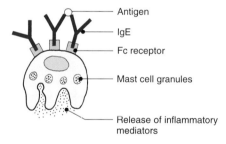

- Antigen
- IgE
- Fc receptor
- Mast cell granules
- Release of inflammatory mediators

Type II (antibody-dependent cytotoxicity)

IgG antibodies directed against an antigen on target skin cells or structures induce cytotoxicity by killer T cells or by complement activation. For example, IgG pemphigus antibodies directed against desmoglein on the keratinocyte surface result in activation of complement, attraction of effector cells and the lysis of the keratinocytes. Intraepidermal blisters result. Haemolytic anaemia and thyroid disease are other examples of type II hypersensitivity. Some of these conditions are 'autoimmune'.

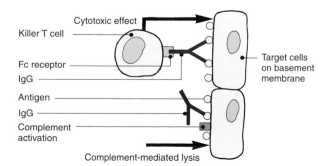

- Cytotoxic effect
- Killer T cell
- Fc receptor
- IgG
- Antigen
- IgG
- Complement activation
- Target cells on basement membrane
- Complement-mediated lysis

Type III (immune complex disease)

Immune complexes formed by the combination of antigen and IgG or IgM antibodies in the blood are deposited in the walls of small vessels, often those of the skin. Complement activation, platelet aggregation and the release of lysosomal enzymes from polymorphs cause vascular damage. This *leucocytoclastic vasculitis* is seen, for example, with systemic lupus erythematosus and dermatomyositis, but also occurs with microbial infections such as infective endocarditis. The 'Arthus reaction' is due to immune complex formation at a local site. It can be induced in the skin by an intradermal injection, and is maximal at 4–10 h after injection.

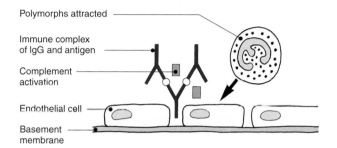

- Polymorphs attracted
- Immune complex of IgG and antigen
- Complement activation
- Endothelial cell
- Basement membrane

Type IV (cell mediated or delayed)

Specifically sensitized Th1 lymphocytes have secondary contact with the antigen when it is presented on the surface of antigen-presenting cells (APCs). Cytokine release produces T-cell activation and amplifies the reaction by recruiting other T-cells and macrophages to the site. Tissue damage results, which is maximal at 48–72 h. Allergic contact dermatitis (see p. 32) and the tuberculin reaction to intradermally administered antigen are both forms of type IV reaction. The responses to skin infections such as leprosy or tuberculosis are granulomatous variants of the reaction.

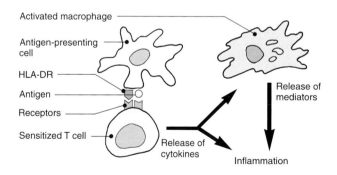

- Activated macrophage
- Antigen-presenting cell
- HLA-DR
- Antigen
- Receptors
- Sensitized T cell
- Release of cytokines
- Release of mediators
- Inflammation

Immunology

- Skin provides a physical barrier to infection and possesses antimicrobial peptides.

- Langerhans cells form outposts of the cellular immune system and can present antigens to immunocompetent cells, e.g. T lymphocytes.

- T cells circulate through normal skin and form part of the skin-associated lymphoid tissue. They are localized by adhesion molecules.

- Keratinocytes can be immunologically active cells.

- All four types of hypersensitivity reaction occur in the skin.

- Genetic factors modulate immunological responses. Certain HLA antigens are associated with increased risk of skin disease, e.g. HLA-DRw4 with pemphigus.

http://www.eucerin.co.uk/skin/physio_7.html

Molecular genetics and the skin

Recent and rapid advances in genetics have had an impact on our understanding of skin diseases. The Human Genome Project has now mapped all human genes, of which there are about 35 000. Genetics has been found to be more complicated than the original Mendelian concept, and common conditions such as atopy occur as a result of a complex interaction between multiple susceptibility genes and the environment. An average pregnancy carries a 1% risk of a single gene disease and a 0.5% risk of a chromosome disorder, but genetically influenced traits, e.g. atopy, are much more common.

The human chromosomes

The human genome comprises 23 pairs of chromosomes that are numbered by size (Fig. 1). Chromosomes are packets of genes with support proteins in a large complex. The karyotype is an individual's number of chromosomes plus their sex chromosome constitution, i.e. 46XX for females and 46XY for males. The phenotype is the expression at a biological level of the genotype, e.g. blue eyes or atopy.

Genes and DNA

A gene is a segment of deoxyribonucleic acid (DNA) that encodes for ribonucleic acid (RNA), which is translated into a protein. A DNA molecule is composed of multiple variable subunits of four nucleotides (two pyrimidines and two purines) on a pentose phosphate support structure. The bases pair in a consistent way: cytosine with guanine and thymine with adenine. The two DNA strands of the double helix are linked by hydrogen bonds between the complementary basepairs. RNA copies are made, and the order of the bases determines the amino acid content of the final protein.

The human genome contains about 35 000 genes. The mapping of disease-associated genes is often based on observing when two genes adjacent on a chromosome are inherited together (linkage) and using probes to identify markers, preferably in several members

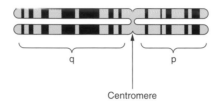

Fig. 1 Chromosome 2. Divided by the centromere into the shorter (p) and the longer (q) arms, showing banding with the Giemsa stain.

of an affected family. The sites of genes responsible for several diseases are now known.

Molecular methods

In the laboratory, DNA can be cut by restriction enzymes at specific sites, and DNA segments can be multiplied many times by the polymerase chain reaction (PCR). Fragments of DNA are identified according to size by gel electrophoresis (Fig. 2). Variations in the DNA sequence for a gene are called polymorphisms and are present in 2% of a stable population. Molecular techniques can be used to:

- detect small amounts of DNA, e.g. of human papilloma virus within a skin cancer
- amplify DNA from a 'candidate' section of an individual's chromosome and compare the base sequences with family members similarly affected by a disorder, thus mapping a specific gene polymorphism characteristic for that disease (Table 1).

Table 1 **Skin conditions or characteristics with definite or probable gene localities on the chromosomes**	
Chromosome site	**Disease or characteristic**
1p34	Porphyria cutanea tarda: enzyme (p. 44)
2q31	Ehlers–Danlos syndrome: collagen III (p. 91)
3p21.3	Dystrophic epidermolysis bullosa: collagen VII (p. 89)
4, 4p	Red hair colour, psoriasis (Psors3 gene)
6p21.3	Psoriasis (Psors1 gene: 30% of susceptibility)
9p21	Familial malignant melanoma: kinase inhibitor (p. 96)
9q22.3	Xeroderma pigmentosum (p. 91)
9q34	Tuberous sclerosis: hamartin (p. 90)
11q12	Atopy: asthma and rhinitis: IgE response (p. 34)
12q13	Epidermolysis bullosa simplex: keratin 5 (p. 89)
12q23	Darier's disease: adenosine triphosphatase (p. 88)
14q11.2	Ichthyosis: transglutaminase (p. 88)
15q11.2	Oculocutaneous albinism: homologue (p. 72)
17q11.2, 17q25	Neurofibromatosis NF1, psoriasis (Psors2)
17q21.31	Ehlers–Danlos syndrome: collagen I (p. 91)
19	Green/blue eye colour, brown hair colour
21 trisomy	Down syndrome (p. 91)
Xq28	Incontinentia pigmenti: nuclear factor (NF)-κB modulator (p. 91)
Xq22.32	X-linked ichthyosis: steroid sulphatase (p. 88)

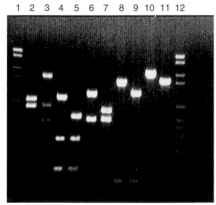

1 2 3 4 5 6 7 8 9 10 11 12

Fig. 2 Agarose gel electrophoresis, showing migration of DNA after cutting with enzymes, screening for mutations in a keratin gene.

Forms of inheritance

An individual with two different genes (alleles) at a particular locus is heterozygous, and one who has identical alleles is homozygous. Genes borne on chromosomes other than X and Y are autosomal, whereas those on X and Y are sex linked. Factors governing genetic penetrance are unclear. Heredity is complex and more than simply dominant or recessive.

- *Dominant.* Affected individuals (both sexes) are heterozygous for the gene, will have an affected parent (except

for new mutations) and have a 50% chance of passing it to their children (Fig. 3).
- *Recessive.* An affected individual (of either sex) is homozygous for the gene, and both parents will be carriers and healthy. Consanguinity increases the risk. Recessive disorders are often severe. There is a 25% chance of heterozygotes passing the gene to the next generation.
- *X-linked recessive.* Only affects males, as females are healthy carriers.
- *X-linked dominant.* Affects males and females, although some disorders, e.g. incontinentia pigmenti, are lethal in males.

- *Mosaicism.* In mosaicism, an individual has two or more genetically different cell lines. The somatic (post-conceptional) mutation of a single cell in an embryo results in a clone of subtly distinct cells. In the skin, this is revealed by the developmental growth pattern of Blaschko's lines (Fig. 4). Certain dermatoses, e.g. naevi and incontinentia pigmenti (Fig. 5), follow these lines, resulting in streaky or whorled patterns where the abnormal clone meets normal cells. A dermatomal distribution (Fig. 6) suggests nerve involvement.
- *Imprinting.* Imprinting involves the differential switching off of genes according to whether they have come from the father or the mother. It may be caused by methylation of DNA.

Inheritance of specific skin disorders

In psoriasis (p. 28) and atopic eczema (p. 34), a family history is common, but the exact mode of inheritance is unclear. Psoriasis may be inherited polygenically or by an autosomal dominant gene with incomplete penetrance. Paternal heredity seems to be more important than maternal. In contrast, in atopic eczema, maternal genes may have a predominant effect. An atopy gene is located on chromosome 11. Inheritance patterns in the rarer conditions are often clearer (Table 2). Epidermolysis bullosa simplex and dystrophica (p. 89), the porphyrias (p. 44), the Ehlers–Danlos syndromes (p. 91) and some other conditions may be dominantly or recessively inherited.

Some dermatoses are associated with polymorphisms in the human leucocyte antigen (HLA) complex on chromosome 6 (p. 11). These tend to show polygenic inheritance and an association with autoimmunity.

Gene therapy

DNA-based prenatal diagnosis is possible in several genodermatoses (p. 89). Recessive disorders in which there is a single gene defect, e.g. steroid sulphatase deficiency in X-linked ichthyosis or recessive epidermolysis bullosa due to a defect in collagen VII, offer scope for genetic treatment. Keratinocytes and fibroblasts are easily cultured, and a normal gene can be inserted into the cellular DNA. It remains to be seen whether this will work in practice.

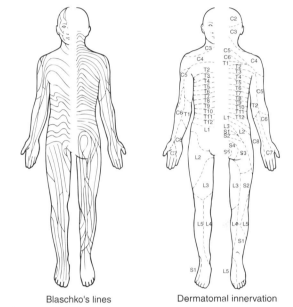

normal
carrier
affected

Fig. 3 **Autosomal dominant and recessive patterns of inheritance.**

Autosomal dominant   Autosomal recessive

Blaschko's lines   Dermatomal innervation

Fig. 4 **Blaschko's lines represent the growth trends of embryonic tissue, whereas the dermatomes map out areas of skin innervation.**

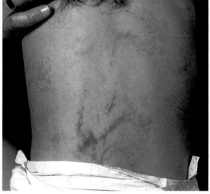

Fig. 5 **Incontinentia pigmenti.** Streaks and whorls follow the lines of Blaschko.

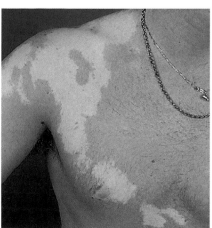

Fig. 6 **Segmental vitiligo.** Rather than follow Blaschko's lines, this occurs in a dermatomal distribution, suggesting a relationship with skin innervation.

Table 2 **The inheritance of selected skin disorders**

Inheritance	Disorder
Autosomal dominant	Darier's disease (p. 88)
	Dysplastic naevus syndrome (p. 97)
	Ichthyosis vulgaris (p. 88)
	Neurofibromatosis NF1 (p. 90)
	Palmoplantar keratoderma (p. 88)
	Peutz–Jeghers syndrome (p. 73)
	Tuberous sclerosis (p. 90)
Autosomal recessive	Acrodermatitis enteropathica (p. 83)
	Non-bullous ichthyosiform erythroderma (p. 88)
	Phenylketonuria (p. 82)
	Pseudoxanthoma elasticum (p. 91)
	Xeroderma pigmentosum (p. 91)
X-linked recessive	X-linked ichthyosis (p. 88)
X-linked	Incontinentia pigmenti (p. 91)

Molecular genetics and the skin

- The human genome of 23 chromosomes (karyotype 46XY or 46XX) contains 35 000 genes, all of which have been mapped. Additionally, mitochondria code 37 genes for oxidative enzymes.
- DNA segments can be amplified by PCR and demonstrated by gel electrophoresis.
- The chromosomal location of the marker gene has been mapped for several skin diseases.
- Dominant, recessive and X-linked inheritances are seen, but heredity is still unclear in several disorders.
- A dermatosis caused by mosaicism, due to a mutation producing more than one cell line, may appear in Blaschko's lines.
- Gene therapy should be possible for some recessive single gene disorders.

http://www.ncbi.nlm.nih.gov/entrez/query.fcgi?db=OMIM

Terminology of skin lesions

Dermatology has a vocabulary that is quite distinct from other medical specialties and without which it is impossible to describe skin disorders. A *lesion* is a general term for an area of disease, usually small. An *eruption* (or *rash*) is a more widespread skin involvement, normally composed of several lesions, which may be the primary pathology (e.g. papules, vesicles or pustules) or due to secondary factors such as scratching or infection (e.g. crusting, lichenification or ulceration).

   Below is a selection of other commonly encountered dermatological terms.

Macule

A macule is a localized area of colour or textural change in the skin. Macules can be hypopigmented, as in vitiligo; pigmented, as in a freckle (**a**); or erythematous, as in a capillary haemangioma (**b**).

Papule

A papule is a small solid elevation of the skin, generally defined as less than 5 mm in diameter. Papules may be flat topped, as in lichen planus; dome shaped, as in xanthomas; or spicular if related to hair follicles.

Nodule

Similar to a papule but larger (i.e. greater than 5 mm in diameter), nodules can involve any layer of the skin and can be oedematous or solid. Examples include a dermatofibroma (below) and secondary deposits.

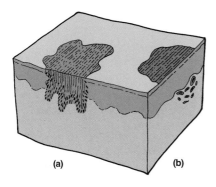

(a)   (b)

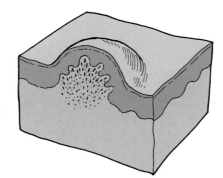

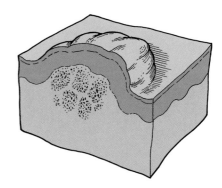

Bulla

A bulla is similar to a vesicle but larger: greater than 5 mm in diameter. The blisters of bullous pemphigoid (**a**) and pemphigus vulgaris (p. 76) are examples.

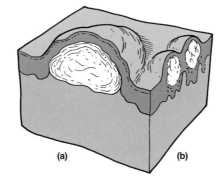

(a)   (b)

Vesicle

A vesicle is a small blister (less than 5 mm in diameter) consisting of clear fluid accumulated within or below the epidermis. Vesicles may be grouped as in dermatitis herpetiformis (subepidermal). Intraepidermal vesicles are shown in the figure left (**b**).

Glossary of other dermatological terms

- **Abscess:** A localized collection of pus formed by necrosis of tissue.
- **Alopecia:** Absence of hair from a normally hairy area.
- **Atrophy:** Loss of epidermis, dermis or both. Atrophic skin is thin, translucent and wrinkled with easily visible blood vessels.
- **Burrow:** A tunnel in the skin caused by a parasite, particularly the acarus of scabies.
- **Callus:** Local hyperplasia of the horny layer, often of the palm or sole, due to pressure.
- **Carbuncle:** A collection of boils (furuncles) causing necrosis in the skin and subcutaneous tissues.
- **Cellulitis:** A purulent inflammation of the skin and subcutaneous tissue.
- **Comedo:** A plug of sebum and keratin in the dilated orifice of a pilosebaceous gland.

- **Crust:** Dried exudate (normally serum, blood or pus) on the skin surface.
- **Ecchymosis:** A macular red or purple haemorrhage, more than 2 mm in diameter, in the skin or mucous membrane.
- **Erosion:** A superficial break in the epidermis, not extending into the dermis, which heals without scarring.
- **Erythema:** Redness of the skin due to vascular dilatation.
- **Excoriation:** A superficial abrasion, often linear, which results from scratching.
- **Fissure:** A linear split in the epidermis, often just extending into the dermis.
- **Folliculitis:** An inflammation of the hair follicles.
- **Freckle:** A macular area in which there is increased pigment formation by melanocytes.

Pustule

A pustule is a visible collection of free pus in a blister. Pustules may indicate infection (e.g. a furuncle), but not always, as pustules seen in psoriasis, for example, are not infected.

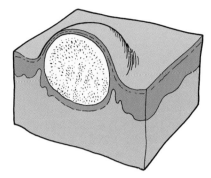

Cyst

A cyst is a nodule consisting of an epithelial-lined cavity filled with fluid or semisolid material. An epidermal ('sebaceous') cyst is shown below.

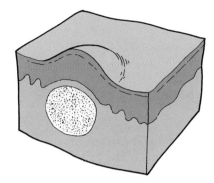

Wheal

A wheal is a transitory, compressible papule or plaque of dermal oedema, red or white in colour and usually signifying urticaria.

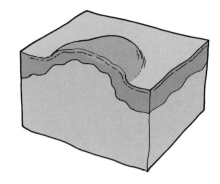

Plaque

A plaque is a palpable, plateau-like elevation of skin, usually more than 2 cm in diameter. Plaques are rarely more than 5 mm in height and can be considered as extended papules. Certain lesions of psoriasis (below) and mycosis fungoides are good examples.

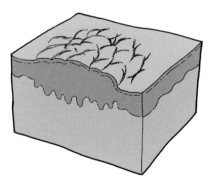

Scale

A scale is an accumulation of thickened, horny layer keratin in the form of readily detached fragments. Scales usually indicate inflammatory change and thickening of the epidermis. They may be fine, as in 'pityriasis'; white and silvery, as in psoriasis (below); or large and fish like, as seen in ichthyosis.

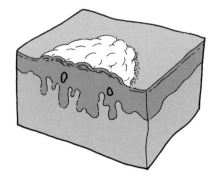

Ulcer

An ulcer is a circumscribed area of skin loss extending through the epidermis into the dermis. Ulcers are usually the result of impairment of the vascular or nutrient supply to the skin, e.g. as a result of peripheral arterial disease.

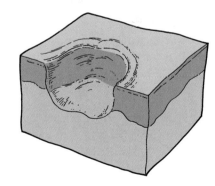

Glossary of other dermatological terms

- **Furuncle:** A pyogenic infection localized in a hair follicle.
- **Hirsuties:** Excessive male pattern hair growth.
- **Hypertrichosis:** Excessive hair growth in a non-androgenic pattern.
- **Keloid:** An elevated and progressive scar not showing regression.
- **Keratosis:** A horn-like thickening of the skin.
- **Lichenification:** Chronic thickening of the skin with increased skin markings, as a result of rubbing or scratching.
- **Milium:** A small white cyst containing keratin.
- **Papilloma:** A nipple-like projection from the skin surface.
- **Petechia:** A haemorrhagic punctuate spot measuring 1–2 mm in diameter.

- **Poikiloderma:** A combination of hyperpigmentation, telangiectasia and atrophy seen together in a dermatosis.
- **Purpura:** Extravasation of blood resulting in red discoloration of the skin or mucous membranes.
- **Scar:** The replacement of normal tissue by fibrous connective tissue at the site of an injury.
- **Stria:** An atrophic linear band in the skin – white, pink or purple in colour. The result of connective tissue changes.
- **Telangiectasia:** Dilated dermal blood vessels giving rise to a visible lesion.

Taking a history

The truism that 'there is no substitute for a good history' is just as applicable in dermatology as in any other branch of medicine. The time needed to take a history depends on the complaint. For example, the history in a patient with hand warts can usually be completed quickly, but more time and detailed questioning are required for the patient with generalized itching.

History taking in dermatology can be divided into four basic investigations: the presenting complaint, past medical history, social and family history, and drug history.

Presenting complaint

Before any diagnosis, it is essential to find out when, where and how the problem started, what the initial lesions looked like and how they evolved and extended. Symptoms, particularly itching, the prime dermatological complaint, must be recorded along with any aggravating or exacerbating factors, such as sunlight. It is useful to gauge the effect of the eruption on the patient's ability to perform everyday tasks. For chronic conditions, it is helpful to assess the effect on the patient's quality of life and mental well-being. Specific scoring systems can record these effects.

Case history 1

An 18-year-old male bank clerk developed a scaly erythematous plaque on the left elbow (Fig. 1) 6 months before presentation. It spread to involve the other elbow and both knees, but was not itchy. He developed scaliness in the scalp and nail dystrophy. His mother once had a similar rash.

Diagnosis: psoriasis (p. 28).

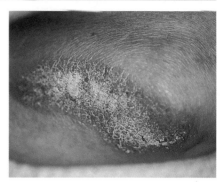

Fig. 1 **Psoriasis plaque on elbow.**

Past medical history

Patients must be asked about any previous skin disease or atopic symptoms, such as hay fever, asthma or childhood eczema. Internal medical disorders may be relevant; these can involve the skin directly or may be associated with certain skin diseases. Prescribed or self-administered drugs may also cause an eruption. Dietary history is occasionally important, e.g. in some patients with atopic eczema (p. 34), but diet is often erroneously blamed for skin disease.

Case history 2

A 29-year-old woman was referred from the department of respiratory medicine where she had recently been diagnosed as having pulmonary sarcoidosis. Three weeks previously, she had developed tender, warm erythematous nodules (Fig. 2) on the shins. She was on no medication. An incisional biopsy confirmed the clinical impression.

Diagnosis: erythema nodosum (p. 81).

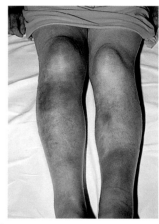

Fig. 2 **Erythema nodosum on the lower legs.**

Social and occupational history

Many social factors can cause or influence a patient's skin complaint. Occupational factors can induce contact dermatitis or other skin changes, and it is often necessary to ask the patient to explain exactly what he or she does. If the eruption improves when the patient is away from work, occupational factors should be suspected. Hobbies may also involve contact with objects or chemicals that could produce contact dermatitis.

Knowledge of the patient's living conditions and home background can be helpful in understanding a problem and deciding on treatment. Alcohol intake should be noted (especially if the use of potentially hepatotoxic drugs is being considered), as well as other factors. Living or travelling in warm climates potentially exposes an individual to a wide range of tropical and subtropical infections, and to strong sunlight.

Case history 3

A 45-year-old male printer engineer gave a 6-month history of hand dermatitis (Fig. 3). A few months previously, he had started to use the solvent trichloroethylene in his job. Patch testing was negative. On substituting a different solvent, the eruption cleared.

Diagnosis: irritant contact dermatitis (p. 32).

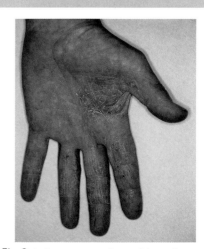

Fig. 3 **Irritant contact dermatitis on the palm of the hand.**

Family history

A full family history is essential. Some disorders with prominent skin signs are genetically inherited, e.g. tuberous sclerosis. Others, such as psoriasis or atopic eczema, have a strong hereditary component. In addition to genetic syndromes, a family history may reveal that other family members have had a recent onset of an eruption similar to that of the patient, suggesting an infection or infestation. It is sometimes also necessary to enquire about sexual contacts.

Case history 4

An 18-year-old male student gave a 3-month history of an intensely itchy papular eruption affecting the hands, wrists and penis (Table 1). Several lesions were excoriated (Fig. 4). Treatment with a potent topical steroid was of little benefit. His girlfriend had also recently developed itchy lesions. Close examination showed burrows in the skin.

Diagnosis: scabies (p. 61).

Case history 5

A 25-year-old female shop assistant complained of brownish macules over her back (Fig. 5) and chest, which had first appeared in childhood and had gradually increased in number and size. During her teens, she had developed several soft pinkish, painless nodules on the trunk, some of which had become pedunculated. Her father had developed a few similar nodules in later life, and one of her two brothers had brown patches on his skin.

Diagnosis: von Recklinghausen's neurofibromatosis (NF-1; p. 90).

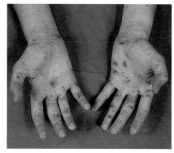
Fig. 4 **Excoriated lesions of scabies.**

Table 1 **Itchy eruption: diagnosis**	
Symptom	**Intensely itchy eruption**
Possible diagnosis	Scabies
	Lichen planus
	Dermatitis herpetiformis
	Urticaria
	Eczema
	Insect bites

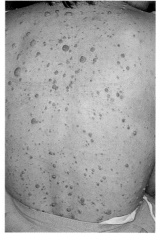
Fig. 5 **Multiple neurofibromas on the back.**

Drug history

Both prescribed and self-administered medicaments can result in a 'drug eruption'. Almost all patients try an over-the-counter topical preparation (or a friend or relative's ointment) on rashes, and many have had a variety of treatments prescribed that may be inappropriate or may cause irritant or allergic reactions. It is important to quiz the patient about all medicament use, including the use of over-the-counter tablets or creams that the patient may well not think relevant.

Cosmetics, cleansing wipes and moisturizing creams can cause dermatitis, and it is often necessary to ask specifically about their use.

Case history 6

A 68-year-old woman had a minor irritating eruption on her forehead. She applied an antihistamine-containing cream that she bought in a pharmacy. Within 24 h of applying it, her face became severely swollen (Fig. 6). Patch testing carried out later showed an allergic reaction to the cream.

Diagnosis: medicament dermatitis (p. 33).

Case history 7

An 18-year-old female secretary was given griseofulvin for a fungal infection. She went sunbathing and, 12 h later, developed an eruption with a distribution in light-exposed areas (Fig. 7).

Diagnosis: phototoxic drug eruption (p. 45).

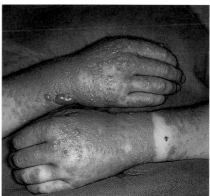
Fig. 7 **Acute phototoxic drug eruption.**

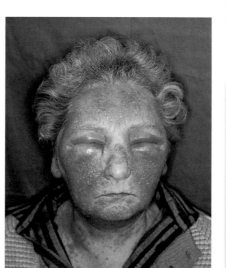
Fig. 6 **Acute allergic contact dermatitis to a topical antihistamine cream.**

Taking a history

- Elicit the nature and temporal course of the eruption or lesion.
- Enquire about atopic symptoms, general medical conditions and foreign travel.
- Take a social, occupational and family history – it may be relevant. Ask about eczema or psoriasis in relatives.
- Identify any impairment of the illness on day-to-day functions.
- Record the recent use of drugs and medications, including topical agents.
- Ask about the use of cosmetics and, in relevant cases, exposure to sun or ultraviolet radiation (e.g. sunbeds).

Examining the skin

The skin needs to be examined in good, preferably natural, light. The whole of the skin should be examined, ideally; this is essential for atypical or widespread eruptions (Fig. 1). Looking at the whole skin often reveals diagnostic lesions that the patient is unaware of or may think unimportant. In the elderly, thorough skin examination often allows the early detection of unexpected but treatable skin cancers.

Skin examination is difficult for the non-dermatologist, and the novice needs a pattern to follow. It is important to:

- note the distribution and colour of the lesions
- examine the morphology of individual lesions, their size, shape, border changes and spatial relationship;

touch the skin – palpation reveals the consistency of a lesion
- assess the nails, hair and mucous membranes, sometimes in combination with a general examination (e.g. for lymphadenopathy)
- wear gloves when examining the mouth, genitals and perineum or if lesions may be infected
- use special techniques, e.g. dermoscopy, microscopy of scrapings to look for fungal elements, or the use of Wood's (ultraviolet) light, where applicable.

Distribution

Stand back from the patient and observe the pattern of the eruption (Fig. 1). Determine whether it is localized (e.g. a tumour) or widespread (e.g. a rash). If the latter, determine whether the eruption is symmetrical and, if so, peripheral or central. Note whether it involves the flexures (e.g. atopic eczema) or the extensor aspects (e.g. psoriasis). Is it limited to sun-exposed areas? Is it linear?

Dermatomal patterns are also seen. Herpes zoster (shingles) is the commonest example of this, but some naevi also appear in this guise or follow Blaschko's lines (p. 13). Regional patterns (Fig. 1), e.g. involvement of the groin or axilla, will suggest certain diagnoses to the experienced physician. For example, guttate psoriasis and tinea versicolor tend to occur on the trunk,

whereas lichen planus often occurs around the wrists, and contact dermatitis frequently affects the face or hands. The factors resulting in these patterns are complex but include skin anatomy, e.g. blood vessels, nerves, appendages or embryonic lines, and environment, e.g. moist conditions in the axillae, chemical contacts and sun exposure.

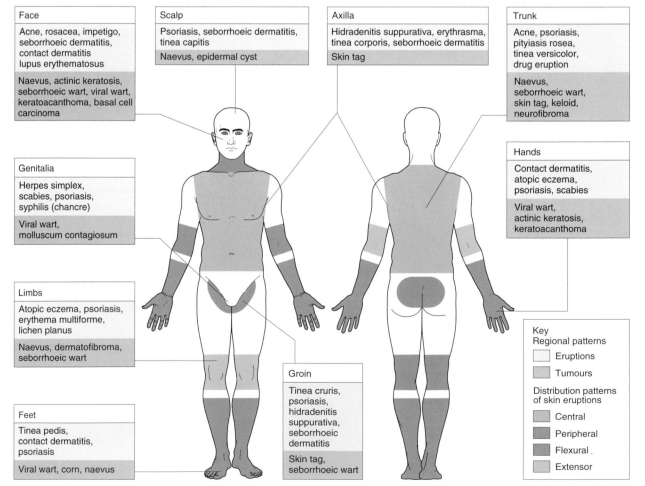

Face
Acne, rosacea, impetigo, seborrhoeic dermatitis, contact dermatitis lupus erythematosus

Naevus, actinic keratosis, seborrhoeic wart, viral wart, keratoacanthoma, basal cell carcinoma

Scalp
Psoriasis, seborrhoeic dermatitis, tinea capitis

Naevus, epidermal cyst

Axilla
Hidradenitis suppurativa, erythrasma, tinea corporis, seborrhoeic dermatitis

Skin tag

Trunk
Acne, psoriasis, pityiasis rosea, tinea versicolor, drug eruption

Naevus, seborrhoeic wart, skin tag, keloid, neurofibroma

Genitalia
Herpes simplex, scabies, psoriasis, syphilis (chancre)

Viral wart, molluscum contagiosum

Hands
Contact dermatitis, atopic eczema, psoriasis, scabies

Viral wart, actinic keratosis, keratoacanthoma

Limbs
Atopic eczema, psoriasis, erythema multiforme, lichen planus

Naevus, dermatofibroma, seborrhoeic wart

Groin
Tinea cruris, psoriasis, hidradenitis suppurativa, seborrhoeic dermatitis

Skin tag, seborrhoeic wart

Feet
Tinea pedis, contact dermatitis, psoriasis

Viral wart, corn, naevus

Key
Regional patterns
- Eruptions
- Tumours

Distribution patterns of skin eruptions
- Central
- Peripheral
- Flexural
- Extensor

Fig. 1 **Regional dermatology.**

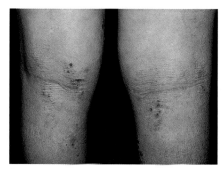

Fig. 2 **Atopic eczema affecting the popliteal fossae.**

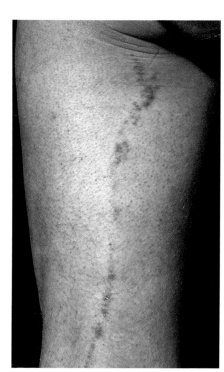

Fig. 3 **Lichen striatus affecting the left leg.**

Individual lesional morphology

A hand lens (or dermoscope) is often helpful in looking at individual lesions. Palpation (often neglected by medical students) is also important to determine the consistency, depth and texture. Definitions of lesions are given on page 14.

Lesions may be monomorphic (e.g. guttate psoriasis) or pleomorphic (e.g. chickenpox). There may also be secondary changes on top of primary lesions. The local configuration of lesions is often of diagnostic help (Table 1). Determine whether the lesions are grouped, linear or annular, or if they show the Koebner phenomenon (p. 28), whereby lesions appear in an area of trauma which is often linear, e.g. a scratch.

Table 1 **Configuration of lesions**	
Configuration	Condition
Linear	Psoriasis, lichen striatus, linear epidermal naevus, lichen planus, morphoea
Grouped	Dermatitis herpetiformis, insect bites, herpes simplex, molluscum contagiosum
Annular	Tinea corporis (ringworm), mycosis fungoides, urticaria, granuloma annulare, annular erythemas
Koebner phenomenon	Lichen planus, psoriasis, viral warts, molluscum contagiosum, sarcoidosis

Nails, hair and mucous membranes

The nails, scalp and hair frequently show diagnostic and even pathognomonic signs (p. 66). With any unusual or atypical eruption, the mucous membranes of the mouth and genitalia may show important changes, such as oral involvement by Wickham's striae in lichen planus, oral lesions in Kaposi's sarcoma or vulval involvement with lichen sclerosus.

General examination

Palpation of lymph nodes is important in patients with skin malignancy. In patients with a skin lymphoma, a full examination is needed, looking particularly for lymphadenopathy and hepatosplenomegaly. Palpation of pedal pulses is vital in patients with leg ulcers.

Special techniques and assessment of disease morbidity

The diagnoses of many skin conditions can be helped by special techniques, detailed on page 20. Photography is often used to record the state of a patient's skin disease and allows comparisons at follow-up visits.

In the current management of skin diseases, it is sometimes necessary to make a quantitative evaluation of the disease and its impact on a patient's life. For example, the National Institute for Health and Clinical Excellence (NICE) states that a patient's psoriasis must be of a certain severity, according to the psoriasis area and severity index, before treatment with a biological agent is recommended (p. 111).

- **Psoriasis Area and Severity Index** (PASI). The PASI is a numerical score of the extent and activity of a patient's psoriasis. It is calculated by a reproducible formula based on the surface area and cutaneous features of the disease.
- **Severity Scoring for Atopic Dermatitis** (SCORAD). The SCORAD gives a numerical value to the severity of a patient's atopic eczema.
- **Dermatology Life Quality Index** (DLQI). The DLQI is a measure of the impact of a skin disease on a patient's social, work and personal activities over the preceding week.

Examining the skin

- Examine the entire skin surface.
- Use a hand lens and adequate illumination. Consider dermoscopy (p. 20).
- Gently palpate lesions to assess texture.
- Look at the nails, hair and mucous membranes (oral and genital).
- Observe for distribution, individual lesion morphology and configuration.
- Always microscope scrapings if a fungal infection is a possibility.

http://www.merck.com/pubs/mmanual/section10/chapter109/109a.htm

Practical clinic procedures

Dermatologists make use of several diagnostic and therapeutic procedures in their everyday clinical practice.

Diagnostic procedures

The ability to diagnose a skin disease is improved by the use of better methods of observing lesions and by appropriate use of samples for laboratory investigation. Patch tests and prick tests are described on page 122.

Dermoscopy

A hand lens helps when looking at small lesions such as nits on hair shafts (Fig. 1) or scabetic burrows, but dermoscopy gives added information, especially for pigmented lesions. Dermoscopy employs a ×10 magnification illuminated lens system, which can visualize a lesion after the application of a drop of oil between the skin and the applied lens. Detailed visualization of the epidermal structures is possible, particularly the pigment network (Fig. 2). Analysis takes account of:

- the symmetry of the lesion
- patterns of pigmentation
- blue–white structures in the pigment network.

Dermoscopy allows an opinion to be made about the nature and malignant potential of the lesion.

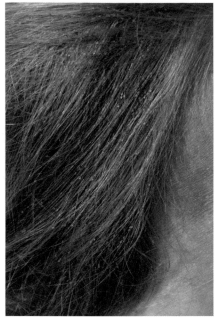

Fig. 1 **Head lice and nits are evident on a hair shaft, best visualized using a hand lens.**

Microbiology samples

Swabs for bacterial and viral culture should be sampled from areas showing pus or exudation. Scrapings for fungal microscopy and culture are obtained by the following technique:

- the active scaly edge of an eruption is sampled using a disposable scalpel blade held vertically to the skin

- nail samples are taken from the distal portion or from debris beneath the nail using clippers or a scalpel
- hair sampling requires plucking of hairs as the hair root is often infected (a scalp scraping is also worthwhile).

Samples are taken onto a small sheet of black paper or a microscope slide (Fig. 3). Direct microscopy of scrapings mounted in 20% potassium hydroxide solution will show hyphae (Fig. 4).

Demonstrating the acarus of scabies

Dermatologists sometimes need to demonstrate the mite to themselves or their patients (p. 60). This can be achieved by:

- removing the acarus using a small needle (the end of the burrow with the mite in can be difficult to see) and mounting it on a microscope slide
- visualizing the acarus by dermoscopy, where it appears as a dark triangle
- taking a superficial scalpel scraping which is examined by microscopy.

Wood's light examination

Wood's light is a handheld ultraviolet (UV) source that can be shone on the skin in a darkened room to diagnose certain skin diseases that show particular patterns of fluorescence in UV radiation. It is used especially for:

(i)

(ii)

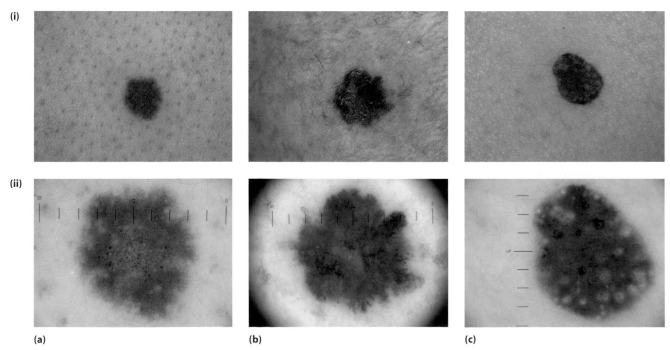

(a)   (b)   (c)

Fig. 2 **Use of the dermoscope in (a) a benign melanocytic naevus, (b) a malignant melanoma, (c) a seborrhoeic wart.** Comparison of the macroscopic **(i)** and dermoscopic **(ii)** appearances in each case.

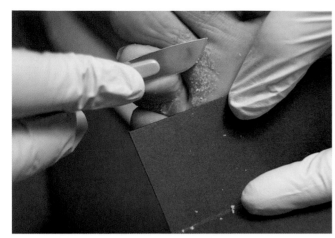

Fig. 3 **Take a scraping from the edge of an area of suspected fungal infection by using a disposable scalpel blade.**

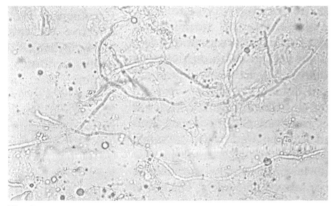

Fig. 4 **Microscopic appearance of skin scrapings showing fungal hyphae.**

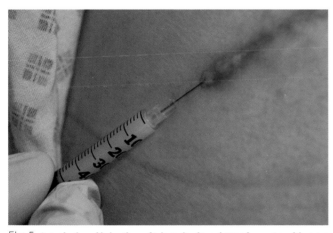

Fig. 5 **Intralesional injection of triamcinolone into a hypertrophic scar.**

- determining the extent of vitiligo
- showing the hypopigmented macules in tuberous sclerosis
- diagnosing bacterial infections such as erythrasma (p. 48)
- diagnosing tinea capitis due to *Microspora* species.

Dermographism
Stroking the skin in patients with symptomatic dermographism will induce whealing (p. 74). Cold-induced urticaria can be provoked by the application of an ice cube to the skin. Rubbing a lesion of urticaria pigmentosa will produce a localized wheal (p. 112).

Doppler studies
The measurement of the ankle/brachial blood pressure index (ABPI) is essential in the management of patients with leg ulcers (p. 71).

Therapeutic procedures
Dermatologists use some non-surgical techniques in their clinical work. Surgical methods and cryotherapy are dealt with elsewhere (p. 107).

Intralesional steroid injection
The injection of steroid into the skin is useful in the management of several diseases, including:

- alopecia areata
- keloid or hypertrophic scars
- acne cysts
- granuloma annulare
- hypertrophic lichen planus
- prurigo nodularis
- nail psoriasis.

Triamcinolone acetonide (10 mg/mL) is normally used in an insulin syringe, which has an integral needle. An injection of 0.1–1.0 mL of the solution is given into the mid- or deep dermis (Fig. 5). The main side-effects are skin atrophy, hypopigmentation and telangiectasia. Occasionally, injection of other substances into the skin is used, e.g. bleomycin for viral warts (p. 51).

Paring of skin
The paring down of hyperkeratotic areas on the hands or feet using a disposable scalpel often helps in:

- **diagnosis**, as it can reveal the underlying lesion, e.g. the punctate thrombosed capillaries of a viral wart or a small haematoma within the epidermis (such as that produced by the friction of shoes on the heel)
- **therapy**, e.g. for callosities under the metatarsals, by reducing the pressure that results from the callus.

On the feet, callosities often develop as a result of the interaction of external forces and an abnormal anatomy of the foot. The advice of a chiropodist or podiatrist will usually be helpful.

Use of caustics
Xanthelasma around the eyes (p. 82) can be treated by the careful application of the caustic trichloroacetic acid (30–50%) solution on an almost dry cotton applicator. Great care is needed to protect the eyes. The treatment should only be carried out by those experienced in the procedure. The xanthelasma turns white with 'frosting' within seconds of application of the acid, and subsequently the treated skin peels off over a period of days.

> ### *Procedures in the skin clinic*
>
> - **Dermoscopy** is useful in deciding whether or not a pigmented lesion might be a malignant melanoma.
> - **Skin scrapings for mycology** should be taken from the edge of a suspect area using a disposable scalpel blade onto a piece of black paper.
> - **Wood's light** can show the extent of vitiligo or diagnose erythrasma or tinea capitis.
> - **Intralesional triamcinolone** is a useful treatment for alopecia areata, keloid, acne cysts and other diseases. Skin atrophy is a potential side-effect.
> - **Paring of skin** can reveal the underlying condition, e.g. a viral wart, or be a treatment for callosity.
> - **Application of caustic:** trichloroacetic acid is used with care in the treatment of xanthelasma.

Basics of medical therapy

The treatment of skin disease includes topical, systemic, intralesional, radiation and surgical modalities. Specific treatments are detailed below. First is an overview of dermatological therapies.

Topical therapy

Topical treatment has the advantage of direct delivery and reduced systemic toxicity. It consists of a *vehicle* or base, which often contains an active ingredient (Table 1).

Vehicles are defined as follows:

- **Lotion.** A liquid vehicle, often aqueous or alcohol based, which may contain a salt in solution. A *shake lotion* contains an insoluble powder (e.g. calamine lotion).
- **Cream.** A semisolid emulsion of oil-in-water; contains an emulsifier for stability and a preservative to prevent overgrowth of microorganisms.
- **Gel.** A transparent semisolid, non-greasy aqueous emulsion.
- **Ointment.** A semisolid grease or oil, containing little or no water but sometimes with added powder. No preservative is usually needed. The active ingredient is suspended rather than dissolved.
- **Paste.** An ointment base with a high proportion of powder (starch or zinc oxide) producing a stiff consistency.

Therapeutic properties of the vehicle

Lotions evaporate and cool the skin and are useful for inflamed/exudative conditions, e.g. for wet wraps (p. 35). The high water content of a cream means that it mostly evaporates; it is also non-greasy and easy to apply or remove. Ointments are best for dry skin conditions such as eczema. They rehydrate and occlude, but (being greasy) are difficult to wash off and are less acceptable to patients than creams. Pastes are ideal for applying to well-defined surfaces, such as psoriatic plaques, but are also hard to remove.

Quantities required

One application to the whole body requires 15–20 g of ointment. The adult face or neck requires 1 g, trunk (each side) 3 g, arm 0.5 g, hand 0.5 g, leg 3 g and foot 1 g. A useful guide for patients is the 'fingertip unit' (FTU) – the amount of cream or ointment that can be applied to the terminal phalanx of the index finger (Fig. 1). One FTU equals 0.5 g. The weekly amount required for the twice-daily use of an emollient in an adult is 250 g. Doctors often underestimate the quantities needed.

The safe maximum amount varies with the strength of the steroid, the age of the patient and the length of treatment. For 1% hydrocortisone, adults can use 150–200 g/week, but children can use only 60 g and babies as little as 20 g. Creams/ointments are applied twice daily except for mometasone, fluticasone and tacalcitol, which are used once daily.

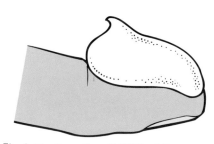

Fig. 1 **The fingertip unit (FTU) = 0.5 g.**

Pharmacokinetics

The ability of a drug to penetrate the epidermis depends on several factors. These include:

- the drug's molecular size and structure and its lipid/water solubility
- the vehicle used and whether application is occluded
- the site on the body – absorption is greatest through the eyelid and genitalia
- whether or not the skin is diseased.

Emollients

Emollients help dry skin conditions such as eczema and ichthyosis by re-establishing the surface lipid layer and enhancing rehydration of the epidermis. Common emollients include emulsifying ointment, aqueous cream, Aveeno, Diprobase, Doublebase, E45, Hydromol, Ultrabase and Unguentum M creams. Sometimes emollients contain urea (Aquadrate, Eucerin) or antimicrobials (Dermol). Oils added to bath water can also help, e.g. Alpha Keri, Aveeno, Balneum, Dermol, Emulsiderm, Hydromol and Oilatum.

Table 1 **An overview of topical medicaments**		
Drug	**Indications**	**Pharmacology**
Corticosteroids	Eczemas, psoriasis, lichen planus, discoid lupus erythematosus, sunburn, pityriasis rosea, mycosis fungoides, photodermatoses, lichen sclerosus	Mode of action is through vasoconstrictive, anti-inflammatory and antiproliferative effects; medication is available in different strengths; side-effects need to be considered
Antiseptics	Skin sepsis, leg ulcers, infected eczema	Chlorhexidine, benzalkonium chloride, silver nitrate and potassium permanganate are used
Antibiotics	Acne, rosacea, folliculitis, impetigo, infected eczema	Chlortetracycline, neomycin, bacitracin, gramicidin, polymixin, sodium fusidate and mupirocin; resistance and sensitization are problems. Metronidazole is used for rosacea
Antifungals	Fungal infections of the skin, *Candida albicans* infections	Nystatin, clotrimazole, miconazole, econazole, terbinafine, ketoconazole, sulconazole and amorolfine
Antiviral agents	Herpes simplex, herpes zoster	Aciclovir, penciclovir
Parasiticidals	Scabies, lice	Benzyl benzoate, permethrin and malathion for scabies; malathion, permethrin and carbaryl for lice – applied as a lotion or shampoo
Coal tar	Psoriasis, eczema	Presumed anti-inflammatory and antiproliferative effects; available as creams, shampoos and in paste bandages
Dithranol	Psoriasis	Antiproliferative effects; available as creams, pastes and ointments
Vitamin D analogues	Psoriasis	Calcitriol, calcipotriol and tacalcitol inhibit keratinocyte proliferation and promote differentiation
Keratolytics	Acne, scaly eczemas	Salicylic acid, benzoyl peroxide and tretinoin
Retinoids	Acne, psoriasis	Isotretinoin (acne), tazarotene (psoriasis), bexarotene (cutaneous T-cell lymphoma)
Calcineurin inhibitors	Atopic eczema	Tacrolimus and pimecrolimus

Dressings and hospital admission

Many departments have treatment centres where daily dressings and ultraviolet (UV) treatments are given. If outpatient management is unsuccessful, hospital admission may be needed. Dressings, for either the outpatient or the inpatient, consist of stockinette gauze applied to the trunk or limbs after the ointments have been put on. These must be changed once or twice a day. Leg ulcer dressings may be changed less frequently, depending on the type of application used.

Bandages impregnated with tar are sometimes helpful for leg ulcers and eczema. Many types of paraffin gauze, hydrocolloid and alginate dressings are now available for leg ulcers (p. 71).

Topical steroids

A summary of the indications for topical treatment with corticosteroids is given in Table 1. The relative potencies of the more commonly prescribed preparations are shown in Table 2.

Side-effects of topical steroid therapy

The use of topical steroids carries the potential for harmful side-effects. These include:

- atrophy of the skin – thinning, erythema, telangiectasia, purpura and striae (p. 110)
- induction of acne or perioral dermatitis, and exacerbation of rosacea
- atypical fungal infection (tinea incognito); bacterial or viral infections may be potentiated
- allergic contact dermatitis, resulting from a component of the preparation or the steroid itself
- systemic absorption – suppression of the pituitary–adrenal axis, Cushingoid appearance, growth retardation
- tachyphylaxis – reduced responsiveness to the steroid after prolonged use.

Systemic therapy

Systemic treatments are used when topical treatment is ineffective, for serious skin diseases and for infections. Details are given in Table 3.

Other treatments

A wide variety of other, more specialized treatments exist for specific skin conditions. Corticosteroids are sometimes

injected directly into lesions (e.g. to treat keloids). Certain disorders are responsive to ultraviolet B or photochemotherapy (p. 45).

In the past, X-irradiation was used to treat a wide range of skin conditions including psoriasis, acne, tinea capitis and tuberculosis of the skin and hand eczema. There are now very few

indications for X-ray treatment of non-malignant disease, although irradiation is of great value in several types of skin tumour.

Cryotherapy, in which liquid nitrogen is applied to the skin, is extensively used in dermatology (p. 107). It is mainly employed for the treatment of benign or premalignant skin tumours.

Table 2 Relative potencies of topical steroids

Potency	Example (generic name)	Proprietary name (UK)
Mild	Hydrocortisone 1% and 2.5%	Efcortelan, Mildison (Cort-Dome USA)
Moderately potent	Clobetasone butyrate 0.05%	Eumovate (UK and USA)
	Fluodroxycortide 0.0125%	Haelan
	Alclometasone dipropionate 0.05%	Modrasone (Aclovate USA)
Potent	Betamethasone valerate 0.1%	Betnovate (Valisone USA)
	Beclomethasone dipropionate 0.025%	Propaderm (UK and Canada)
	Betamethasone dipropionate 0.05%	Diprosone (UK and USA)
	Fluocinolone acetonide 0.025%	Synalar (UK and USA)
	Fluocinonide 0.05%	Metosyn (Lidex USA)
	Fluticasone propionate 0.05%	Cutivate (UK and USA)
	Hydrocortisone butyrate 0.1%	Locoid (UK and USA)
	Mometasone furoate 0.1%	Elocon (UK and USA)
	Triamcinolone acetonide 0.1%	Adcortyl (Aristocort, Kenalog USA)
Very potent	Clobetasol propionate 0.05%	Dermovate (Temovate USA)
	Diflucortolone valerate 0.3%	Nerisone Forte (UK and Canada)
	Halcinonide 0.1%	Halciderm Topical (Halog USA)

Table 3 An overview of systemic therapy

Group	Drug	Indications
Corticosteroids	Prednisolone usually	Bullous disorders, connective tissue disease, vasculitis
Cytotoxics	Methotrexate	Psoriasis, sarcoidosis
	Hydroxyurea	Psoriasis
	Azathioprine	Bullous disorders, chronic actinic dermatitis, atopic eczema
Biologicals	Etanercept, infliximab, efalizumab	Psoriasis unresponsive to other systemic agents
Immunosuppressants	Ciclosporin	Psoriasis, atopic eczema, pyoderma gangrenosum
	Gold	Bullous disorders, lupus erythematosus
Retinoids	Acitretin	Psoriasis, other keratinization disorders
	Isotretinoin	Acne
Antifungals	Griseofulvin, terbinafine	Fungal infection
	Ketoconazole	Fungal infection (*Candida albicans* too)
	Itraconazole, fluconazole	Fungal infection, candidiasis
Antibiotics	Various	Skin sepsis, acne, rosacea
Antivirals	Aciclovir, valaciclovir	Herpes simplex, herpes zoster
	Famciclovir	Herpes zoster, genital herpes simplex
Antihistamines	H1 blockers	Urticaria, eczema
Antiandrogens	Cyproterone	Acne (females only)
Antimalarials	Hydroxychloroquine	Lupus erythematosus, porphyria cutanea tarda
Antileprotic	Dapsone	Dermatitis herpetiformis, leprosy, vasculitis

Basics of medical therapy

- Correct diagnosis is essential to ensure appropriate treatment.
- When using topical steroids:
  - use the lowest potency that is effective
  - look out for side-effects, especially atrophy of the skin
  - emollients can help reduce the amount of topical steroid required.
- Explain the treatment to the patient and preferably give a written handout; this aids compliance. The fingertip unit is a convenient way to indicate the amount of cream the patient should apply.
- Use the simplest treatment possible; patients easily get mixed up if they have several different tubes to use.
- Prescribe adequate amounts. Patients are often given too little, 'run out' of their creams and return to the clinic no better because the treatment has been inadequate.

http://www.merck.com/pubs/mmanual/section10/chapter110/110a.htm ■ http://www.dermnetnz.org ■ http://www.drugs.com

Epidemiology of skin disease

Skin disease is very common. About 10% of a general practitioner's workload and 6% of hospital outpatient referrals can be accounted for by skin problems. Skin disease is also economically significant; it is a major occupational cause of loss of time from work and the second most common industrial disease (p. 120).

In any discussion of epidemiology, it is important first to define the terms used:

- *prevalence* refers to the proportion of a defined population affected by a disease at any given time
- *incidence* is defined as the proportion of a population experiencing the disorder within a stated period of time (usually 1 year).

The type, prevalence and incidence of skin disease all depend on social, economic, geographical, racial, cultural and age-related factors.

Skin disease in the general population

Reliable population statistics are difficult to obtain, but it appears that, in Europe, the prevalence of skin disease needing some sort of medical care is about 20%. Eczema, acne and infective disorders (including warts) are the commonest complaints (Fig. 1). Only a minority seek medical advice.

Skin disease in community and specialized clinics

The precise proportion of skin disorders seen in a community setting (Fig. 2) will vary with the age structure of the population served, the amount and type of industry in the area and socioeconomic factors. Demographic studies may reveal a trend; for example, for unknown reasons, atopic eczema has become more common over the last 20 years.

Patients seen in a specialist dermatology clinic are a selected population (Fig. 3). In some countries, e.g. the UK, a general practitioner will have referred them; in other places, self-referral may depend on the availability of medical insurance. Referral patterns vary between different regions, depending on local facilities, interests and customs. In Europe, within a year, just over 1% of the population is referred for a dermatological opinion. In the mid-2000s, a quarter of all new referrals required a surgical procedure.

Socioeconomic factors

Improvements in the standard of living resulting from the nineteenth-century industrialization of Europe were accompanied by a fall in the incidences of most infectious diseases and a decline in the infant mortality rate. Better nutrition, improved living conditions and the introduction of hygienic measures are thought to have been important. Most forms of infectious disease, including those of the skin, are now more common in the developing world than in western countries, and it would seem that the poorer standards of living are a cause of this.

However, industrialization brings its own problems. Occupational dermatitis is quite common in industrialized countries, and mild cases are often not reported. Increased sophistication in western countries also means that patients now want something done about disorders or minor imperfections that would not have bothered past generations.

Changes in social fashion have also brought about changes in skin disease. For example, the habit of sunbathing, which became popular in the 1970s, seems to have resulted in an increase in the incidence of malignant melanoma from the 1980s to the present.

The media have also had an effect: the numerous articles and programmes on the potential problems associated with a change in pigmented naevi have produced a flood of referrals of worried patients seeking reassurance about their lesions! However, it is still true that many people with minor skin problems do not consult a doctor.

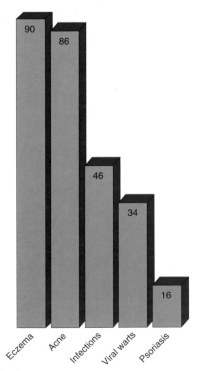

Fig. 1 **Prevalence per 1000 population for skin disease of any severity.**

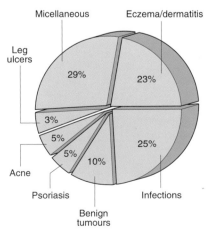

Fig. 2 **Breakdown of skin diseases seen in general practice (% of total).**

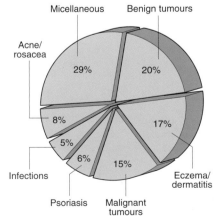

Fig. 3 **Breakdown of skin diseases seen in a hospital dermatological clinic (% of total).**

Geographical factors

Humid conditions found in hot countries predispose to fungal and bacterial infections, and to other conditions such as 'prickly heat' (an itchy eruption due to blocked sweat ducts). Ultraviolet radiation in sunny climes will result in actinic damage and malignant change in the skin of non-pigmented migrants to the area.

Figure 4 shows a comparison between some common complaints in different geographical locations. The rates for bacterial and fungal infections show variation, and skin cancers are more common in Australia. However, the figures for eczema/dermatitis are remarkably constant.

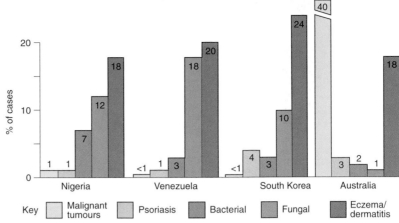

Fig. 4 **Geographical variations in hospital attendances (%) with some common dermatological disorders.**

Racial and cultural factors

Quite apart from the obvious differences in pigmentation, the skin structure varies between the different races (p. 118). For example, hair is often spiral in black Africans but straight in mongoloids. In caucasians, hair is more variable and may be straight, wavy or helical. Skin tumours and actinic damage are seen more in caucasians than in black Africans, with mongoloids showing an intermediate incidence. Keloids and hair problems, such as pseudofolliculitis (p. 119), are more common in black Africans, whereas mongoloid skin has a tendency to become lichenified and acne may be less frequent. Vitiligo appears to have a similar incidence in all races, but is more conspicuous and may have a greater psychological impact in those with a dark skin.

Cultural factors may bring problems. For example, tight braiding of the hair, practised by some Afro-Caribbeans, may result in alopecia, whereas the use of certain traditional oils or cosmetics can produce dermatitis or a change in pigmentation.

Age and sex prevalence of dermatoses

Different disorders are associated with different times of life (Table 1). Some disorders occur throughout life but are more common at certain ages, whereas others are almost exclusively encountered in defined age groups. For example, atopic eczema is most common in infants, acne is mainly seen in adolescents, and psoriasis has its peak onset in the second and third decades of life. Certain disorders tend to appear in middle age, e.g. pemphigus and malignant melanoma. In old age, degenerative and malignant skin conditions are often found. Thus, the age structure of the population will influence the type of dermatology practised.

Some conditions are more common to a specific gender (Table 2).

Table 1	**Age-related onset of selected skin disorders**
Age	**Disorder**
Childhood	Port wine stain and strawberry naevi, ichthyosis, erythropoietic protoporphyria, epidermolysis bullosa, atopic eczema, infantile seborrhoeic dermatitis, urticaria pigmentosa, viral exanthems, viral warts, molluscum contagiosum, impetigo
Adolescence	Melanocytic naevi, acne, psoriasis (notably guttate), seborrhoeic dermatitis, vitiligo, pityriasis rosea
Early adulthood	Psoriasis, seborrhoeic dermatitis, lichen planus, dermatitis herpetiformis, lupus erythematosus, vitiligo, tinea versicolor
Middle age	Porphyria cutanea tarda, lichen planus, rosacea, pemphigus vulgaris, venous ulceration, malignant melanoma, basal cell carcinoma, mycosis fungoides
Old age	Asteatotic eczema, generalized pruritus, bullous pemphigoid, venous and arterial ulcers, seborrhoeic warts, solar keratosis, solar elastosis, Campbell-de-Morgan spots, basal cell carcinoma, squamous cell carcinoma, herpes zoster

Table 2	**Skin disorders with a male or female preponderance**
Sex	**Disorder**
Female	Palmoplantar pustulosis, lichen sclerosus, lupus erythematosus, systemic sclerosis, morphoea, rosacea, dermatitis artefacta, venous ulceration, *in situ* squamous cell carcinoma, malignant melanoma
Male	Seborrhoeic dermatitis, dermatitis herpetiformis, porphyria cutanea tarda, polyarteritis nodosa, pruritus ani, tinea pedis and cruris, mycosis fungoides, squamous cell carcinoma, actinic keratosis

Epidemiology

- The commonest skin diseases in the general community are eczema, acne and infections, including viral warts.

- About 20% of the general population have some sort of skin disorder requiring medical attention.

- Skin disease accounts for 10% of all consultations in general practice.

- Better living conditions reduce skin infection, but excess sun on a white skin predisposes to skin cancer.

Body image, the psyche and the skin

The stress of having skin disease

The potentially harsh psychological effects of having chronic skin disease tend to be underestimated. Up to 30% of skin outpatients suffer 'psychological distress' from their condition. This is particularly understandable in the teenager with acne, or in someone who has extensive psoriasis or eczema. In both these situations, the individual's devalued body image may be out of proportion to the objective severity of his or her skin problem. Skin diseases can thus make patients into 'social lepers' who feel that their social lives are restricted because other people do not want to mix with them. These effects on 'quality of life' can be assessed by specific questionnaires, e.g. the Dermatology Life Quality Index (DLQI).

Patients sometimes feel that their disorder is either caused directly by, or exacerbated by, 'stress'. This is difficult to prove, as it is often impossible to differentiate reactive from aetiological states. Many dermatologists believe that psychological factors can, for example, make eczema and psoriasis worse, but most would also agree that these are stressful conditions in their own right. However, it is accepted that there are a small number of conditions that are of psychogenic origin. Management with a liaison psychiatrist can be helpful.

Skin disorders of psychogenic origin

Dermatitis artefacta

Dermatitis artefacta (Fig. 1) should be suspected from the presence of lesions with bizarre shapes (often linear or angular and in accessible sites) that do not conform to natural disease. The lesions are often ulcerated or crusted and do not heal as expected, although they do heal if occluded. Blisters or bruises are also sometimes found.

The condition tends to occur in young women. Confrontation is not recommended, as this may lead to an angry denial. Management is aimed at excluding genuine disease, establishing a rapport with the patient and gently trying to investigate the presence of psychological stresses, e.g. in the home or work environment or in social or sexual relationships.

Delusions of body image

Patients may present with no objective skin disease but still complain of symptoms such as burning or redness of the face, or display a preoccupation with an imagined problem such as excessive facial hair. This condition, sometimes known as dysmorphophobia, is usually seen in women, although it does occur in men, who may complain of a burning scrotum. Most of these patients are depressed, although some may show signs of schizophrenia. Psychiatric referral is needed for those with true delusions.

Delusions of parasitosis

Patients with this condition are convinced that their skin is infested with parasites, and they often bring collections of keratin and debris to support their contention. Self-induced excoriation of the skin may be seen. It mainly occurs in women over the age of 40 years. Most patients do not have an organic psychosis, but they are often obsessional and do have a monosymptomatic hypochondriasis. Treatment is difficult. It is necessary to exclude a true parasitosis. The antipsychotic drug pimozide (in a dose of 2–10 mg daily) is helpful in some patients but requires electrocardiogram (ECG) monitoring.

Trichotillomania

Rubbing, pulling and twisting the hair is not uncommon in children and results in thinning of scalp hair, which recovers spontaneously. When the condition occurs in adults, the hair may be cut using scissors or a razor, and the prognosis is not so good.

Neurogenic excoriations

Accessible areas of the skin, particularly the forearms and back of the neck, are commonly involved in this condition, with excoriated lesions in a variety of stages of evolution from ulcers to healed scars (Fig. 2). The damage is inflicted as a result of an uncontrollable itch, but there is no primary lesion. Effective occlusion will allow healing. *Acne excoriée* is a variant seen in young women who squeeze and pick their acne lesions, resulting in artefactual erosions.

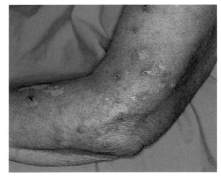

Fig. 2 **Neurogenic excoriations on the arm.** Some have healed to leave hypopigmented scars.

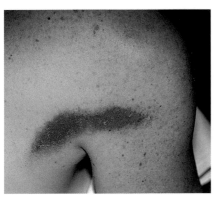

Fig. 1 **Dermatitis artefacta: a linear lesion.**

> ### Body image, the psyche and the skin
>
> - Psychological stress is commonly associated with skin disease, and the patient's psychological state should be routinely assessed. Quality of life questionnaires are available.
> - Some skin disorders (e.g. eczema and psoriasis) may get worse at times of stress in certain patients. It may be helpful for the patient to recognize this.
> - A small number of skin diseases are psychogenic in origin. A liaison psychiatrist may offer assistance.

Diseases

Psoriasis – Epidemiology, pathophysiology and presentation

Definition
Psoriasis is a chronic, non-infectious, inflammatory dermatosis characterized by well-demarcated erythematous plaques topped by silvery scales (Fig. 1).

Epidemiology
Psoriasis affects 1.5–3% of the population in Europe and North America, but is less common in Africa and Japan. The sex incidence is equal. The condition may start at any age, even in the elderly. The two peaks of onset are the second–third and sixth decades. It is unusual in children under 8 years old.

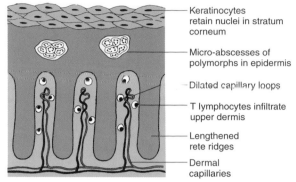

Keratinocytes retain nuclei in stratum corneum

Micro-abscesses of polymorphs in epidermis

Dilated capillary loops

T lymphocytes infiltrate upper dermis

Lengthened rete ridges

Dermal capillaries

Fig. 1 **Histopathology of psoriasis.**

Aetiopathogenesis

Genetics
Inherited factors predispose to the development of psoriasis, and candidate genes have been detected (p. 12). About 35% of patients show a family history, and identical twin studies show a concordance of 64%. There is a 14% probability that a child with one parent who has psoriasis will be affected, but this increases to 41% if both parents have psoriasis. There are strong correlations with the human leucocyte antigens (HLAs) Cw6, B13 and B17. Environmental factors are thought to trigger the disease in susceptible individuals.

Epidermal kinetics and metabolism
The number of cycling epidermal cells is increased sevenfold in psoriasis because of an increase in the proliferating cell compartment of the basal and suprabasal layers. The cell cycle time is not reduced. Growth factors, especially transforming growth factor-α, seem to mediate these events. The upper dermal capillary plexus is expanded. At least eight possible chromosomal loci for psoriasis have been found, e.g. *PSOR1* at 6q21.3 (p. 12).

Precipitating factors
A number of precipitating factors are associated with the disorder:

■ *Koebner phenomenon*. Trauma to the epidermis and dermis, such as a scratch or surgical scar (p. 19), can precipitate psoriasis in the damaged skin (see Fig. 2).
■ *Infection*. Typically, a streptococcal sore throat may precipitate guttate psoriasis.

■ *Drugs*. Beta-blockers, lithium and antimalarials can make psoriasis worse or precipitate it.
■ *Sunlight*. Exposure to sunlight can aggravate psoriasis (in about 6%), although it has a beneficial effect in the majority.
■ *Psychological stress*. The effects are difficult to assess; most clinicians believe it can exacerbate psoriasis.
■ *Cigarettes and alcohol*. These seem to make psoriasis worse.

Pathology
The epidermis is thickened, with keratinocytes retaining their nuclei (Fig. 1). There is no granular layer, and keratin builds up loosely at the horny layer. The rete ridges are elongated, and polymorphs infiltrate up into the stratum corneum where they form micro-abscesses. Capillaries are dilated

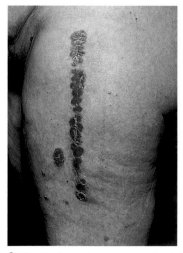

Fig. 2 **The Koebner phenomenon.** Psoriasis has developed in a surgical scar.

in the papillary dermis. T lymphocytes are seen infiltrating the earliest psoriatic lesions and may initiate several of the changes observed.

Clinical presentation
Psoriasis varies in severity from the trivial to the life threatening. Its appearance and behaviour also range widely from the readily recognizable chronic plaques on the elbows to the acute generalized pustular form. Psoriasis can be confused with other conditions (see Table 1).

Presentation patterns of psoriasis include:

■ plaque
■ guttate
■ flexural
■ localized forms
■ generalized pustular
■ nail involvement
■ erythroderma (p. 42).

Plaque
Well-defined, raised disc-shaped plaques (Fig. 3) involving the elbows, knees, scalp hair margin or sacrum are the classic presentation (see also p. 16; Fig. 1). The

Table 1 **Differential diagnosis of psoriasis**	
Variant of psoriasis	**Differential diagnosis**
Plaque psoriasis	Psoriasiform drug eruption (due to beta-blockers) Hypertrophic lichen planus
Palmoplantar psoriasis	Hyperkeratotic eczema Reiter's disease
Scalp psoriasis	Seborrhoeic dermatitis
Guttate psoriasis	Pityriasis rosea
Flexural psoriasis	Candidiasis of the flexures
Nail psoriasis	Fungal infection of the nails

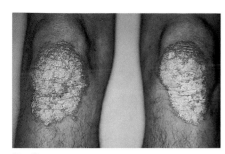

Fig. 3 **Typical scaly plaques of psoriasis on the knees.**

plaques are usually red and covered by waxy white scales, which, if detached, may leave bleeding points. Plaques vary in diameter from 2 cm or less to several centimetres, and are sometimes pruritic.

Guttate

Guttate psoriasis is an acute symmetrical eruption (a 'flurry') of 'drop-like' lesions with little scale in the early stage, usually on the trunk and limbs. This form mostly occurs in adolescents or young adults and may follow a streptococcal throat infection (Fig. 4).

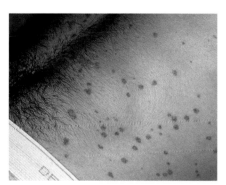

Fig. 4 **The drop-like lesions of guttate psoriasis.**

Flexural

This variant of psoriasis affects the axillae, submammary areas, groin and natal cleft (Fig. 5). Plaques are smooth and often glazed. It is mostly found in the elderly.

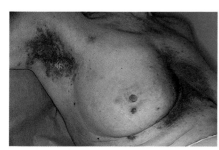

Fig. 5 **Smooth non-keratotic involvement in flexural psoriasis.**

Localized forms

Psoriasis can also present in a number of localized forms:

- *Palmoplantar pustulosis* is characterized by yellow- to brown-coloured sterile pustules on the palms or soles (Fig. 6). A minority of subjects have classic plaque psoriasis elsewhere. It is most common in middle-aged women who are cigarette smokers, and it follows a protracted course.
- *Acrodermatitis of Hallopeau* is an uncommon indolent form of pustular psoriasis affecting the digits and nails (see p. 31, Fig. 3).
- *Scalp psoriasis* may be the sole manifestation of the disease (see p. 31, Fig. 2). It can be confused with dandruff but is generally better demarcated and more thickly scaled.
- *Napkin psoriasis* is a well-defined psoriasiform eruption in the nappy

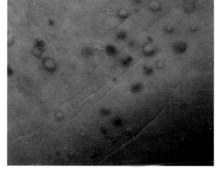

Fig. 6 **Palmoplantar pustulosis: a localized variant of psoriasis on the sole of the foot.**

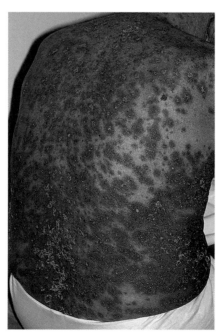

Fig. 7 **Generalized pustular psoriasis in an elderly patient.**

area of infants, few of whom later develop true psoriasis.

Generalized pustular

Generalized pustular is a rare but serious and even life-threatening form of psoriasis. Sheets of small, sterile yellowish pustules develop on an erythematous background and may spread rapidly (Fig. 7). The onset is often acute. The patient is unwell, with fever and malaise, and requires hospital admission.

Nail involvement

Psoriasis affects the matrix or nail bed in 25–50% of cases (Fig. 8). Thimble pitting is the commonest change, followed by *onycholysis* (separation of the distal edge of the nail from the nail bed). An oily or salmon pink discoloration of the nail bed is seen, often adjacent to onycholysis. Subungual hyperkeratosis, with a build-up of keratin beneath the distal nail edge, mostly affects the toenails. Nail changes are frequently associated with psoriatic arthropathy. Treatment is often difficult.

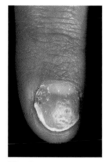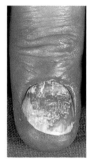

Fig. 8 **Nail involvement in psoriasis: pitting (left) and subungual hyperkeratosis with onycholysis (right).**

> ## Psoriasis
>
> - Psoriasis affects 1.5–3% of the population.
> - Inheritance is polygenic: 35% have a family history.
> - Geneticists have identified loci for possible psoriasis genes, e.g. *PSOR1* with chromosome locus 6q21.3.
> - Peaks of onset are in the second–third and the sixth decades.
> - The number of proliferating keratinocytes is increased sevenfold, but the epidermal cell cycle time is not shortened.
> - Presentation is variable: the chronic plaque form affecting the elbows, knees and scalp is the commonest.
> - Precipitating factors include streptococcal infection, drugs, sunlight, alcohol, smoking and psychological stress.
> - Nail involvement is found in 25–50% of cases and is difficult to treat.

http://www.skincarephysicians.com/ ■ http://www.pinch.com/skin/

Psoriasis – Complications and management

Complications

Psoriasis may be complicated by the development of arthropathy, erythroderma and the Koebner phenomenon (p. 28, Fig. 2).

Psoriatic arthropathy

Psoriatic joint disease occurs in 20–30% of psoriasis patients and is associated with more severe skin disease. It shows an equal sex ratio and takes three forms:

- *Asymmetrical arthritis*. A small number of joints are usually involved, with few erosions and good preservation of function.
- *Symmetrical polyarthritis*. This form is associated with erosions, deformity and loss of function (Fig. 1). It is distinguished from rheumatoid arthritis by predominantly affecting distal interphalangeal joints and by the rheumatoid factor test being negative.
- *Predominant spondylitis*. This type is similar to ankylosing spondylitis and may be accompanied by a peripheral arthritis, although it behaves independently of it.

Erythrodermic psoriasis

Inpatient treatment is needed for this condition, often with systemic drugs. Details are given on page 42.

Management

The non-infectious nature of psoriasis, its relapsing nature and the likely need for long-term therapy should be explained. A sympathetic approach is helpful, and patients often obtain support from the self-help group The Psoriasis Association (see p. 128). Treatment is tailored to the patient's particular requirements, taking into account the type and extent of the disease, and the age and social background (Table 1).

Topical therapy

It is usual to prescribe topical agents as the first-line treatment.

Vitamin D analogues

Calcipotriol (Dovonex), *tacalcitol* (Curatoderm) and *calcitriol* (Silkis) are topical synthetic vitamin D analogues for use in mild and moderate chronic plaque psoriasis. They inhibit cell proliferation and stimulate keratinocyte differentiation, correcting some of the epidermal cell proliferation changes in psoriasis. Patient acceptability is good as the preparations do not smell or stain, are easy to apply and do not have the risk of skin atrophy seen with topical steroids. Skin irritation may be a problem. Efficacy is commensurate with dithranol or topical steroids.

Hypercalcaemia is possible if the maximum dose is exceeded. Calcipotriol cream can be used up to 100 g/week (40% of the body surface on a twice-daily basis), and tacalcitol ointment up to 35 g/week (20% of body surface as a once-daily dose). Tacalcitol is tolerated on the scalp and face, where calcipotriol tends to irritate. Calcipotriol is available as a scalp preparation. Vitamin D analogues are often used in alternation with a topical steroid, and in combination with ultraviolet B or psoralen plus ultraviolet A (PUVA) therapy.

Topical corticosteroids

Topical steroids have the advantage of being clean, non-irritant and easy to use. However, against this must be balanced the risk of side-effects (p. 23) and of precipitating an unstable form of psoriasis, especially on their withdrawal. Topical steroids are the treatment of choice for face, genitalia and flexures, and are useful for stubborn plaques on hands, feet and scalp. Potent steroids should not be applied to the face, although they may be used judiciously on palms and soles. Elsewhere, moderately potent steroids normally suffice. Their use must be monitored carefully. Creams are often preferred to ointments. Lotions and gels are available for the scalp.

Coal tar preparations

Coal tar distillates have been used for decades to treat psoriasis. They are safe and seem to act by inhibiting DNA synthesis. The main disadvantages of tar are that it smells and is messy. Despite this, it can be useful for inpatient care, e.g. combined with ultraviolet B – the Goeckermann regimen. Refined tar (1–10%) is available in a cream or lotion base for outpatient use (e.g. Alphosyl, Carbo-Dome, Exorex). These preparations are suitable for chronic plaque psoriasis or guttate psoriasis once the acute phase is past.

Dithranol (Anthralin)

Dithranol has an antimitotic effect and is irritant to normal skin. It cannot be used on the face or genitalia, and it stains skin, hair, linen, clothes and bathtubs a purple–brown colour. For inpatient use, the usual base is Lassar's paste (zinc and salicylic acid paste BP). It is applied to the plaques of psoriasis initially in the 0.1% strength, increasing up to 2% if necessary. The surrounding skin is protected with a bland preparation such as white soft paraffin, and the treated area is covered with tube gauze. The combination of this with a daily tar bath and

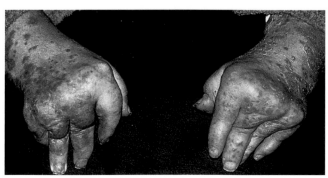

Fig. 1 **Severe mutilating symmetrical arthritis with widespread psoriasis.**

Table 1 **A guide to psoriasis therapy**	
Type of psoriasis	**Treatment options**
Stable plaque	Vitamin D analogue with topical steroid Dithranol (short contact), coal tar, tazarotene Narrow-band ultraviolet B
Extensive plaque	Narrow-band ultraviolet B (plus topicals) Methotrexate, ciclosporin, PUVA or Re-PUVA Biologicals
Guttate	Topical steroids (mild/moderate), coal tar Narrow-band ultraviolet B
Facial/flexural	Topical steroids (mild/moderate); tacalcitol
Palmoplantar	Topical steroids (potent) Acitretin, PUVA or Re-PUVA
Generalized pustular/ erythrodermic	Acitretin, methotrexate, ciclosporin Biologicals

ultraviolet B is called the Ingram regimen. Psoriasis clears within 3 weeks in most patients on this treatment.

The 'short contact regimen', in which dithranol is applied for 30 min each day, is suitable for outpatients with stable plaque psoriasis. The dithranol is best washed off in a shower. Dithrocream is a suitable preparation and comes in concentrations from 0.1% to 2%.

Retinoids
A topical retinoid, tazarotene (0.05% and 0.1%; Zorac gel), is effective for chronic plaque psoriasis. It may irritate and is often used alternating with a topical steroid.

Keratolytics and scalp preparations
Hyperkeratotic psoriasis of the palms and soles can be treated with 5% salicylic acid ointment. Scalp psoriasis (Fig. 2) responds to 3% salicylic acid in a cream base (sometimes with 3% precipitated sulphur) applied daily or every 2 or 3 days, and is used in combination with a tar-containing shampoo (e.g. Alphosyl, Capasal, Polytar, T/Gel). Coconut oil compound (e.g. Cocois) also helps scaly scalps.

Systemic therapy
Psoriasis that is life threatening, unresponsive to adequate topical treatment or restricting the ability to work (Fig. 3) may require systemic therapy. Benefits must be weighed against side-effects. The use of potentially toxic drugs is justified by their ability to transform a patient's life from severely restricted to nearly normal. Phototherapy and photochemotherapy are outlined on page 102.

Methotrexate
The folate antagonist methotrexate is well established as an effective treatment for severe psoriasis and may have anti-inflammatory as well as immune modulatory effects. It is given once a week orally as a single dose (usually 7.5–15 mg), although it can be given intramuscularly (or intravenously). Normal liver, kidney and bone marrow function must be established before starting methotrexate, and these functions must be monitored during treatment. Liver disease, alcoholism and acute infection are contraindications to methotrexate, and drug interaction (e.g. with aspirin, non-steroidal anti-inflammatory drugs or co-trimoxazole) must be avoided. Improvement is seen within 2–4 weeks. Minor side-effects (e.g. nausea) are common, but liver fibrosis or cirrhosis is a risk long term. Liver damage can be monitored using the serum procollagen III aminopropeptide, but some centres still recommend liver biopsy after every 1.5-g cumulative dose. Methotrexate is also a teratogen.

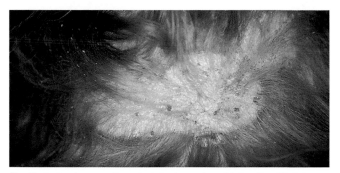

Fig. 2 **Scaly plaques of psoriasis in the scalp, with localized hair loss.**

Retinoids
The vitamin A derivative acitretin (Neotigason) is particularly effective in treating pustular psoriasis and in thinning hyperkeratotic plaques. Acitretin may be used with topical therapies or with UVB or PUVA ('Re-PUVA'), when it allows a more rapid clearance at a lower total dose of UV. Most patients develop minor side-effects, such as dry mucous membranes, itching and peeling skin. More serious complications include hyperostosis, abnormal liver function, hyperlipidaemia and teratogenicity. The last virtually precludes the use of acitretin in women of child-bearing age. Although acitretin has a half-life of 50 days, in some patients it is metabolized to etretinate, a retinoid that takes 2 years to be excreted.

Ciclosporin
Ciclosporin (Neoral), an immunosuppressant widely used to prevent rejection of organ transplants, is effective in severe psoriasis. It acts by inhibiting T-lymphocyte activation and interleukin-2 production. Dose-dependent reversible nephrotoxicity is a side-effect. Blood pressure and kidney function are monitored during treatment. There may be a risk of skin cancers or lymphoma, and concomitant UV treatment is avoided.

Biologic agents and other systemic treatments
Other immunosuppressive drugs can control psoriasis, but they are not as potent as methotrexate. Hydroxyurea has the advantage of not affecting the liver, but it can suppress the bone marrow. Fumaric acid esters are effective in some cases (p. 110). Biological agents offer great promise but are expensive (see p. 110).

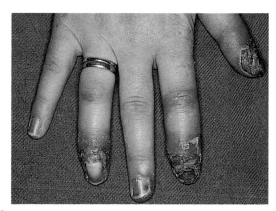

Fig. 3 **Acrodermatitis continua variant of psoriasis.** Sterile pustular changes with dactylitis are present on three fingers.

> ### *Treatment of psoriasis*
> Side-effects are often the limiting factor in psoriasis treatment.
>
> **Topical treatment** is usually the first approach:
> - *Steroids*: popular and effective but beware of side-effects.
> - *Vitamin D analogues*: clean, effective, but may irritate.
> - *Coal tar*: safe but messy and not very popular with patients.
> - *Dithranol*: effective, irritant, rather impractical for home use.
> - *Keratolytics*: useful for scalp disease combined with tar or sulphur.
>
> **Systemic treatment** is used for serious or severe psoriasis:
> - *PUVA*: popular but long-term risk of skin cancer.
> - *Retinoids*: good for pustular psoriasis and as Re-PUVA; teratogenic.
> - *Methotrexate*: a well-established systemic drug; hepatotoxic.
> - *Ciclosporin*: effective but potentially nephrotoxic.
> - *Biologicals*: offer potential for targeted therapy. Expensive.

http://www.psoriasis.org/   ■   http://www.psoriasis-association.org.uk/

Eczema – Basic principles/contact dermatitis

Definition

Eczema is a non-infective inflammatory skin condition that shows itching, redness and scaling. The term 'eczema' literally means 'to boil over' (Greek), and this well describes the acute eruption in which blistering occurs.

Eczema represents a reaction pattern to a variety of stimuli, some of which are recognized but many of which are unknown. Eczema and dermatitis mean the same thing and may be used interchangeably. However, to patients, the term 'dermatitis' often implies an occupational causation, and its use may unnecessarily raise the question of litigation and compensation.

Classification

The current classification of eczema is unsatisfactory in that it is inconsistent. However, it is difficult to provide a suitable alternative as the aetiology of most eczemas is not known. Different types of eczema may be recognized by morphology, site or cause. A division into endogenous (due to internal or constitutional factors) and exogenous (due to external contact agents) is convenient (Table 1). However, in clinical practice, these distinctions are often blurred and, not infrequently, the eczema cannot be classified. A further division into acute (Fig. 1) and chronic (Fig. 2) eczema can be made in many

Table 1 **A classification of eczema**	
Type	**Variety**
Exogenous (contact)	Allergic, irritant
	Photoreaction
Endogenous	Atopic
	Seborrhoeic
	Discoid (nummular)
	Venous (stasis, gravitational)
	Pompholyx
Unclassified	Asteatotic (eczéma craquelé)
	Lichen simplex
	(neurodermatitis)
	Juvenile plantar dermatosis

cases according to the morphology of the eruption.

Acute eczema

In acute eczema, epidermal oedema (spongiosis), with separation of keratinocytes, leads to the formation of epidermal vesicles (Fig. 3a). Dermal vessels are dilated, and inflammatory cells invade the dermis and epidermis.

Chronic eczema

In chronic eczema, there is thickening of the prickle cell layer (acanthosis) and stratum corneum (hyperkeratosis) with retention of nuclei by some corneocytes (parakeratosis) (Fig. 3b). The rete ridges are lengthened, dermal vessels dilated, and inflammatory mononuclear cells infiltrate the skin.

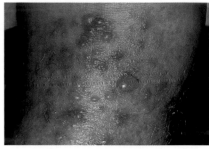

Fig. 1 **Acute dermatitis (eczema).** Erythema and oedema are seen with papules, vesicles and sometimes large blisters. Exudation and crust formation follow. The eruption is painful and pruritic. This case resulted from a contact allergy to a locally applied cream.

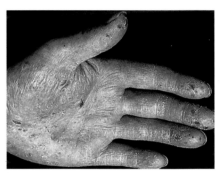

Fig. 2 **Chronic dermatitis (eczema).** Lichenification, scaling and fissuring of the hands due to repeated exposure to irritants. Allergic contact dermatitis cannot be excluded on the appearance alone.

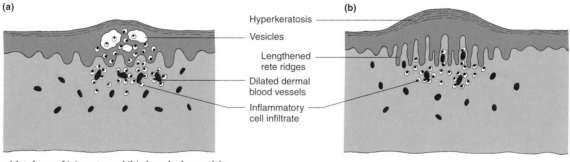

(a) **(b)**

Hyperkeratosis
Vesicles
Lengthened rete ridges
Dilated dermal blood vessels
Inflammatory cell infiltrate

Fig. 3 **The histology of (a) acute and (b) chronic dermatitis.**

Contact dermatitis

Definition

Dermatitis precipitated by an exogenous agent, often a chemical, is known as contact dermatitis. It is particularly common in the home, among women with young children and in industry, where it is a major cause of loss of time from work (see p. 120).

Aetiopathogenesis

Irritants cause more cases of contact dermatitis than allergens, although the clinical appearances are often similar. Often, there is an inherited susceptibility to react to irritants. Allergic contact dermatitis is an example of type IV hypersensitivity (p. 11).

Irritants cause dermatitis in a number of different ways, but usually by a direct noxious effect on the skin's barrier function. The most important irritants are:

- water and other fluids
- abrasives, i.e. frictional irritancy
- chemicals, e.g. acids and alkalis
- solvents, soaps and detergents.

A strong irritant causing necrosis of epidermal cells will produce a reaction within hours but, in most cases, the effect is more chronic. Repetitive and cumulative exposure over several months or years to water, abrasives and chemicals can induce dermatitis, commonly on the hands. Individuals with a history of atopic eczema are more susceptible to irritants.

Clinical presentation

Contact dermatitis may affect any part of the body, although the hands and face are common sites. The appearance of a dermatitis at a particular site (Fig. 4) suggests contact with certain objects. For example, an eczema on the wrist of a woman with a history of reacting to cheap earrings suggests a nickel allergic response to a watchstrap buckle (Fig. 5). Diagnosis is often not easy as a history of irritant or allergen exposure is not always forthcoming. Knowing the patient's occupation, hobbies, past history and use of cosmetics or medicaments helps in listing possible causes.

Nickel sensitivity is the commonest contact allergy, affecting 10% of women and 1% of men. Usually, it causes only an inconvenient eczema at jewellery or metal contact sites, but an industrial

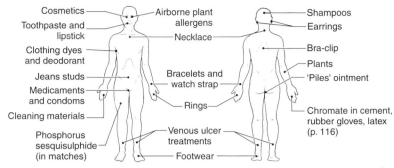

Fig. 4 **Distribution clues for contact dermatitis.**

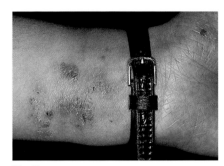

Fig. 5 **Allergic contact dermatitis to nickel in a watchstrap buckle.**

dermatitis can result, e.g. in nickel platers or metal machinists.

Environmental sources of common allergens are shown in Table 2. Medicaments (p. 17) and cosmetics (p. 104) can also induce allergic or irritant reactions. Allergic contact dermatitis occasionally becomes generalized by secondary 'autosensitization' spread. Activation by ultraviolet (UV) radiation of a topical agent, e.g. UV sunscreen filters or previously some perfumes, produces a photocontact reaction in sun-exposed sites (p. 44).

Differential diagnosis

Contact dermatitis of the hands needs to be differentiated from endogenous eczema, latex contact urticaria (p. 120), psoriasis and fungal infection. Acute

contact dermatitis of the face may resemble angioedema or erysipelas.

Management

The management of contact dermatitis is not always easy because of the many and often overlapping factors that can be involved in any one case. The *identification* of any offending allergen or irritant is the overriding objective. *Patch testing* (p. 122) helps to identify any allergens involved and is particularly useful in dermatitis of the face, hands and feet. The exclusion of an offending allergen from the environment is desirable and, if this can be achieved, the dermatitis may clear.

However, it is difficult to fully eliminate all contact with ubiquitous allergens such as fragrance or colophonium. Similarly, irritants are often impossible to exclude. Some contact with irritants may be inevitable owing to the nature of certain jobs, but occupational hygiene can often be improved. Unnecessary contact with irritants should be limited, protective clothing worn (notably nitrile gloves) and adequate washing and drying facilities provided. *Barrier creams* are seldom the answer, although they do encourage personal skin care. *Topical steroids* (moderately potent or potent) help in contact dermatitis, but avoidance measures should predominate.

Table 2	**The sources of common allergens**
Allergen	**Source**
Chromate	Cement, tanned leather, primer paint, anticorrosives
Cobalt	Pigment, paint, ink, metal alloys
Colophonium	Glue, plasticizer, adhesive tape, varnish, polish
Epoxy resins	Adhesive, plastics, mouldings
Fragrances	Cosmetics, creams, soaps, deodorants, aromatherapy
Nickel	Jewellery, zips, fasteners, scissors, instruments
Paraphenylenediamine	Dye (clothing, hair), shoes, colour developer
Plants	*Primula obconica*, chrysanthemums, garlic, poison ivy/oak (USA)
Preservatives	Cosmetics, creams and oils
Rubber chemicals	Gloves, clothing, shoes, masks, tyres, condoms

Contact dermatitis

- **Irritant factors of various types** cause more contact dermatitis than allergens.

- **Irritant contact dermatitis,** in many cases, can be difficult to distinguish from allergic or endogenous eczema on morphological grounds alone.

- **Atopics and those with 'a sensitive skin'** are more susceptible to the effects of irritants.

- **Patch testing** is helpful to confirm allergic contact dermatitis, particularly of the face, hands and feet. Specific immunoglobulin (IgE) tests or prick tests may also be needed, e.g. for latex.

- **Common allergens:** nickel, rubber chemicals, fragrances, chromate, cobalt, colophonium, preservatives, plant allergens and paraphenylenediamine.

- **Common irritants:** water, frictional abrasives, chemicals (especially alkalis), solvents, oils, detergents, soaps, low humidity and temperature extremes.

- **Elimination and avoidance** of allergens and irritants are useful, although prevention is the ideal.

www.eczema.org/ ■ http://www.emedicine.com/emerg/topic131.htm

Eczema – Atopic eczema

Definition

Atopic eczema is a chronic pruritic inflammation of the epidermis and dermis, often associated with a personal or family history of asthma, allergic rhinitis, conjunctivitis or atopic eczema. Uncontrollable scratching is prominent, and the course is remitting.

Aetiopathogenesis

'Atopy' defines an inherited tendency (p. 12), present in 15–25% of the population, to develop one or more of the aforementioned disorders and to produce high levels of circulating immunoglobulin (Ig)E antibodies, commonly to inhalant allergens (e.g. house dust mite). A T-helper (Th) 2 cell response seems to be predominant over Th1 (p. 10), and the resultant cytokine profile favours IgE production. However, the serum IgE is normal in 20% of atopic eczema subjects. There is evidence that Th1 cell immunity directed against house dust mite antigen may be important in atopic eczema, although the basic cause of these immune defects is still unclear.

Incidence

About 12–15% of infants are affected. It usually starts within the first 6 months of life and, by 1 year, 60% of those likely to develop atopic eczema will have done so. Two-thirds have a family history of atopy. Remission occurs within 10–20 years in 40–60%, although some relapse later.

Clinical presentation

The appearance of atopic eczema differs depending on the age of the patient.

Infancy

Babies develop an itchy vesicular exudative eczema on the face (Fig. 1), head and hands, often with secondary infection. About half continue to have eczema beyond 18 months.

Childhood

After 18 months, the pattern often changes to the familiar involvement of the antecubital and popliteal fossae, neck, wrists and ankles (Figs 2 and 3). The face often shows erythema and infraorbital folds. Lichenification, excoriations and dry skin (Fig. 4) are common, and palmar markings may be increased. Post-inflammatory

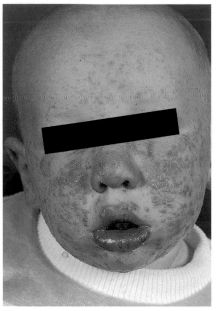

Fig. 1 **Atopic eczema in an infant.** Secondary bacterial infection was present.

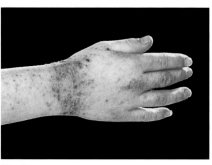

Fig. 2 **Atopic eczema in a child, showing excoriations and lichenification at the wrist.**

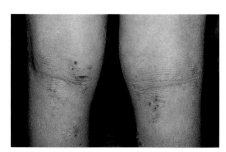

Fig. 3 **Atopic eczema involving the popliteal fossa in a child.**

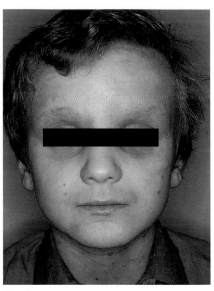

Fig. 4 **A 'dry' pruritic type of atopic eczema.** Note the loss of eyebrows due to constant rubbing of the face.

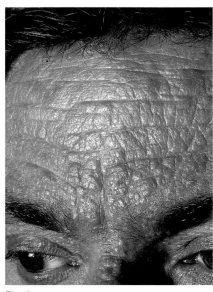

Fig. 5 **Grossly lichenified and nodular atopic eczema on the face of an adult.**

hyperpigmentation occurs in those with a pigmented skin. Scratching or rubbing cause most of the clinical signs and are a particular problem at night when they can interfere with sleep. Behavioural difficulties can occur, and a child's eczema can disrupt family life. Schoolchildren with eczema may be teased or rejected by their classmates. Occasionally, a 'reverse pattern' of

eczema is seen, with involvement of the extensor aspects of the knees and elbows.

Adults

The commonest manifestation in adult life is hand dermatitis, exacerbated by irritants, in someone with a past history of atopic eczema. However, a small number of adults have a chronic severe form of generalized and lichenified atopic eczema (Fig. 5), which may interfere with their employment and social activities. Stressful situations, such as examinations or marital problems, often coincide with exacerbations.

Differential diagnosis

Infantile flexural eczema (p. 112) may sometimes develop into the atopic variety and, occasionally, the distinction from scabies is necessary. Rarely, infants with immune deficiency syndromes (e.g. Wiskott–Aldrich) or with Langerhans cell histiocytosis (p. 112) have an eczematous eruption.

Investigations

Prick tests or the allergen-specific IgE tests to inhalant and (sometimes) food allergens are frequently positive, although the relevance is often unclear unless there is a confirmatory history. Total serum IgE levels are raised in 80% of patients. These tests are rarely needed to make the diagnosis. Swabs for bacterial and viral culture may be helpful during an exacerbation.

Complications

Atopic eczema is subject to several complications – some common and some rare:

- *Bacterial infection.* Secondary infection usually with *Staphylococcus aureus* (a 'superantigen', p. 47) commonly causes an exacerbation.
- *Viral infection.* Patients have an increased susceptibility to infection with molluscum contagiosum and possibly with viral warts.
- *Eczema herpeticum.* There is a propensity to develop widespread lesions with herpes simplex (Fig. 6).
- *Cataracts.* A specific form of cataract infrequently develops in young adults with severe atopic eczema.
- *Growth retardation.* Children with severe atopic eczema may have short stature. The cause is usually unknown.
- *Ichthyosis vulgaris.* This is more common in patients with atopic eczema.

Management

A strategy should be discussed with the patient and carers. General measures

include explaining the disorder and its treatment to the patient and the parents, stressing the normally good prognosis. A child should wear loose cotton clothing and avoid wool (which irritates) and excessive heat. Nails should be kept short. Cats and dogs cause exacerbations in some patients and are best kept away. The exclusion of house dust mite from the home environment is difficult. Careers advice is also important. Wet work jobs (e.g. nursing, hairdressing, cleaning) and industrial work with exposure to irritant oils should be avoided. Some sufferers obtain support from groups such as the National Eczema Society (p. 128). Specialist nurses are skilful in managing eczema patients.

Specific treatments for atopic eczema are summarized in Table 1.

Table 1	**Treatment of atopic eczema**
Treatment	**Indication**
Emollients	Most eczema; ichthyosis
Topical steroids	Most types of eczema
Topical tacrolimus	Steroid-resistant eczema
Tar bandage	Lichenified/excoriated eczema
Oral antihistamine	Pruritus
Oral antibiotic	Bacterial superinfection
Exclusion diet	Food allergy/resistant eczema
UVB, ciclosporin and azathioprine	Resistant and severe eczema unresponsive to topical therapy

Topical therapy

Emollients

Emollients such as aqueous cream and emulsifying ointment (p. 22) should be used regularly on the skin and as soap substitutes. They moisturize the dry skin, diminishing the desire to scratch and reducing the need for topical steroids. Bath oil emollients may also help.

Topical steroids and tacrolimus

The rule is to prescribe the least potent strength steroid that is effective. In children, 1% hydrocortisone ointment applied twice a day is usually adequate (ointments are generally preferred to creams for eczema). Sometimes, it is necessary to use a moderately potent steroid for a short time in children with resistant eczema, and for rather more prolonged periods in adults with established and severe eczema. Tacrolimus ointment (Protopic: 0.03% children, 0.1% adults) or pimecrolimus (Elidel, 1%) are alternatives to steroids, especially in facial and hand eczema.

Topical antibiotics or antiseptics

Topical antiseptics, or a 7-day course of a topical antibiotic, may be used for

infected eczema, in combination with a steroid (e.g. Fucibet cream) or separately (e.g. Bactroban or Fucidin ointment).

Coal tar or ichthammol paste

Coal tar or ichthammol paste is useful for lichenified or excoriated eczema, used as an occlusive medicated bandage (e.g. Coltapaste or Ichthopaste) normally left on overnight.

Wet wrap technique

Wet wraps are often required for a short time on an exudative eczema.

Systemic therapy

A sedative antihistamine, such as promethazine or alimemazine, given at night, helps to reduce the desire to scratch in both children and adults. Infected exacerbations frequently require the intermittent use of an antibiotic by mouth, and flucloxacillin is often selected. Eczema herpeticum is usually an indication for admission to hospital (with appropriate isolation of the patient); treatment is with aciclovir. Patients with severe and resistant forms of atopic eczema may be treated with narrow-band UVB (p. 102), azathioprine or ciclosporin (p. 23), initially given as an 8-week course.

Dietary manipulation

Some children with atopic eczema give a history that suggests food allergy (e.g. urticaria of the mouth on contact with the food, or gastrointestinal symptoms), and it is clear that the offending food should be avoided. Otherwise, dietary treatment is reserved for a minority who have not improved with standard therapy. Diets free from cows' milk or eggs may be tried, supervised by a dietician to ensure exclusion and to prevent nutritional deficiencies.

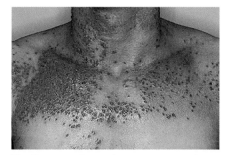

Fig. 6 **Eczema herpeticum.** Herpes simplex infection complicating atopic eczema.

> ### Atopic eczema
>
> - Affects 12–15% of infants: onset at less than 1 year in 60% of cases.
> - Aetiology is not well understood but immune function is disturbed.
> - Classically affects the face in infants, later knee and elbow flexures.
> - Itch–scratch cycle induces lichenification.
> - Exacerbations are often due to infection, particularly staphylococcal.
> - Treatment involves emollients, topical steroids, tacrolimus, tar bandages, systemic antihistamines and antibiotics.

Eczema – Other forms

The other main types of eczema are seborrhoeic, discoid, venous, asteatotic and hand dermatitis.

Seborrhoeic dermatitis

Seborrhoeic dermatitis is a chronic, red, scaly, inflammatory eruption usually affecting the scalp and face (Table 1).

Aetiopathogenesis

Sebum production is normal, but the eruption often occurs in the sebaceous gland areas of the scalp, face and chest. Endogenous and genetic factors, and an overgrowth of the commensal yeast *Malassezia* (previously *Pityrosporum ovale*) are involved. The condition is severe in some patients with human immunodeficiency virus (HIV) infection.

Clinical presentation

There are four common patterns:

- *Scalp and facial involvement.* Excessive dandruff, with an itchy scaly erythematous eruption affecting the sides of the nose, scalp margin, eyebrows and ears (Fig. 1). Blepharitis may occur. Most common in young adult males.
- *Petaloid.* A dry, scaly patch of eczema over the presternal area.
- *Pityrosporum folliculitis.* An erythematous follicular eruption with papules or pustules over the back (Fig. 2).

- *Flexural.* Involvement of the axillae, groins and submammary areas by a moist intertrigo, often secondarily colonized by *Candida albicans*. Seen in the elderly (do not confuse with the similarly named infantile eruption, p. 112).

Management

The scalp lesions require the use of a medicated shampoo (e.g. containing coal tar, selenium sulphide or ketoconazole), either alone or following the application of 2% sulphur and 2% salicylic acid cream left on for several hours. Facial, truncal and flexural involvement responds to an imidazole or antimicrobial, often combined with 1% hydrocortisone, in a cream or ointment base (e.g. Daktacort and Vioform-Hydrocortisone). Oral itraconazole is also effective. Recurrence is common and repeated treatment often necessary.

Table 1 **Differential diagnosis of seborrhoeic dermatitis**	
Site of seborrhoeic dermatitis	**Differential diagnosis**
Face	Psoriasis, contact dermatitis, rosacea
Scalp	Psoriasis, fungal infection
Trunk	Psoriasis, pityriasis versicolor, fungal infection

Discoid (nummular) eczema

Discoid eczema is an eczema of unknown aetiology characterized by coin-shaped lesions on the limbs; it typically affects middle-aged or elderly men (Fig. 3). Younger subjects may have atopic eczema.

Clinical presentation

The coin-shaped eczema lesions are often symmetrical and can be intensely itchy. The eczema may be vesicular or chronic and lichenified. It may clear after a few weeks, but tends to recur. Secondary bacterial infection is common.

Management

The condition can often be confused with tinea corporis and contact dermatitis. A potent or very potent topical steroid, often combined with an antimicrobial or antibiotic, is helpful.

Venous (stasis) eczema

Venous eczema affects the lower legs (Fig. 4) and is associated with underlying venous disease (p. 70). Incompetence of the deep perforating veins increases hydrostatic pressure in dermal capillaries. Pericapillary fibrin deposition impedes oxygen diffusion and leads to clinical changes.

Clinical presentation

Most patients are middle-aged or elderly women. Leashes of venules and haemosiderin pigmentation around

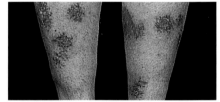

Fig. 3 **Discoid eczema of the lower leg.**

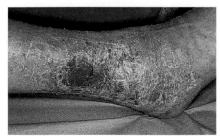

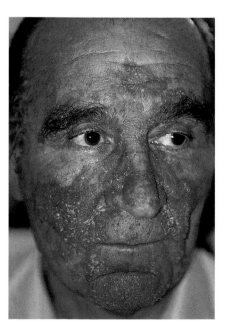

Fig. 1 **Seborrhoeic dermatitis affecting the face.**

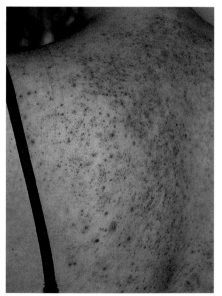

Fig. 2 **Seborrhoeic dermatitis of the *Pityrosporum* folliculitis type affecting the back.**

Fig. 4 **Venous eczema.**

the ankles are early signs. Eczema develops, sometimes with fibrosis of the dermis and subcutaneous tissue (lipodermatosclerosis) and ulceration. Contact allergy to an applied medicament can complicate the picture.

Management
An emollient, alone or with a mild or moderately potent steroid ointment, is needed. Tar-impregnated bandages (e.g. Ichthopaste or Coltapaste) applied once or twice a week, are useful especially when ulceration coexists. Venous disease or ulceration is treated on its own merit (p. 70).

Hand dermatitis
Hand dermatitis is a common, often recurrent condition that varies from being acute and vesicular to chronic, hyperkeratotic and fissured. The condition results from a variety of causes, and several factors are often involved. In children, hand dermatitis is mostly due to atopic eczema. An atopic predisposition often underlies adult hand dermatitis, especially if caused by repeated exposure to irritants.

Allergic causes need excluding, and most adults with hand dermatitis require patch testing. Fungal infection is ruled out by microscopy and culture, especially in unilateral hand dermatitis, and the feet are examined because tinea pedis can provoke a hand dermatitis as an 'id' phenomenon (p. 56). A core of patients is left who have an endogenous recurrent hand dermatitis often characterized by sago-like vesicles on the sides of the fingers, on the palms and sometimes on the soles.

Clinical presentation
Hand dermatitis often presents as a chronic eczema, but may appear as a

vesicular eruption known as *pompholyx*. Vesicles may be seen with atopic eczema or contact dermatitis but, in pompholyx, there is usually no associated disorder. The onset is in young adults, particularly in warm weather, and it is often recurrent. Involvement can be confined to a few microvesicles on the fingers, or it can be extensive with bullae affecting the whole hand (Fig. 5). Some of these patients are nickel sensitive.

Management
Acute pompholyx requires drainage of large blisters and the application (once or twice a day) of wet dressings (e.g. immersed in 0.01% aqueous potassium permanganate or Burow's solution of 0.65% aqueous aluminium acetate). Oral antibiotics are given if bacterial infection is present. Some dermatologists prescribe systemic steroids, but these are usually not necessary. Once the acute stage settles, potent or highly potent steroid lotions or creams are used with cotton gloves. For chronic or subacute cases, a steroid ointment and emollients are helpful. Advice for patients with hand dermatitis is given in Table 2.

Asteatotic eczema (eczéma craquelé)
Asteatotic eczema is a dry eczema with fissuring and cracking of the skin, often affecting the limbs in the elderly (Fig. 6).

Overwashing of patients in institutions, a dry winter climate,

hypothyroidism and the use of diuretics can contribute to eczema in the atrophic skin of old people. The skin of the limbs and trunk is erythematous, dry and itchy and shows a fine crazy-paving pattern of fissuring. Emollients applied to the skin and used in the bath often suffice to clear up the condition, but sometimes a mild steroid is necessary.

Other eczemas
Other types of eczema are occasionally encountered. They include: lichen simplex chronicus, lichen striatus, juvenile plantar dermatosis (p. 112) and napkin (diaper) eruption (p. 112).

Lichen simplex chronicus (neurodermatitis)
Neurodermatitis is an area of lichenified eczema due to repeated rubbing or scratching, as a habit or due to 'stress'. It usually occurs as a single plaque on the lower leg, back of the neck or in the perineum (*pruritus vulvae/ani*: p. 117). The skin markings are exaggerated, and pigmentation may occur. Asians and Chinese are particularly susceptible. Sometimes a nodular lichenification known as *prurigo nodularis* develops on the shins and forearms. Emollients, topical steroids, weak tar paste and tar-impregnated bandages are the mainstay of treatment.

Lichen striatus
Lichen striatus is a rare self-limiting linear eczema affecting a limb and occurring in adolescents (p. 19).

Table 2 **Hints on hand care for hand dermatitis patients**
Hand washing
Use warm water and unscented soap; avoid paper towels and hot air dryers; instead use a dry cotton towel
Protection
Avoid wet work if possible, or otherwise wear cotton gloves under vinyl or nitrile gloves; wear gloves in cold weather and for dusty work
Medicaments
Use emollients regularly throughout the day; apply steroid ointments twice a day
Avoid handling
Shampoos, hair preparations, detergents, solvents, polishes, certain vegetables (e.g. tomatoes, potatoes), peeling fruits (e.g. oranges) and cutting raw meat

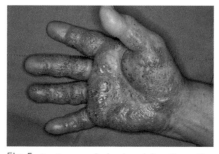

Fig. 5 **Acute pompholyx involving the entire palmar surface of the hand in a nickel-sensitive woman.**

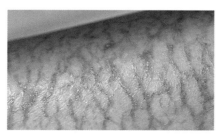

Fig. 6 **Asteatotic eczema.**

Eczema

- **Seborrhoeic dermatitis** commonly affects the scalp and face. It responds to combined antimicrobial/hydrocortisone creams.

- **Discoid eczema** often presents as coin-shaped lesions on limbs of the middle-aged or elderly. It improves with moderate potency topical steroids.

- **Venous eczema** is associated with venous disease. It responds to emollients and low or moderate potency topical steroids.

- **Hand dermatitis:** multiple and mixed aetiology; determine causes by exclusion.

- **Asteatotic eczema:** the eczéma craquelé of elderly skin. Treat with emollients or low potency topical steroids.

- **Lichen simplex chronicus:** an area of lichenified eczema induced by persistent scratching, often found on the posterior neck or lower leg.

- **Lichen striatus:** a rare linear eczema.

Lichenoid eruptions

Lichen planus and other disorders with a lichenoid appearance of shiny flat-topped papules are presented here.

Lichen planus

Lichen planus is a relatively common pruritic papular dermatosis involving the flexor surfaces, mucous membranes and genitalia.

The cause is unknown, but an immune pathogenesis for lichen planus is suspected as T cells infiltrate the skin, immunoglobulin (Ig)M is found at the dermoepidermal junction, a lichenoid eruption is part of graft-versus-host disease (p. 81), and there is an association with some autoimmune diseases.

Pathology

In lichen planus, the granular layer is thickened, basal cells show liquefaction degeneration and lymphocytes infiltrate the upper dermis in a band-like fashion (Fig. 1).

Clinical presentation

Two-thirds of cases occur in the 30- to 60-year-old age group. It is uncommon at the extremes of age, and the sex incidence is equal. Lichen planus tends to start on the limbs. It may spread rapidly to become generalized within 4 weeks, but the commoner localized forms progress more slowly. Typical lesions are very itchy flat-topped polygonal papules, a few millimetres in diameter, which may show a surface network of delicate white lines (Wickham's striae). Initially, the papules are red, but they become violaceous (Fig. 2).

The eruption is symmetrical and affects:

- forearms and wrists
- lower legs and thighs
- genitalia, mucous membranes
- palms and soles.

Mucous membrane involvement, especially of the buccal mucosa, occurs in up to two-thirds of cases, and may be present without skin lesions (Fig. 3). Lichen planus also shows the Koebner phenomenon (p. 19). Follicular and other variants are found (see below). In most cases, papules flatten after a few months to leave pigmentation, but some become hypertrophic. Half of all

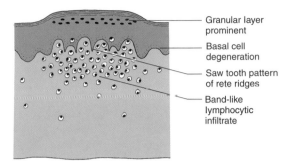
Fig. 1 **Histopathology of lichen planus.**

- Granular layer prominent
- Basal cell degeneration
- Saw tooth pattern of rete ridges
- Band-like lymphocytic infiltrate

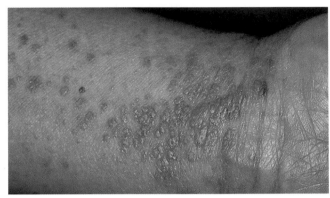
Fig. 2 **Typical violaceous papules of lichen planus at the wrist.**

patients are clear within 9 months, but 15% have continuing symptoms even after 18 months. Up to 20% have a further attack. Lichen planus may be confused with other conditions, as shown in Table 1.

Variants of lichen planus

A number of variants of lichen planus exist:

- *Annular.* Found in 10% of cases, commonly on the glans penis.
- *Atrophic.* Rare, may be seen with hypertrophic lesions.
- *Bullous.* Blisters appear infrequently in lichen planus.
- *Follicular.* May occur with typical lichen planus; can affect the scalp alone (scarring alopecia; p. 65).

- *Hypertrophic.* Verrucous plaques affect the lower legs or arms (Fig. 4); may persist for years.
- *Mucous membrane.* Any mucosal surface may be affected, with or without lesions elsewhere. In the mouth, may represent contact allergy to mercury in amalgam fillings (Fig. 3).

Complications

Lichen planus may be complicated by:

- *Nail involvement.* Found in 10% of patients. Longitudinal grooving and pitting are reversible, but dystrophic/atrophic lesions can produce scarring or permanent nail loss.
- *Scalp lesions.* May be follicular, but pseudopelade-like permanent

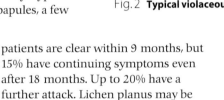

Table 1 **Differential diagnosis: lichen planus**	
Type of lichen planus	**Differential diagnosis**
Generalized	Lichenoid drug eruption
	Guttate psoriasis
	Atypical pityriasis rosea
Genital	Psoriasis, scabies
	Lichen sclerosus
Hypertrophic	Lichen simplex

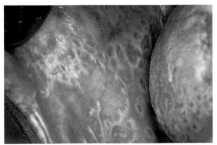
Fig. 3 **White lace-like Wickham's striae on the buccal mucosa.**

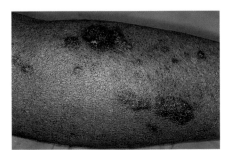
Fig. 4 **Hypertrophic lichen planus showing hyperpigmentation.**

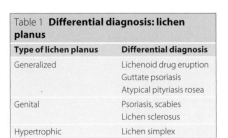

scarring alopecia is more common (p. 65).

- *Malignant change*. Very infrequent.

Management
Lichen planus disease is self-limiting in most patients. Moderate to high potency topical steroids usually produce symptomatic improvement. Oral lesions are helped by a steroid-containing paste (e.g. Adcortyl in Orabase). Hypertrophic lichen planus may require highly potent topical steroids, sometimes under occlusion, or intralesional steroid injection. Extensive involvement, ulcerative mucous membrane lesions or a potentially scarring nail dystrophy warrant a trial of oral prednisolone (in a dose of 10–20 mg/day) for 1–3 months. Long-term systemic steroids are not justified. Acitretin or psoralen with ultraviolet A (PUVA) may help resistant cases.

Lichen sclerosus
Lichen sclerosus is an uncommon disorder typified by white lichenoid atrophic lesions on the genitalia. Although associated with autoimmune disease, the cause is unknown.

Pathology
The epidermis may be thickened, thinned or hyperkeratotic. The upper dermis is oedematous with few cells: collagen is hyalinized. Lymphocytes infiltrate the lower dermis.

Clinical presentation
Lichen sclerosus occurs 10 times more frequently in women. It is commonest in middle age, although it may develop in childhood (with a better prognosis). Genital lesions are almost invariable, but involvement of the trunk or arms is seen. Individual lesions are a few millimetres in diameter, porcelain white and slightly atrophic, and may aggregate into wrinkled plaques (Fig. 5). Hyperkeratosis, telangiectasia, purpura and even blistering occur. Vulval and perianal lesions cause itching and

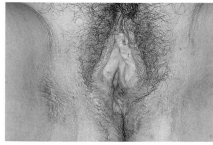

Fig. 5 **Lichen sclerosus of the vulva.**

soreness. Involvement in the male results in urethral stricture and phimosis (balanitis xerotica obliterans). Occasionally, lesions are found in the mouth. Lichen sclerosus is chronic and usually permanent in adults. Spontaneous resolution is most likely at puberty in childhood cases.

Differential diagnosis
Female genital involvement may resemble lichen simplex chronicus (p. 37), Bowen's disease (p. 100) and extramammary Paget's disease. Male genital lesions mimic lichen planus, psoriasis and some rare inflammatory and premalignant forms of balanitis (p. 117).

Complications
Shrinkage of the vulva occurs, and dyspareunia is a problem in females. Males may experience recurrent balanitis and ulceration of the glans. Squamous cell carcinoma develops infrequently in the longstanding lesions of both sexes.

Management
Non-genital lesions require no treatment. In female genital involvement, a moderate or potent strength steroid cream will reduce the itch and prevent scarring. Vulvectomy is contraindicated in uncomplicated cases.

Treatment is similar for the male genital lesions, although circumcision

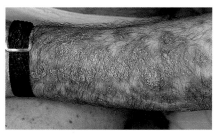

Fig. 6 **A lichenoid drug eruption, here due to quinine.**

Type of agent	Drug
Antiarthritic	Gold, penicillamine, non-steroidal anti-inflammatory drugs
Antibiotic	Streptomycin, tetracyclines
Antimalarial	Chloroquine, mepacrine, quinine
Antituberculous	Isoniazid, ethambutol
Diuretic	Thiazides, furosemide
Angiotensin-converting enzyme inhibitor	Captopril, enalapril
Antidiabetic	Tolbutamide, chlorpropamide
Antipsychotic	Phenothiazines, lithium

Table 2 **Drugs causing a lichen planus-like eruption**

is performed if phimosis develops. Both sexes need long-term follow-up and biopsy of any suspicious areas.

Lichen nitidus
Lichen nitidus is an uncommon eruption of minute monomorphic flesh-coloured papules. The aetiology is unknown. Histology reveals a lymphohistiocytic infiltrate, which expands a single dermal papilla.

Clinical presentation and management
The eruption is asymptomatic, often noticed by chance, and usually occurs in children or young adults. Uniform pinhead-sized papules, which may be grouped, are seen on the forearms, penis, abdomen and buttocks. The main differential diagnosis is lichen planus (with which it may coexist) and keratosis pilaris (p. 88).

Treatment is usually unnecessary. Lichen nitidus may resolve in weeks or persist indefinitely.

Lichen planus-like drug eruption
An eruption resembling lichen planus can follow the ingestion of several drugs.

Clinical presentation
A lichen planus-like rash has been recognized with gold and mepacrine therapy for many years. The eruption, which can be severe, is often more hypertrophic and hyperpigmented than true lichen planus (Fig. 6) and, on histology, shows a greater number of eosinophils. Resolution after withdrawal of the drug is often slow. Table 2 lists some of the drugs responsible.

Lichenoid eruptions

- **Lichen planus** is a relatively common pruritic papular eruption, which resolves in most cases within 18 months.

- **Lichen planus-like drug eruption** resembles lichen planus but is more persistent; it is seen, for example, with gold, chloroquine and thiazides.

- **Lichen nitidus** is a rare, asymptomatic eruption of fine monomorphic papules on the abdomen, arms and penis.

- **Lichen sclerosus** is most common in women, and frequently affects the genitalia. Vulval shrinkage may occur. Topical steroids are helpful. There is a risk of malignant change.

Papulosquamous eruptions

Papulosquamous eruptions are raised, scaly and marginated, and include psoriasis, lichen planus and other conditions listed in Table 1. Eczema is not included as it does not usually have a sharp edge. These eruptions are not related aetiologically. Several are characterized by fine scaling and have the prefix 'pityriasis', which means 'bran-like scale'.

Table 1 **Papulosquamous eruptions**	
Chronic superficial dermatitis	Pityriasis rubra pilaris (p. 42)
Drug eruption (p. 84)	Pityriasis versicolor
Lichen planus (p. 38)	Psoriasis (p. 28)
Pityriasis alba	Reiter's disease
Pityriasis lichenoides	Secondary syphilis
Pityriasis rosea	Tinea infection (p. 56)

Pityriasis rosea

Pityriasis rosea is an acute, self-limiting disorder probably infective in origin, characterized by scaly oval papules and plaques that occur mainly on the trunk.

Clinical presentation

The generalized eruption is preceded in most patients by the appearance of a single lesion, 2–5 cm in diameter, known as a 'herald patch' (Fig. 1). Some days later, many smaller plaques appear, mainly on the trunk but also on the upper arms and thighs. Individual plaques are oval, pink and have a delicate peripheral 'collarette' of scale. They are distributed parallel to the lines of the ribs, radiating away from the spine. Itching is mild or moderate. The eruption fades spontaneously in 4–8 weeks. It tends to affect teenagers and young adults. The cause is unknown, but epidemiological evidence of 'clustering' suggests an infective aetiology.

Differential diagnosis and management

Guttate psoriasis, pityriasis versicolor and secondary syphilis may cause confusion. A serological test for syphilis is needed in doubtful cases. The condition is self-limiting, and treatment does not hasten clearance, although a moderate potency topical steroid can help to relieve pruritus.

Pityriasis (tinea) versicolor

Pityriasis versicolor is a chronic, often asymptomatic, fungal infection characterized by pigmentary changes and involving the trunk.

Clinical presentation

The condition is caused by overgrowth of the mycelial form of the commensal yeast *Malassezia* (previously *Pityrosporum ovale*) and is particularly common in humid or tropical conditions. In Europe, it mainly affects young adults, appearing on the trunk and proximal parts of the limbs (Fig. 2). In untanned, white caucasians, brown or pinkish oval or round superficially scaly patches are seen, but, in tanned or racially pigmented skin, hypopigmentation is found as a result of the release by the organism of dicarboxylic acids that inhibit melanogenesis.

Differential diagnosis

Differentiation from vitiligo is important: usually pityriasis versicolor has a fine scale, and scrapings readily show the 'grapes and bananas' appearance of the spores and short hyphae on microscopy. Pityriasis rosea and tinea corporis may occasionally appear similar.

Management

Treatment involves either the topical application of one of the imidazole antifungals (e.g. Canesten or Daktarin cream) or the use of 2.5% selenium sulphide (Selsun) shampoo applied for 30 min (or ketoconazole (Nizoral) shampoo applied for 30 min) and showered off (use three times a week for 2 weeks). Itraconazole, 200 mg daily for 7 days, is effective for resistant cases. Recurrences are common, and patients are advised that re-treatment may be required.

Reiter's disease

Reiter's disease is a syndrome of polyarthropathy, urethritis, iritis and a psoriasiform eruption.

Clinical presentation and management

Reiter's disease almost invariably affects males who have the HLA-B27 genotype and commonly follows a genitourinary or bowel infection. The joint and eye changes are often severe. Skin involvement includes a balanitis (p. 117) and red, scaly, pustular, psoriasiform plaques on the feet (keratoderma blenorrhagicum).

Severe skin changes are unresponsive to topical therapy, and methotrexate or acitretin is often needed.

Chronic superficial dermatitis

Previously known as parapsoriasis, a term best avoided, this is an uncommon chronic dermatitis of small scaly pink–brown oval or round-shaped plaques, mainly on the trunk. The variant with larger plaques may proceed to mycosis fungoides (cutaneous T-cell lymphoma) or be this from the onset.

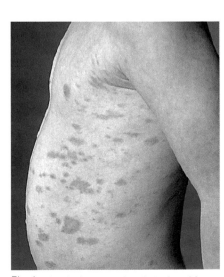

Fig. 1 **Pityriasis rosea, showing a herald patch on the lower abdomen and associated oval scaly plaques.**

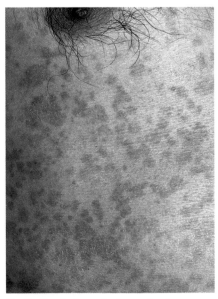

Fig. 2 **Pityriasis versicolor on the chest: brown scaly patches are evident.**

Clinical presentation

In chronic superficial dermatitis, scaly patches develop, usually on the abdomen, buttocks or thighs (Fig. 3). The onset is in young to mid-adult life, and the plaques are indolent. It may be difficult to predict which cases will progress to mycosis fungoides (p. 100), especially as the evolution may take place over many years, but the 'benign' lesions tend to be small and finger-like in shape, whereas the 'premalignant' plaques are larger, asymmetrical, atrophic and can show associated poikiloderma (reticulate pigmentation, telangiectasia and atrophy). Biopsy is necessary to look for the changes of mycosis fungoides (p. 100), and further biopsy of any changed area is required. The disease is often indolent and may persist over a period of several years.

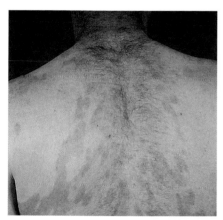

Fig. 3 **Plaques of chronic superficial dermatitis on the back of a middle-aged man.**

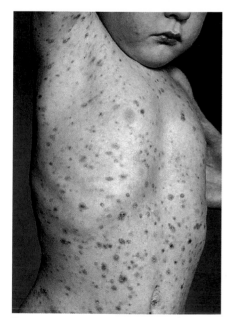

Fig. 4 **Pityriasis lichenoides (acute type) in a child.**

Differential diagnosis and management

Psoriasis, discoid eczema and tinea corporis may need to be considered in the diagnosis, but the plaques of chronic superficial dermatitis are distinguished by being fixed.

The first-line treatment with moderately potent topical steroids is sometimes helpful. Ultraviolet B (UVB) or psoralen with UVA (PUVA) will often be needed for the large plaque variant. Long-term follow-up is recommended.

Other pityriases

Other varieties of pityriasis include:

- *Pityriasis lichenoides*. A rare chronic eruption in which small papules topped by a fine single scale appear on the limbs and trunk. It is seen in adolescents and young adults and may occur in an acute form (Fig. 4), which heals with scarring.
- *Pityriasis rubra pilaris*. A rare, scaly follicular eruption, which may progress to erythroderma (see p. 42).
- *Pityriasis alba*. Occurs in children or young adults and is characterized by fine scaly white patches on the face or arms. It is often seen in atopic patients.

Secondary syphilis

Definition

Secondary syphilis is an inflammatory response in the skin and mucous membranes to the disseminated *Treponema pallidum* spirochaete.

There has been a resurgence of syphilis in recent years.

Clinical presentation

The secondary phase of syphilis (p. 116) starts 4–12 weeks after the appearance of the primary chancre and consists of an eruption, lymphadenopathy and variable malaise. Pink or copper-coloured macules, which later develop into papules, appear in a symmetrical distribution on the trunk and limbs and are non-itchy (Fig. 5). Annular patterns are not uncommon, and involvement of the palms and soles is distinctive. Other signs are moist warty lesions (condyloma lata) in the anogenital area, buccal erosions that may be arcuate (snail-track ulcers) and a diffuse patchy alopecia. Mucosal lesions are infectious. Without treatment, the lesions of secondary syphilis resolve spontaneously in 1–3 months.

Differential diagnosis and management

Pityriasis rosea, psoriasis, drug eruption, infectious mononucleosis, rubella and measles may need to be considered. Treponemal serology is positive in all patients with secondary syphilis. Treatment is with intramuscular procaine benzylpenicillin (p. 116). Patients with syphilis are best managed by physicians familiar with the treatment of genitourinary infections.

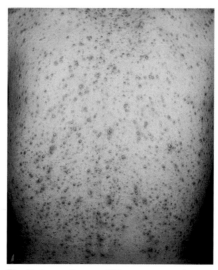

Fig. 5 **Secondary syphilis. Coppery red-coloured macules and papules are evident on the trunk.**

Papulosquamous eruptions

- **Pityriasis rosea** is a fairly common self-limiting eruption that involves the trunk of young adults. Scaly oval plaques follow a herald patch. It may be infective in origin.

- **Pityriasis versicolor** is a common truncal eruption of young adults and is due to *Malassezia*, a commensal yeast. It is often revealed in the summer as pale areas adjacent to tanned skin.

- **Reiter's syndrome** typically affects young males and follows a genitourinary or bowel infection. Keratotic skin lesions are seen with eye and joint changes.

- **Chronic superficial dermatitis** is an uncommon truncal eruption seen in young or middle-aged adults. The large plaque variant may represent early cutaneous T-cell lymphoma.

- **Pityriasis lichenoides** is a rare chronic eruption of scaly-topped papules on the trunk and limbs. An acute form may scar.

- **Secondary syphilis** is a symmetrical, non-itchy truncal eruption with mucosal and palmar or plantar lesions, due to infection with *Treponema pallidum*.

http://www.emedicine.com/derm/topic335.htm ■ http://www.dermis.net/dermisroot/en/32672/diagnose.htm

Erythroderma

Definition
Erythroderma or generalized exfoliative dermatitis defines any inflammatory dermatosis that involves all or nearly all the skin surface (sometimes stated as more than 90%). It is a secondary process and represents the generalized spread of a dermatosis or systemic disease throughout the skin.

Pathology
The duration and severity of the inflammatory process play more of a part in deciding the histology than the underlying cause. In the acute eruption, oedema of the epidermis and dermis is prominent, and there is an inflammatory infiltrate. More chronic lesions show lengthened rete ridges and thickening of the epidermis. Abnormal lymphocytes may eventually be apparent in those cases resulting from lymphoma, and specific changes identified on biopsy of a typical lesion when psoriasis, ichthyosiform erythroderma or pityriasis rubra pilaris is the cause.

Clinical presentation
Erythroderma is an uncommon but important dermatological emergency, as the systemic effects are potentially fatal.

General symptoms and signs
Some features are common to all patients with erythroderma, no matter what the cause. It is twice as common in men and mainly affects the middle-aged and elderly. The condition often develops suddenly, particularly when associated with leukaemia or an eczema. A patchy erythema may rapidly spread to be universal within 12–48 h and be accompanied by pyrexia, malaise and shivering. Scaling appears 2–6 days later and, at this stage, the skin is hot, red, dry and obviously thickened. The patient experiences irritation and tightness of the skin and feels cold. The exfoliation of scales may be copious and continuous. Scalp and body hair is lost when erythroderma has been present for some weeks. The nails become thickened and may be shed. Pigmentary changes occur and, in those with a dark skin, hypopigmentation is seen. The picture is influenced by the patient's general condition and the underlying cause. The commonest causes of erythroderma are eczema, psoriasis and lymphoma (Table 1). Other dermatoses, including drug eruptions and pityriasis rubra pilaris, may also be implicated. Multiple skin biopsies may help in diagnosis.

Eczema
Atopic eczema may become erythrodermic at any age. Erythroderma from eczema is most common in the elderly, in whom the eczema may be unclassified. Itch is often intense.

Psoriasis
At first, the eruption resembles conventional psoriasis but, when the

Table 1 **Causes of erythroderma and their relative frequencies**

Cause	Frequency (%)
Eczema (contact/atopic/ seborrhoeic/unclassified)	40
Psoriasis	25
Lymphoma/leukaemia/ Sézary syndrome	15
Drug eruption	10
Pityriasis rubra pilaris/ ichthyosiform erythroderma	1
Other skin disease	1
Unknown	8

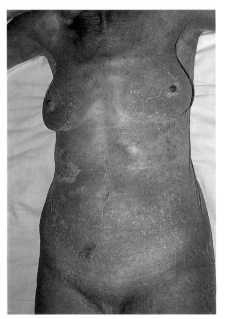

Fig. 1 **Erythrodermic psoriasis.**

exfoliative stage is reached, these specific features are lost (Fig. 1). The withdrawal of potent topical steroids or of systemic steroids, or an intercurrent drug eruption, can precipitate erythrodermic psoriasis. Sterile pinhead-sized pustules sometimes develop, and the condition may progress to generalized pustular psoriasis (p. 29).

Lymphoma/Sézary syndrome
Early biopsies may not be specific, and this may delay diagnosis, although universal erythroderma, infiltration of the skin and severe pruritus are helpful pointers (p. 87). Lymphadenopathy is often prominent, but the nodes are not always involved by lymphoma. Sézary syndrome (Fig. 2) typically occurs in elderly males and is characterized by the presence of abnormal T lymphocytes with large convoluted nuclei (Sézary cells) in the blood and skin. Patients may be stable for a number of years, then deteriorate rapidly.

Drug eruption
An acute drug eruption (p. 84), often of the toxic erythema or morbilliform type, may become erythrodermic (Fig. 3). Carbamazepine, phenytoin, diltiazem, cimetidine, gold, allopurinol and sulphonamides are the commonest culprits.

Pityriasis rubra pilaris
Pityriasis rubra pilaris is a disorder of unknown aetiology that begins in adults with redness and scaling of the scalp and progresses to cover the limbs and trunk (Fig. 4). It is a follicle-based eruption and characteristically shows islands of sparing and a yellow keratotic

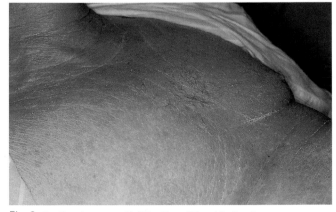

Fig. 2 **Erythroderma and infiltration of the skin due to Sézary syndrome.**

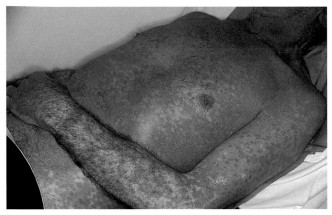

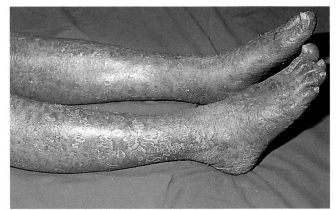

Fig. 3　**An erythrodermic reaction to an anti-inflammatory drug.**

Fig. 4　**Pityriasis rubra pilaris affecting the legs.**

thickening of the palms (Fig. 5). Treatment with acitretin will bring the eruption under control. Clearance occurs spontaneously in 1–3 years. A relapsing childhood type is reported.

Other dermatoses

Ichthyosiform erythroderma is a type of inherited ichthyosis (p. 88) that is present from birth or early infancy. Acute graft-versus-host disease and, very occasionally, severe scabies or extensive pemphigus can cause erythroderma.

In about 10% of cases of erythroderma, no cause is found. The possibility of a latent lymphoma must be considered.

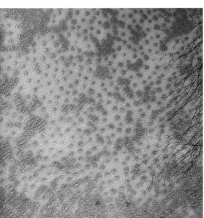

Fig. 5　**Pityriasis rubra pilaris. (a)** Yellowish hyperkeratosis of the palms. **(b)** Typical follicular lesions.

(a)　(b)

Complications

Erythroderma is associated with profound physiological and metabolic changes (Table 2). Cardiac failure and hypothermia are risks, especially in the elderly, and cutaneous or respiratory infection may also occur. Oedema is almost invariable and cannot be regarded as a sign of heart failure. The pulse rate is always increased. Cardiac failure and infection are difficult to diagnose. Blood cultures are easily contaminated with skin microflora. Lymphadenopathy is common and does not necessarily signify lymphoma. In the presteroid era, erythroderma was fatal in one-third of cases, largely due to cardiac failure or infection.

Management

Inpatient treatment and skilled nursing care is mandatory. The patient is nursed in a comfortably warm room at a steady temperature (preferably 30–32°C), and the pulse, blood pressure, temperature and fluid balance are regularly monitored. A pressure-relieving mattress is sometimes used. Soothing emollient

Table 2　**Pathophysiology of erythroderma**	
Clinical complication	**Pathophysiology**
Cardiac failure	Increased skin blood flow
	Increased plasma volume
Cutaneous oedema	Increased capillary permeability
	Increased plasma volume
	Hypoalbuminaemia
Hypoalbuminaemia	Increased plasma volume
	Reduced albumin synthesis, increased metabolism
	Protein loss in scaling
Dehydration	Increased transepidermal water loss
	Increased capillary permeability
Impaired temperature regulation	Excess heat loss
	Failure to sweat
Dermatopathic lymphadenopathy	Cutaneous inflammation and infection

creams and topical steroids are a mainstay of local treatment and are often adequate. Systemic steroids are life saving in severe cases. The maintenance of normal haemodynamics, attention to electrolyte equilibrium and adequate

nutritional support (particularly with regard to minimizing protein losses) are vital for severely ill patients. Cardiac failure and intercurrent infections are treated as necessary.

Erythroderma

■ A rare but potentially fatal eruption, often of sudden onset, showing near-universal skin involvement.

■ Commonest causes: eczema, psoriasis, lymphoma and drug eruption.

■ Characterized by hot, red, oedematous, dry and exfoliating skin.

■ Complications include cardiac failure, hypothermia, infection and lymphadenopathy.

■ Inpatient management and close supervision are required.

■ Treatment consists initially of bland emollients and topical steroids. Systemic steroids and full supportive therapy may be needed in life-threatening cases.

Photodermatology

Photodermatoses – idiopathic

Polymorphic light eruption

Polymorphic light eruption is a dermatosis of unknown aetiology characterized by pruritic papules, plaques and sometimes vesicles that last for days in light-exposed areas.

Clinical presentation

This is the commonest photodermatosis, and women are affected twice as frequently as men. Pruritic urticated papules, plaques and vesicles develop on light-exposed skin usually about 24 h after sun or artificial ultraviolet (UV) exposure (Fig. 1). It starts in the spring and may persist throughout the summer. The degree of severity is variable.

Differential diagnosis and management

Photoallergic contact dermatitis, drug-induced photosensitivity and lupus erythematosus may need to be considered in the diagnosis of polymorphic light eruption.

The first-line therapy is to use sunscreens and protective measures. A short course of psoralen with UVA (PUVA) in the late spring can 'harden' the skin so that the patient is able to have a disease-free summer.

Chronic actinic dermatitis (actinic reticuloid)

Chronic actinic dermatitis is a rare UV-induced disease of unknown cause affecting middle-aged or elderly men who develop thick plaques of dermatitis on sun-exposed skin.

Histologically, the skin shows a dense lymphocytic infiltrate. Some of the lymphocytes may be atypical and suggest lymphoma (hence the name).

Clinical presentation

There is often a long history of a chronic dermatitis that evolves into a photodermatitis, or a photoallergic contact dermatitis may have been present from the outset. Lichenified plaques of chronic dermatitis form on light-exposed sites and beyond, and are worse in the summer, although the eruption tends to become perennial (Fig. 2). The patients are sensitive to the UVA and UVB wavelengths and often to

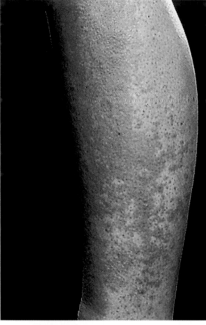

Fig. 1 **Polymorphic light eruption affecting the lower legs.**

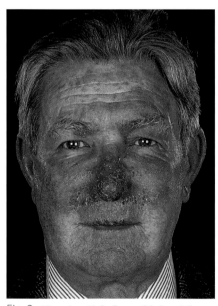

Fig. 2 **Chronic actinic dermatitis involving the light-exposed areas of the face.**

visible light as well. They may also have a contact or photocontact sensitivity to plant sesquiterpene lactones (airborne allergens) or to cosmetic ingredients, although the contribution of this to the overall picture is unclear.

Differential diagnosis and management

Airborne contact dermatitis or drug-induced photosensitivity may need to be considered, but there is normally little doubt about the diagnosis. Phototesting is helpful.

Light avoidance, sunscreens and topical steroids are used at first in the management of chronic actinic dermatitis. Subsequently, azathioprine, ciclosporin, mycophenolate or systemic steroids may be necessary.

Solar urticaria and actinic prurigo

Solar urticaria and actinic prurigo are rare conditions. In solar urticaria, wheals appear within minutes of exposure to sunlight. Differentiation is required from erythropoietic protoporphyria (p. 45), especially in childhood. Actinic prurigo starts in childhood and is characterized by papules and excoriations, mainly on sun-exposed sites.

Photodermatoses – other causes

Genetic disorders

Certain rare genetic disorders show photosensitivity. They may have chromosome instability (e.g. Bloom syndrome) or defective DNA repair (e.g. xeroderma pigmentosum, p. 91).

Metabolic disorders

Porphyrias

Porphyrins are important in the formation of haemoglobin, myoglobin and cytochromes. The porphyrias are rare, mostly inherited, metabolic disorders in which deficiencies of enzymes in the porphyrin biosynthetic pathway lead to accumulations of intermediate metabolites (p. 82). The metabolites are detectable in the urine, faeces and blood, are toxic to the nervous system and cause photosensitivity in the skin.

The main cutaneous porphyrias are:

- *Erythropoietic protoporphyria.* Autosomal dominant and starting in childhood, this is a painful red blistering eruption. Pitted linear scars are left on the nose and hands.
- *Porphyria cutanea tarda.* This is the commonest porphyria, often associated with liver disease and frequently alcohol related. Sun-induced subepidermal blisters on the face and hands (Fig. 3) leave fragile,

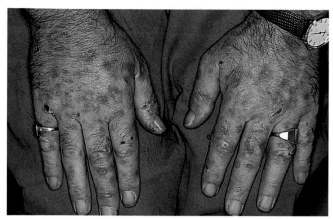

Fig. 3 **Porphyria cutanea tarda.** Changes can be seen on the dorsal aspects of the hands.

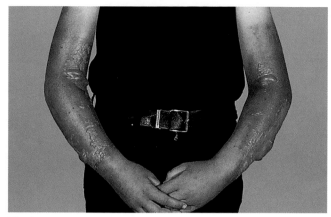

Fig. 4 **Phytophotodermatitis to common rue.** The patient had been gathering the plant in the bright sunlight and developed an extreme bullous reaction. The mechanism is toxic, i.e. irritant, rather than allergic.

scarred and hairy skin. Alcohol and aggravating drugs (e.g. oestrogens) are avoided. Venesection or low-dose chloroquine therapy may be used.

■ *Variegate porphyria*. Autosomal dominant and common in South Africa, the skin signs are like porphyria cutanea tarda. However, acute attacks with abdominal pain and neuropsychiatric symptoms resemble *acute intermittent porphyria*, which has no skin features.

Pellagra

Dietary deficiency of vitamin B3 (nicotinic acid) may give a photosensitive dermatitis in association with diarrhoea and dementia.

Due to drugs or chemicals

Drug induced

Several drugs may produce an eruption in light-exposed areas by either toxic (dose-dependent) or allergic mechanisms. The morphology may be eczematous, blistering (e.g. griseofulvin, p. 17), pigmented (e.g. amiodarone, p. 84) or an exaggerated sunburn reaction. Rarely, photo-onycholysis can occur (e.g. with tetracycline). Common photosensitizing drugs are shown in Table 1.

Topically applied chemicals

The commonest topical photosensitizers (i.e. allergens) are sunscreen agents (e.g. benzophenones), non-steroidal anti-inflammatory drugs (NSAIDs), coal tar derivatives and fragrances. Topical phototoxicity (with an irritant mechanism) is usually due to plant-derived psoralens, as found for example in carrot, celery, fennel, parsnip, common rue and giant hogweed. Phytophotodermatitis describes a photocontact dermatitis that results from the local photosensitization of the skin through contact with psoralens from a plant (Fig. 4). In Berloque dermatitis, streaky pigmentation, often on the sides

of the neck, results from the application of perfumes containing psoralens, usually oil of Bergamot (p. 104).

Dermatoses improved or worsened by sunlight

UV improves certain conditions (Table 2) and is used as a treatment as natural sunlight, UVB or PUVA. However, benefit is not observed in every case, and UV can, for example, make a patient's psoriasis or atopic eczema worse. The sun may even precipitate psoriasis. The sun can aggravate several other conditions, listed in Table 2

Table 2 **Dermatoses improved or aggravated by sunlight**

Improved	Worsened or provoked
Acne	Darier's disease
Atopic eczema	Herpes simplex
Mycosis fungoides	Lupus erythematosus
Pityriasis rosea	Porphyrias
Psoriasis	Rosacea
Uraemic pruritus	Vitiligo

Photodermatology

■ In normal skin, sunlight can cause tanning, sunburn and, in time, photoageing (p. 102).

■ The important idiopathic photodermatoses are polymorphic light eruption, chronic actinic dermatitis (actinic reticuloid) and solar urticaria.

■ Dermatoses worsened by sunlight include Darier's disease, herpes simplex, lupus erythematosus, cutaneous porphyrias, rosacea and vitiligo.

■ Dermatoses improved by sunlight include acne, atopic eczema, mycosis fungoides, pityriasis rosea, psoriasis and the pruritus of renal failure.

■ Drugs that are not infrequent causes of photosensitivity include tetracyclines, phenothiazines, angiotensin-converting enzyme (ACE) inhibitors, non-steroidal anti-inflammatory drugs (NSAIDs), furosemide and thiazides.

Table 1 **Drugs causing photosensitivity**

Amiodarone	Non-steroidal anti-inflammatory drugs
Angiotensin-converting enzyme inhibitors	Nifedipine
Ciprofloxacin	Phenothiazines
Furosemide	Tetracyclines
Nalidixic acid	Thiazides

http://www.emedicine.com/derm/topic324.htm   http://www.dermnet.org.nz/dna.pmle/pmle.html

Bacterial infection – Staphylococcal and streptococcal

The skin is a barrier to infection but, if its defences are penetrated or broken down, numerous microorganisms can cause disease (Table 1).

The normal skin microflora

Normal skin has a resident flora of usually harmless microorganisms, including bacteria, yeasts and mites. The bacteria are mostly staphylococci (e.g. *Staphylococcus epidermidis*), micrococci, corynebacteria (diphtheroids) and propionibacteria. They cluster in the stratum corneum or hair follicles, and their number varies between individuals and between different sites on the body. Micrococci, for example, number 0.5 million/cm² in the axilla but only 60/cm² on the forearm. Some individuals are high carriers.

Staphylococcal infections

A third of people intermittently carry *Staphylococcus aureus* in the nose or, less often, the axilla or perineum. Staphylococci can infect the skin directly or secondarily, as in eczema or psoriasis.

Impetigo

Impetigo is a contagious superficial skin infection caused by either staphylococci or streptococci, or both.

Clinical presentation

Impetigo is now relatively uncommon in the UK, mainly because of improved social conditions, but it is endemic in developing countries. It generally occurs in children and presents as thin-walled easily ruptured vesicles, often on the face, which leave areas of yellow-crusted exudate (Fig. 1). Lesions spread rapidly and are contagious. A bullous form, with blisters 1–2 cm in diameter, is seen in all ages and affects the face or extremities. Atopic eczema, scabies, herpes simplex and lice infestation may all become impetiginized. Impetigo can be confused with herpes simplex or a fungal infection.

Management

Most localized cases respond to the removal of the crusts with saline soaks and the application of a topical antibiotic (e.g. mupirocin, fusidic acid or neomycin/ bacitracin). Systemic flucloxacillin or erythromycin is given for widespread infection. Impetigo caused by *Streptococcus pyogenes* may result in glomerulonephritis, a serious complication. Methicillin-resistant *Staph. aureus* (MRSA) carriage (and infection) has increased with the widespread use of antibiotics.

Ecthyma

Ecthyma is characterized by circumscribed, ulcerated and crusted infected lesions that heal with scarring. An insect bite or neglected minor injury may become infected with staphylococci or streptococci (or both). Ecthyma mostly occurs on the legs (Fig. 2) and may be seen in drug addicts or debilitated patients. Treatment is with systemic and topical antibiotics.

Table 1 **Bacterial diseases of the skin**	
Organism	**Infection**
Commensals	Erythrasma, pitted keratolysis, trichomycosis axillaris
Staphylococcal	Impetigo, ecthyma, folliculitis, secondary infection
Streptococcal	Erysipelas, cellulitis, impetigo, ecthyma, necrotizing fasciitis
Gram-negative	Secondary infection, folliculitis, cellulitis
Mycobacterial	TB (lupus vulgaris, warty tuberculosis, scrofuloderma), fish tank granuloma, Buruli ulcer, leprosy
Spirochaetal	Syphilis (e.g. primary, secondary), Lyme disease (erythema chronicum migrans)
Neisseria	Gonorrhoea (pustules), meningococcaemia (purpura)
Others	Anthrax (pustule), erysipeloid (pustule)

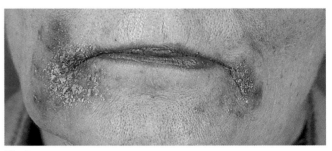

Fig. 1 **Impetigo of the face due to *Staphylococcus aureus*.**

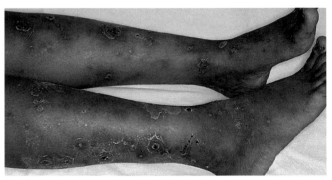

Fig. 2 **Ecthyma, due to a streptococcus, affecting the lower legs.**

Folliculitis and related conditions

Infection can affect hair follicles. *Folliculitis* is an acute pustular infection of multiple hair follicles; a *furuncle* is an acute abscess formation in adjacent hair follicles; and a *carbuncle* is a deep abscess formed in a group of follicles giving a painful suppurating mass.

Clinical presentation

Follicular pustules are seen in hair-bearing areas, e.g. the legs, scalp or face. In men, folliculitis may affect the beard area (sycosis barbae). In women, it may occur on the legs after hair removal by shaving or waxing. *Staph. aureus* is usually, but not invariably, responsible. A Gram-negative folliculitis (e.g. with *Pseudomonas*) may occur with prolonged antibiotic treatment for acne. *Pityrosporum folliculitis* is a separate condition due to a commensal yeast (p. 36).

Furuncles (boils) present as tender red pustules that suppurate and heal with scarring. They often occur on the face, neck, scalp, axillae and perineum. Some patients have recurrent staphylococcal boils of the axillae or perineum. Large suppurating carbuncles (Fig. 3) due to *Staph. aureus* may cause systemic upset.

Management
Swabs for bacterial culture are taken from the lesion and from carrier sites, e.g. the nose, axilla and groin. Obesity, diabetes mellitus and occlusion from clothing are predisposing factors. Acute staphylococcal infections are treated with antibiotics, both systemic (e.g. flucloxacillin or erythromycin) and topical (e.g. fusidic acid, mupirocin or neomycin/bacitracin). Chronic and recurrent cases are more difficult. Carrier sites, e.g. the nose, need treatment with a topical antibiotic (e.g. mupirocin). General measures such as improved hygiene, regular

bathing or showering, the use of antiseptics in the bath and on the skin (e.g. chlorhexidine) can help, but courses of oral antibiotics may be needed. Carbuncles often need prompt surgical drainage. An infrequent complication is thrombosis in the cavernous sinus, associated with facial infection.

Staphylococcal scalded skin syndrome
Staphylococcal scalded skin syndrome is an acute toxic illness, usually of infants, in which there is shedding of sheets of epidermis associated with localized staphylococcal infection in the skin or elsewhere. Large sheets of superficial epidermis are shed, resembling a scald, leaving denuded erythematous areas. Phage group II staphylococci release into the bloodstream epidermolytic toxins, which cause the epidermis to split. A related

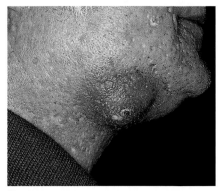
Fig. 3 **A carbuncle.** This required surgical drainage. The patient had had previous staphylococcal infection.

condition in adults is mostly drug induced (p. 85).

Although a serious condition requiring inpatient treatment, the prognosis is good when systemic flucloxacillin or erythromycin is prescribed.

Streptococcal infections

Strep. pyogenes, the principal human skin pathogen, is occasionally found in the throat and may persist after an infection. It is sometimes carried in the nose and can contaminate and colonize damaged skin.

Erysipelas
Erysipelas is an acute infection of the dermis by *Strep. pyogenes*. It shows well-demarcated raised erythema, oedema and skin tenderness.

Clinical presentation
The skin lesions may be preceded by fever, malaise and 'flu-like' symptoms. Erysipelas usually affects the face (where it may be bilateral) or the lower leg, and appears as a painful hot red swelling (Fig. 4). The lesion has a well-defined edge and may blister. Cellulitis may coexist. The streptococci usually gain entry to the skin via a fissure, e.g. behind the ear, or associated with tinea pedis between the toes.

Differential diagnosis and complications
On the face, erysipelas may be confused with angioedema or allergic contact dermatitis, but the condition is usually distinguishable as it causes tenderness and systemic upset. Recurrent attacks in the same place can result in lymphoedema due to lymphatic damage. A fatal streptococcal septicaemia can occur in debilitated patients. Guttate psoriasis

(p. 28) and acute glomerulonephritis may follow a streptococcal infection.

Management
A good response is usually seen with prompt treatment. Topical therapy is inappropriate, and penicillin should be prescribed. *Strep. pyogenes* is nearly always sensitive. Intravenous treatment is needed at first for a severe infection, usually with benzylpenicillin for 2 or so days. Oral penicillin V can then be given for 7–14 days. In less severe cases, penicillin V is adequate. Erythromycin is used if there is penicillin allergy. Recurrent erysipelas, i.e. more than two episodes at one site, requires prophylactic long-term penicillin V (250 mg once or twice a day), with attention to hygiene at potential portals of entry.

Necrotizing fasciitis
Necrotizing fasciitis is an acute and serious infection. It usually occurs in otherwise healthy subjects after minor

trauma. An ill-defined erythema, often on the head or limbs and associated with a high fever, rapidly becomes necrotic. Early surgical debridement and systemic antibiotics are essential.

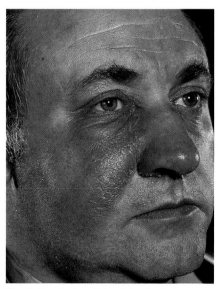
Fig. 4 **Erysipelas of the right cheek due to a streptococcal infection.**

Staphylococcal and streptococcal infections

- **Normal skin microflora** includes staphylococci, micrococci, corynebacteria and propionibacteria, and may number 0.5 million/cm². Some individuals are higher carriers than others.

- **Staphylococcal infection** of the skin may be primary, e.g. impetigo, ecthyma or folliculitis, or secondary, e.g. superinfection of eczema, psoriasis or leg ulcers.

- **Streptococcal infections** may also be primary, e.g. erysipelas or cellulitis, or secondary, e.g. infection of dermatoses or leg ulcers.

Other bacterial infections

Diseases due to commensal overgrowth

Sometimes, 'normal' commensals can result in disease. Among the most common are:

- *Pitted keratolysis.* Overgrowth of resident microorganisms, which digest keratin, occurs with occluding footwear and sweaty feet (Fig. 1). Malodorous pitted erosions and punched out, discoloured areas result. Better hygiene, topical neomycin or soaks with 0.01% aqueous potassium permanganate or 3% aqueous formaldehyde usually help.
- *Erythrasma.* A dry, reddish-brown, slightly scaly and usually asymptomatic eruption that affects the body folds (Fig. 2). It fluoresces coral pink with Wood's light, owing to the production of porphyrins by the corynebacteria. Imidazole creams,

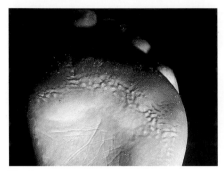

Fig. 1 **Pitted keratolysis, due to overgrowth of resident microorganisms.**

topical fusidic acid or oral erythromycin are effective.
- *Trichomycosis axillaris.* Overgrowths of corynebacteria form yellow concretions on axillary hair. Topical antimicrobials usually effect a cure.

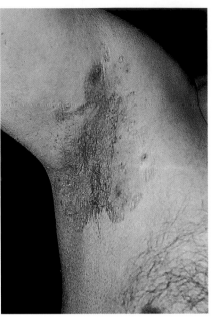

Fig. 2 **Erythrasma affecting the axilla.** This was caused by overgrowth of corynebacteria.

Mycobacterial infections

Mycobacterium tuberculosis and *M. leprae* (p. 58) are the most important mycobacteria in human disease, although other species can cause infections. In western countries, tuberculosis (TB) has recently shown resurgence, related to immigration, and co-infection with human immunodeficiency virus (HIV). In the developing world, 50% of HIV-infected individuals also have TB. TB can produce a number of cutaneous manifestations (Table 1).

Table 1 **Skin manifestations of tuberculosis**
Lupus vulgaris: reddish-brown plaques, e.g. on the neck
Tuberculides: cutaneous hypersensitivity reactions
Scrofuloderma: skin involved from underlying node
Warty tuberculosis: warty plaques, e.g. on buttock

Lupus vulgaris

Reddish-brown plaques, often on the head or neck, characterize lupus vulgaris. It is the commonest *M. tuberculosis* skin infection.

Clinical presentation

Lupus vulgaris follows primary inoculation and develops in individuals with some immunity. It begins as painless reddish-brown nodules that slowly enlarge to form a plaque (Fig. 3),

leaving scarring and sometimes destruction of deeper tissues such as cartilage. Presentation in the elderly is often due to reactivation of inadequately treated pre-existing disease.

Differential diagnosis and complications

Papules of lupus vulgaris typically show an 'apple-jelly' colour when compressed with a glass slide (diascopy). A biopsy will reveal tuberculoid granulomata with a few bacilli. The Mantoux test is positive. Sometimes it is necessary to consider:

- morphoeic basal cell carcinoma
- sarcoidosis or leprosy
- discoid lupus erythematosus.

Squamous cell carcinoma may develop in longstanding scarred lesions. The presence of *M. tuberculosis*

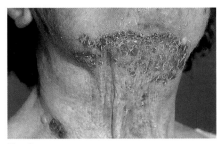

Fig. 3 **Lupus vulgaris, due to *M. tuberculosis.***

somewhere in the body can induce cutaneous reactions called 'tuberculides'. *Erythema nodosum* (p. 81) is the best known example. Another is *erythema induratum*, which occurs as painful ulcerating nodules on the lower legs of women and is thought to be a hypersensitivity response to TB.

Management

Four drugs, normally rifampicin, isoniazid, pyrazinamide and ethambutol, are given for the initial 8 weeks. After this, isoniazid and rifampicin are continued to complete a 6-month course. Directly observed therapy, in which ingestion of drugs is witnessed, improves cure rates if compliance could be a problem. Adverse reactions to TB drugs are common.

Scrofuloderma

A tuberculous lymph node or joint can directly involve the overlying skin, often on the neck and in children. Fistulae and scarring result.

Warty tuberculosis

A warty reddish or brown plaque, frequently on the hands, knees or buttock, results from inoculation of TB bacilli into the skin of someone with immunity from previous infection. It is rare in western countries, but is a common form of cutaneous TB in the developing world.

Other cutaneous mycobacterial infections

Fish tank granuloma
Typically, this is a reddish, slightly scaly plaque on the hand or arm of someone who keeps tropical fish. It is due to *Mycobacterium marinum*, which infects fish and is also found in swimming pools, sea water and fresh water.

Buruli ulcer
In tropical zones, *Mycobacterium ulcerans* – acquired from vegetation or water after trauma – produces a painless erythematous nodule usually on the leg or forearm. The nodule becomes necrotic and ulceration results.

Disseminated infection with *Mycobacterium avium* complex is seen in patients with HIV infection (p. 54).

Spirochaetal infections

Spirochaetes are thin, spiral and motile organisms. Syphilis (p. 116), due to *Treponema pallidum*, is the best known spirochaetal disease, but other spirochaetes, e.g. *Borrelia burgdorferi*, can be pathogenic.

Non-venereal treponemal infections
Non-venereal treponemal infections are endemic in tropical and subtropical areas where people live in conditions of extreme poverty. They are caused by spirochaetes that are very similar to *T. pallidum*. Serological tests for syphilis are positive. All three diseases discussed below respond to long-acting penicillins.

- *Yaws* occurs in central Africa, central America and southeast Asia. In children, the treponeme enters the skin through an abrasion and, after a few weeks, results in an ulcerated papilloma that heals with scarring.

Secondary lesions follow and, in the late stage, bone deformities develop.
- *Bejel* (endemic syphilis), found in rural Middle Eastern tribes living in unhygienic conditions, is similar to yaws but starts around the mouth. It is transmitted by skin contact.
- *Pinta* is confined to central and south America. It results in hyperkeratoses over extensor aspects of joints with both hypo- and hyperpigmentation.

Lyme disease
Lyme disease is a cutaneous and systemic infection caused by the spirochaete *Borrelia burgdorferi* and spread by tick bite. Most cases have been reported in the USA and Europe. At the site of the tick bite, usually a limb, a slowly expanding erythematous ring (erythema chronicum migrans) develops (Fig. 4). Arthritis and neurological and cardiac disease may follow. A response to high-dose amoxicillin or doxycycline is usual.

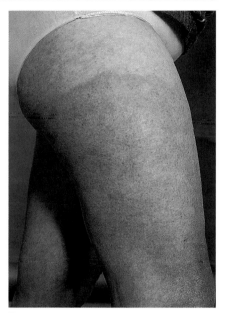
Fig. 4 **Erythema chronicum migrans of Lyme disease.**

Further bacterial infections

Anthrax
A haemorrhagic bulla, associated with oedema and fever, forms at the site of inoculation of the skin with *Bacillus anthracis*, usually from contaminated animal products. It is now rare. Ciprofloxacin or amoxicillin are curative.

Gram-negative infections
Bacilli such as *Pseudomonas aeruginosa* can infect skin wounds, notably leg ulcers. They may also cause folliculitis and cellulitis.

Cellulitis
Cellulitis is an infection of the subcutaneous tissues. It is often due to streptococci, but is deeper and more extensive than erysipelas. The cardinal features are swelling, redness and local pain with systemic upset and fever. The leg is often affected (Fig. 5). The organism may gain entry through fissures between

the toes or via a leg ulcer. Lymphangitis is common, and lymphatic damage may result. Hospital admission is usually indicated, particularly if the leg is involved. Antistreptococcal antibiotics are given for straightforward cases. However, a broad-spectrum antibiotic is prescribed for cellulitis complicating a leg ulcer, because a selection of organisms may be responsible. Blood cultures and ulcer swabs may give some guidance.

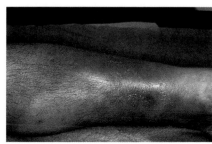
Fig. 5 **Cellulitis affecting the lower leg.**

> ### Other bacterial infections
> - Overgrowth of commensal organisms can result in minor skin 'disease'.
> - Cutaneous mycobacterial infection is mainly due to *M. tuberculosis*, but occasionally 'atypical' mycobacteria such as *M. marinum* cause disease.
> - Non-venereal treponematoses, e.g. yaws, are still important diseases of rural people living in poor conditions in the developing world.
> - Lyme disease is a tick-transmitted infection with *Borrelia burgdorferi*; the skin signs are often associated with arthritis or neurological disease.
> - Cellulitis often affects the leg and is frequently caused by streptococci, although other organisms may be involved.

Viral infections – Warts and other viral infections

Unlike bacteria and yeasts, viruses are not thought to exist on the skin surface as commensals. However, studies in patients with viral warts have shown viral DNA in epidermal cells of seemingly normal skin next to warty areas.

Viral warts

Warts (verrucae) are common and benign cutaneous tumours due to infection of epidermal cells with human papillomavirus (HPV).

Aetiopathogenesis and pathology

Over 80 subtypes of DNA HPV have been identified. The virus infects by direct inoculation and is caught by touch, sexual contact or at the swimming baths. Certain HPV subtypes are associated with specific clinical lesions, e.g. types 2 and 57 with common hand warts, types 1, 2 and 4 with plantar warts, types 3 and 10 with plane warts, types 6, 11, 16 and 18 with genital warts. Genital HPV subtypes cause cytological dysplasia of the cervix, which may be precancerous. Immunosuppressed individuals, such as those with renal transplants, are particularly susceptible to viral warts (p. 55). The epidermis is thickened and hyperkeratotic. Keratinocytes in the granular layer are vacuolated due to being infected with the wart virus.

Clinical presentation

Certain clinical patterns are well recognized:

- *Common warts*. These present as dome-shaped papules or nodules with a papilliferous surface. They are usually multiple, and are commonest on the hands (Fig. 1) or feet in children but also affect the face and genitalia. Their surface interrupts skin lines. Some facial warts are 'filiform' with fine digit-like projections.
- *Plane warts*. These are smooth flat-topped papules, often slightly brown in colour, and commonest on the face (Fig. 2) and dorsal aspects of the hands. They are usually multiple and resist treatment, but eventually resolve spontaneously, often after becoming inflamed. They can show the Koebner phenomenon.
- *Plantar warts*. These are seen in children and adolescents on the soles of the feet; pressure causes them to grow into the dermis. They are painful and covered by callus, which, when pared, reveals dark punctate spots (thrombosed capillaries). Mosaic warts are plaques on the soles that comprise multiple individual warts.
- *Genital warts*. In males, these affect the penis and, in homosexuals, the perianal area. In females, the vulva, vagina and perianal area may be involved (Fig. 3). The warts may be small or may coalesce into large cauliflower-like 'condylomata acuminata'. Proctoscopy (if perianal warts are present) and colposcopy (for female genital warts) are needed to identify and treat any rectal or cervical warts because of the risk of neoplastic change. Sexual partners need to be examined.

Differential diagnosis and complications

The diagnosis of viral warts is usually obvious. Occasionally, corns on the sole or hand, or molluscum contagiosum elsewhere, are confused. With viral warts, under the fingernails and toenails, it is important to consider amelanotic malignant melanoma, periungual fibroma (of tuberous sclerosis, p. 90) and bony subungual exostosis. Genital warts may resemble the condyloma lata of secondary syphilis. HPV types 16 and 18 in genital warts carry a risk of malignant change. HPV infections in renal transplant patients have been linked with skin cancers.

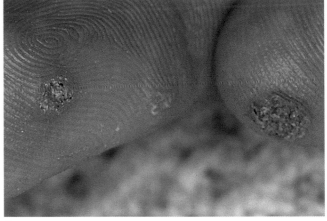

Fig. 1 **Common viral warts on the hand.**

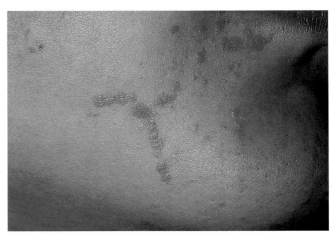

Fig. 2 **Plane viral warts on the face.**

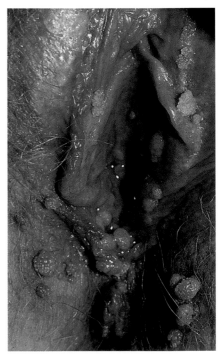

Fig. 3 **Viral warts on the vulva.**

Management

In children, 30–50% of plantar warts disappear spontaneously within 6 months. Hand and foot warts should be pared by a scalpel or using an emery board. This gets rid of keratotic skin and allows easier treatment. Table 1 shows the available treatments. Immunosuppressed patients, especially those with renal transplants, are prone to wart infections. They need special management and should be inspected and treated for warts before being given their grafts.

Other viral infections

Other viral infections include molluscum contagiosum, orf, human immunodeficiency virus (p. 54) and those in Table 2.

Molluscum contagiosum

Molluscum contagiosum are discrete pearly-pink umbilicated papules that are caused by a DNA pox virus. Mollusca mainly affect children or young adults. Spread is by contact, including sexual transmission or on towels. The dome-shaped papule, a few millimetres in diameter, has a punctum and, if squeezed, releases a cheesy material. The lesions are usually multiple and grouped, sometimes with a localized eczema. They are commonest on the face, neck and trunk (Fig. 4). Isolated ones may go unrecognized. Untreated, they may persist for several months.

If natural resolution is slow, imiquimod cream can be helpful. In the adult or older child, curettage under local anaesthesia or cryotherapy is appropriate. These measures are poorly tolerated in young children, and one approach is to instruct the parents to gently express the 'ripe' lesions after the child has bathed.

Orf

Orf usually occurs as a solitary, rapidly growing papule, often on the hand. The orf pox virus is endemic in sheep and

causes a pustular eruption around the muzzle area. Human infection is well recognized in country regions and occurs in shepherds, veterinary surgeons and, typically, the farmer's wife who has been bottle-feeding a lamb.

A solitary red papule appears, usually on a finger, after an incubation period of about 6 days (Fig. 5). It grows rapidly to 1 cm or so in size, evolving into a painful purple pustule, which often has a necrotic umbilicated centre. Erythema multiforme (p. 80) and lymphangitis are complications. Spontaneous resolution takes 2–4 weeks. Secondary infection requires a topical or systemic antibiotic.

Table 1 Treatments for viral warts

Modality	Details	Indication	Contraindications/side-effects
Topical	Salicylic and lactic acids (e.g. Duofilm, Occlusal, Salactol, Salatac)	Hand and foot warts	Facial/anogenital warts, atopic eczema, contact allergy to colophonium in collodion preparations
	Glutaraldehyde (e.g. Glutarol)	Hand and foot warts	Facial/anogenital warts, atopic eczema
	Formaldehyde (e.g. Veracur)	Foot warts	Facial/anogenital warts, atopic eczema
	Podophyllotoxin (0.15%) cream	Anogenital warts	Pregnancy (teratogenic)
	Imiquimod cream	Anogenital warts	Pregnancy; local reaction
Cryotherapy	Applied every 3–4 weeks	Hand and foot, genital warts	Painful; may cause blistering
Curettage and cautery	Local anaesthetic (or general anaesthetic if large)	Solitary filiform warts, especially on face. Large anogenital warts	Not recommended for hand or foot warts as scars may result; warts may recur
Other	Intralesional bleomycin	Resistant hand/foot warts	Procedure can be painful
	Laser surgery	Any type of wart	Post-operative pain; can scar
	Interferon-β or -γ	Resistant (genital) warts	Systemic side-effects

Table 2 Other viral infections

Disorder	Cause	Clinical presentation	Course and management
Fifth disease (erythema infectiosum)	Parvovirus B19	Slapped cheek sign, lace-like erythema over hands, feet or trunk, sometimes arthralgia	Small outbreaks typically affect children aged 2–10 years; fades in 11 days; treatment unnecessary
Gianotti–Crosti syndrome	Hepatitis B and other viruses	Small red lichenoid papules on face, buttocks and extremities	Affects young children (peak 1–12 years); clears in 2–8 weeks
Hand, foot and mouth disease	Coxsackie A16 and others	Oral blisters/ulcers, red-edged vesicles on hands/feet, mild fever	Epidemics in young children; fades in 1 week; no treatment needed
Kawasaki disease	Unknown microorganism: ? response to superantigens	Generalized erythema, peeling of hands/feet, strawberry tongue, fever, myocarditis, lymphadenopathy, coronary artery aneurysms	Affects young children; usually resolves in 2 weeks; investigate for cardiac involvement; treat with intravenous gammaglobulin and aspirin
Measles	RNA morbillivirus	Koplik's spots on buccal mucosa, morbilliform rash	Incubation period 10 days, prodrome; rash fades after 6–10 days

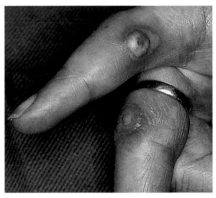

Fig. 5 **Orf on the fingers of a farmer's wife.**

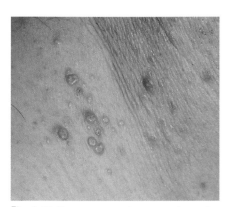

Fig. 4 **Molluscum contagiosum on the neck.**

Warts and other viral conditions

Viral warts
- Hand and foot warts are common: overall, 65% clear spontaneously within 2 years.
- Try wart paints for hand and foot warts before proceeding to cryotherapy.
- Patients with anogenital warts need screening for other genital infections (p. 116).

Molluscum contagiosum
- Caused by a pox virus. Treated by imiquimod cream, curettage or cryotherapy.
- Untreated, the lesions will remit spontaneously, although this may take several months.

Orf
- Found in rural areas, affecting farmers and vets. The condition is endemic in sheep.
- Diagnosis is usually obvious, but treat secondary infection and watch for erythema multiforme.

Viral infections – Herpes simplex and herpes zoster

Herpes simplex

Herpes simplex is a very common, acute, self-limiting vesicular eruption due to infection with *Herpesvirus hominis*.

Aetiopathogenesis and pathology

Herpes simplex virus is highly contagious and is spread by direct contact with infected individuals. The virus penetrates the epidermis or mucous membrane epithelium and replicates within the epithelial cells. After the primary infection, the latent non-replicating virus resides mainly within the dorsal root ganglion, from where it can reactivate, invade the skin and cause recrudescent lesions. There are two types of herpes simplex virus. *Type 1* disease is usually facial or non-genital, and *type 2* lesions are commonly genital, although this distinction is not absolute. The pathological changes of epidermal cell destruction by the herpes virus result in intraepidermal vesicles and multinucleate giant cells. Infected cells may show intranuclear inclusions.

Clinical presentation

Type 1 primary infection usually occurs in childhood and is often subclinical. Acute gingivostomatitis is a common presentation in those with symptoms. Vesicles on the lips and mucous membranes quickly erode and are painful. Sometimes the cornea is involved. The illness is often accompanied by fever, malaise and local lymphadenopathy and lasts about 2 weeks.

Herpetic whitlow is another presentation (Fig. 1). A painful vesicle or pustule is found on a finger in, for example, a nurse or dentist attending a patient secreting the virus. Similar direct inoculation is sometimes seen in

sportsmen such as wrestlers ('herpes gladiatorum').

Type 2 primary infection is normally seen after sexual contact in young adults, who develop acute vulvovaginitis or penile or perianal lesions. Culture-positive genital herpes simplex in a pregnant woman at the time of delivery is an indication for caesarean section, as neonatal infection can be fatal.

Recurrence is a hallmark of herpes simplex infection; it occurs at a similar site each time, usually on the lips, face (Fig. 2) or genitals (Fig. 3). Rarely, herpes simplex may appear in a zosteriform dermatomal distribution. The outbreak of groups of vesicles is often preceded for a few hours by tingling or burning. Crusts form within 24–48 h, and the infection fades after a week. Attacks may be precipitated by respiratory infection (hence 'cold' sore), sunlight or local trauma.

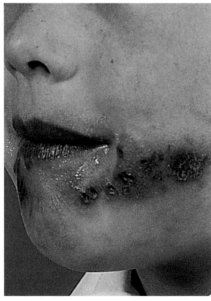

Fig. 2 **Herpes simplex on the cheek of a child.**

Differential diagnosis

Occasionally, herpes simplex can be confused with impetigo but, in recrudescent disease, the recurrent nature usually indicates the diagnosis. If necessary, the virus can be cultured or detected by an immunofluorescent test.

Complications

Complications are infrequent but can be serious. They include:

- *Secondary bacterial infection.* This is usually due to *Staphylococcus aureus*.
- *Eczema herpeticum.* Widespread herpes simplex infection is a serious and potentially fatal complication seen in patients with atopic eczema (p. 34) or Darier's disease (p. 88).
- *Disseminated herpes simplex.* Widespread herpetic vesicles may occur in the newborn or in immunosuppressed patients.
- *Chronic herpes simplex.* Atypical and chronic lesions may be seen in patients with human immunodeficiency virus (HIV) infection.
- *Herpes encephalitis.* This is a serious complication of herpes simplex, not always accompanied by skin lesions.
- *Carcinoma of the cervix.* This is more common in women with serological evidence of infection with type 2 herpes simplex, which may be a predisposing factor.
- *Erythema multiforme.* Herpes simplex infection is the most common cause of recurrent erythema multiforme (p. 80).

Management

Mild herpetic lesions may not require any medication. The treatment of choice for recurrent mild facial or genital herpes simplex is aciclovir (Zovirax) cream (applied five times a day for 5 days), which reduces the length of the attack and the duration of viral shedding, and should preferably be started at the first indication of a recrudescence. More severe episodes warrant oral treatment with aciclovir (200 mg five times a day for 5 days), which shortens the attack. Long-term oral administration is useful in those with frequent recurrent attacks. Intravenous aciclovir may be life saving in the immunosuppressed and in infants with eczema herpeticum. Genital herpes simplex can also be treated with oral

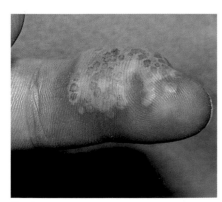

Fig. 1 **Primary herpes simplex occurring as a herpetic whitlow on a finger.**

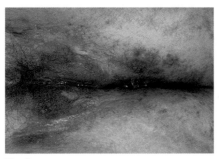

Fig. 3 **Genital lesions of recurrent herpes simplex.**

famciclovir or valaciclovir. In those with genital herpes simplex, barrier contraception methods are advisable during intercourse, and intercourse should be avoided during symptomatic episodes.

Herpes zoster

Herpes zoster (shingles) is an acute, self-limiting, vesicular eruption occurring in a dermatomal distribution; it is caused by a recrudescence of *Varicella zoster* virus.

Aetiopathogenesis and pathology

Herpes zoster nearly always occurs in subjects who have previously had varicella (chickenpox). The virus lies dormant in the sensory root ganglion of the spinal cord but, when reactivated, the virus replicates and migrates along the nerve to the skin, producing pain and ultimately inducing the cutaneous lesions of shingles. A viraemia is frequent, and disseminated involvement may be seen. The pathological changes are identical to those of herpes simplex.

Clinical presentation

Pain, tenderness or paraesthesia in the dermatome may precede the eruption by 3–5 days. Erythema and grouped vesicles follow, scattered within the dermatomal area (Fig. 4). The vesicles become pustular and then form crusts that separate in 2–3 weeks to leave scarring. Secondary bacterial infection may occur. Herpes zoster is normally unilateral and may involve adjacent dermatomes. The thoracic dermatomes are affected in 50% of cases and, in the elderly, involvement of the ophthalmic division of the trigeminal nerve is particularly common (Fig. 5). Two-thirds of patients with herpes zoster are over 50 years of age, and it is uncommon in children. The lesions shed virus, and contacts with no previous exposure may develop chickenpox.

Some scattering of vesicles outwith the dermatomal distribution is not uncommon, but disseminated or unusually haemorrhagic vesicles raise the possibility of immunosuppression or underlying malignancy. Local lymphadenopathy is usual, as is sensory disturbance of varying degree, including pain, numbness and paraesthesia. Shingles is recurrent in 5% of cases.

Differential diagnosis

The prodromal pain of herpes zoster can mimic cardiac or pleural pain, or an acute abdominal emergency. Once the eruption has appeared, the diagnosis is usually obvious, although herpes simplex may infrequently occur in a dermatomal fashion. Viral culture is sometimes needed.

Complications

Serious complications may occur in herpes zoster. These include:

- *Ophthalmic disease.* Corneal ulcers and scarring may result from shingles of the first trigeminal division. Ophthalmological assistance is mandatory.
- *Motor palsy.* Rarely, the viral involvement may spread from the posterior horn of the spinal cord to the anterior horn, and result in a motor disorder. Cranial nerve palsies or paralysis of the diaphragm or other muscle groups may occur.
- *Disseminated herpes zoster.* Immunosuppressed subjects, and patients with Hodgkin's disease in particular, can develop confluent haemorrhagic involvement, which spreads and may become necrotic or gangrenous. Varicella pneumonia or encephalitis are potentially fatal.
- *Post-herpetic neuralgia.* Neuralgia is infrequent in patients under 40 years but is found in a third of those over 60 years. The pain subsides in the majority within 12 months.

Management

In mild shingles, treatment is symptomatic, with rest, analgesia and bland drying preparations such as calamine lotion. Secondary bacterial infection may require a topical antiseptic or antibiotic. More severe cases may be treated, if seen within 48 h of onset, with oral aciclovir (800 mg five times a day for 7 days) or famciclovir (750 mg once daily for 7 days), which promotes resolution, reduces the viral shedding time and may reduce post-herpetic neuralgia. Immunosuppressed patients often require intravenous aciclovir. Oral prednisolone, given early in the course of herpes zoster for 14 days, reduces the incidence of post-herpetic neuralgia, but must not be used if the patient is immunosuppressed. Post-herpetic neuralgia may respond to topical capsaicin (Axsain).

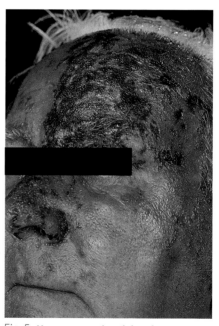

Fig. 5 **Herpes zoster involving the ophthalmic division of the trigeminal nerve.**

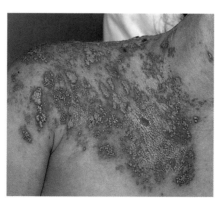

Fig. 4 **Herpes zoster of the C4 dermatome.**

Herpes simplex and herpes zoster

Herpes simplex
- Type 1 infection: usually orofacial, childhood onset.
- Type 2 infection: mostly genital, adult onset.
- Characterized by recurrent bouts at the same locus.
- Aciclovir is an effective topical or systemic treatment.

Herpes zoster
- Recrudescence of dormant *Varicella zoster* virus.
- Dermatomal, especially thoracic and trigeminal distributions.
- Neuralgia may complicate, mainly in the elderly.
- Dissemination suggests underlying immunosuppression.

Human immunodeficiency virus disease and immunodeficiency syndromes

Immunodeficiency results from absence or failure of one or more elements of the immune system. It may be acquired, e.g. acquired immunodeficiency syndrome (AIDS), or inherited, e.g. chronic mucocutaneous candidiasis.

Table 1	**Skin signs and the progressive stages of HIV infection (Centers for Disease Control)**			
Group	I (Primary phase)	II (Early phase: asymptomatic)	III (Persistent generalized lymphadenopathy)	IV (Symptomatic: AIDS)
Skin signs	Transient maculopapular eruption on trunk	Hypersensitivity reactions, onset or worsening of eczemas, psoriasis or folliculitis, wart virus and fungal infections	Herpes zoster, eczemas worsen, candidiasis, Kaposi's sarcoma	Candidiasis, opportunistic infections, Kaposi's sarcoma, lymphoma

Human immunodeficiency virus (HIV) disease

Infection with HIV is a progressive process that mostly leads to the development of AIDS.

Aetiopathogenesis

HIV1 and HIV2 (the latter mainly found in West Africa) are retroviruses containing reverse transcriptase, which allows incorporation of the virus into a cell's DNA. The virus infects and depletes helper/inducer CD4 T lymphocytes, leading to loss of cell-mediated immunity and opportunistic infection, e.g. with *Pneumocystis jiroveci*, mycobacteria or cryptococci. HIV is spread by infected body fluids, e.g. blood or semen. High-risk groups for HIV infection include men who have sex with men, intravenous drug users and haemophiliacs who have received infected blood products.

Clinical presentation

The acute infection may be symptomless but, in a variable proportion of cases, seroconversion is accompanied by a non-specific glandular fever-like illness with a maculopapular exanthem on the trunk. HIV infection may be asymptomatic for several years, although most infected individuals will eventually develop symptoms. In the early stages of symptomatic infection, skin changes, fatigue, weight loss, generalized lymphadenopathy, diarrhoea and fever are present without the opportunistic infections that define AIDS. Opportunistic organisms include the ubiquitous *Mycobacterium avium* complex and *Cryptococcus neoformans*, and toxoplasmosis and cytomegalovirus.

As the disease progresses, the number of CD4$^+$ lymphocytes falls and, when the blood count is below 50 cells/mL in the late phase of HIV infection (AIDS), *M. avium* complex infection, lymphoma and encephalopathy may develop. The mean latent period between infection and the development of AIDS is 10 years. Skin signs include (Table 1):

- *Dry skin.* Skin dryness, often with asteatotic eczema, and seborrhoeic dermatitis (Fig. 1) are common and early findings. Their severity increases as the disease advances.
- *Fungal and papillomavirus infections.* Tinea infections and perianal and common viral warts are seen in early disease.
- *Acne and folliculitis.* These worsen in early and mid-stage disease.
- *Other infections.* Oral candidiasis, oral hairy leukoplakia (thought to be associated with Epstein–Barr virus; Fig. 2) and infection with herpes simplex, herpes zoster, molluscum contagiosum and *Staphylococcus aureus* are increased in advanced disease.
- *Other dermatoses.* Drug eruptions, hyperpigmentation and basal cell carcinomas are more common; psoriasis can get worse and syphilis may coexist.
- *Kaposi's sarcoma.* Kaposi's sarcoma is a multicentric tumour of vascular endothelium seen in a third of patients with AIDS or AIDS-related complex, particularly in male homosexuals. It presents as purplish nodules or macules on the face, limbs, trunk or in the mouth (Fig. 3), but often also involves the internal organs and lymph nodes. Kaposi's sarcoma is due to co-infection with herpes virus 8 infection. A more benign sporadic form, seen in elderly East European Jewish men, is not associated with HIV.
- *Lymphoma.* Lymphomas seen with late-phase HIV infection are often extranodal and sometimes cutaneous.

Management

Clinical diagnosis of HIV infection is confirmed by a blood test for antibodies to the virus. Patients should be managed in departments with special experience

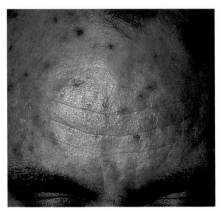

Fig. 1 **Seborrhoeic dermatitis, often seen in early and intermediate HIV infection.**

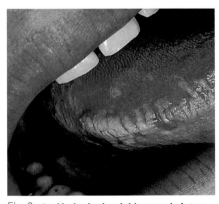

Fig. 2 **Oral hairy leukoplakia, seen in late HIV infection (AIDS).**

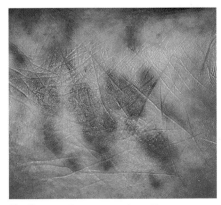

Fig. 3 **Kaposi's sarcoma, found in intermediate and late HIV infection.**

in HIV disease. Infected individuals are counselled and sexual contacts are traced. Without antiretroviral therapy, 5 years after HIV infection, 15% will have progressed to AIDS, but two-thirds of the remainder will be asymptomatic. Ten years after infection, 50% will have developed AIDS, of whom 80% will have died. After AIDS has developed, mortality is high, with 50% dying in 1 year and 85% in 5 years. About 20–50% of infants born to HIV-infected women have HIV disease.

The best predictors of progression are the CD4 count (<250 cells/mL predicts a 66% chance of developing AIDS within 2 years), HIV RNA viral load and the development of oral candidiasis.

Medical intervention is by highly active antiretroviral therapy (HAART, with reverse transcriptase and protease inhibitors), the prophylaxis of opportunistic infection and general support including early treatment of infections. Plasma viral load and blood CD4 counts are monitored. Aerosol pentamidine or oral co-trimoxazole is effective in preventing *P. jiroveci* pneumonia, and ganciclovir is used to control cytomegalovirus infection. Kaposi's sarcoma may be treated with radiotherapy, cytotoxic agents or interferon-α.

Congenital immune deficiency syndromes

Congenital immune deficiency syndromes are divided into:

- *B-cell deficiency*: immunoglobulin deficit; sometimes combined with…
- *T-cell deficiency*: impairment of cell-mediated immunity (see p. 11).
- *Defects in effector mechanisms* such as complement or neutrophils.

Many of these conditions are very rare and present in infancy with failure to thrive. Opportunistic or pyogenic infections that often involve the skin are a feature.

Examples of these include:

- *X-linked agammaglobulinaemia.* Infections occur in infancy once maternal antibodies run out.
- *IgA deficiency.* Affects 1 in 700 caucasians; half have recurrent infections.
- *Severe combined immunodeficiency.* Fatal in infancy because of overwhelming infection unless treated by bone marrow transplant.

- *Wiskott–Aldrich syndrome.* X-linked with T-cell defects, thrombocytopenia and an associated eczema.
- *Chronic mucocutaneous candidiasis.* Seen with severe immune deficiencies, multiple endocrine dysfunction or occurring sporadically; mainly due to a T-cell defect. Candidiasis usually involves the mouth, skin or nails (Fig. 4).
- *Chronic granulomatous disease.* Phagocytosis is defective.

Skin signs of immunosuppression for allografts

The use of corticosteroids, azathioprine and ciclosporin for the suppression of allograft rejection is well established. Cutaneous side-effects include not only drug eruptions and side-effects from the drugs but also infections and tumours, which develop as a result of impairment of immune surveillance, and graft-versus-host disease, which is a manifestation of an immune reaction against the host's body by the grafted tissue (p. 81). Recipients of renal allografts seem to be at particular risk of developing skin cancers. Specific skin problems in immunosuppressed allograft recipients include:

- *Infections and infestations.* Herpes zoster (p. 53), herpes simplex and cytomegalovirus infection may be reactivated with immunosuppressive therapy. Boils and cellulitis are common, and crusted 'Norwegian' scabies (p. 114) may occur.
- *Human papillomavirus infection.* About 50% of renal transplant patients have viral warts (Fig. 5). These may be associated with actinic keratoses or other dysplastic lesions on sun-exposed sites. The human papillomavirus acts as a carcinogen along with sun exposure.

- *Skin cancers.* The risk of skin cancer in renal transplant recipients is increased 20-fold compared with the normal population. Squamous cell carcinomas (Fig. 6) are more common than basal cell carcinomas. The tumours may look banal but behave aggressively.
- *Graft-versus-host disease.* See page 81.

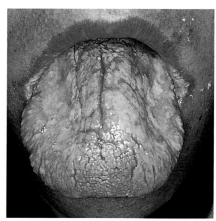

Fig. 4 **Chronic mucocutaneous candidiasis, mainly due to a T-cell defect.**

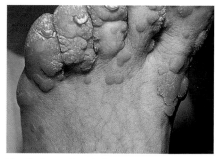

Fig. 5 **Extensive viral warts in an immunosuppressed renal transplant patient.**

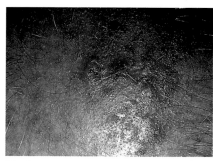

Fig. 6 **Squamous cell carcinoma associated with immunosuppression in a renal transplant recipient.**

HIV disease and immunosuppression

- **HIV infection** may be asymptomatic for several years. Skin signs of early HIV disease include dry skin and seborrhoeic dermatitis; signs of late disease are extensive infections, oral candidiasis and Kaposi's sarcoma. HAART and the prevention of opportunistic infection have transformed the outlook for HIV patients.

- **Congenital immunodeficiency syndromes** are rare, often present with failure to thrive in infancy and are associated with opportunistic or pyogenic infections.

- **Immunosuppression for allografts** is particularly associated with human papillomavirus infection, squamous cell carcinomas or dysplastic lesions and graft-versus-host disease.

http://www.avert.org/ ■ http://www.cdc.gov/az.do#C ■ http://wonder.cdc.gov/wonder/help/AIDS/MMWR-12-18-1992.html

Fungal infections

Fungal infection in humans is common and mainly due to two groups of fungi:

- *dermatophytes* – multicellular filaments or hyphae
- *yeasts* – unicellular forms that replicate by budding.

These are usually confined to the stratum corneum, but deep mycoses invade other tissues (p. 59). Pityriasis versicolor, due to the yeast *Malassezia*, (previously *Pityrosporum ovale*) is described on page 40.

Dermatophyte infections

Dermatophyte fungi reproduce by spore formation. They infect the stratum corneum, nail and hair, and induce inflammation by delayed hypersensitivity or by metabolic effects. There are three asexual genera:

- *Microsporum* infect skin and hair
- *Trichophyton* infect skin, nail and hair
- *Epidermophyton* infect skin and nail.

Thirty species are pathogenic in humans. Zoophilic species (transmitted to humans from animals), e.g. *Trichophyton verrucosum* (Fig. 1), produce more inflammation than anthropophilic (human only) species.

Pathology

Dermatophytes inhabit keratin as branching hyphae, identifiable on microscopy. Skin scrapings, placed on a slide with 10% aqueous potassium hydroxide (to separate the keratinocytes) and a coverslip, are examined microscopically for hyphae (p. 20). The dermatophyte is identified by culturing the scrapings on medium (e.g. Sabouraud's) for 3 weeks.

Clinical presentation

Tinea (Latin: *worm*) denotes a fungal skin infection which is often annular. The exact features depend on the site. The various presentations include:

- **Tinea corporis** (trunk and limbs). Single or multiple plaques, with scaling and erythema especially at the edges, characterize this presentation. The lesions enlarge slowly, with central clearing, leaving a ring pattern, hence 'ringworm' (Figs 1 and 2). Pustules or vesicles may be seen.
- **Tinea cruris** (groin). This is more common in men and is often seen in athletes ('jock itch'), who may also have tinea pedis. It spreads to the upper thigh but rarely involves the scrotum. The advancing edge may be scaly, pustular or vesicular. Causative organisms are shown in Table 1.
- **Tinea incognito.** Fungal infection can be modified in appearance and spread by the anti-inflammatory effect of a topical steroid.
- **Tinea manuum** (hand). Typically, this appears as a unilateral, diffuse powdery scaling of the palm (Fig. 3). *Trichophyton rubrum* is often the cause. Tinea pedis may coexist.
- **Tinea capitis** (scalp/hair). See pages 64 and 110.
- **Tinea unguium** (nails). See page 66.
- **Tinea pedis** (athlete's foot).

Athlete's foot (p. 110) is common in adults (especially young men), rare in children and predisposed to by communal washing, swimming baths, occlusive footwear and hot weather. Itchy interdigital maceration, usually of the fourth/fifth toeweb space, is most frequent, but diffuse 'moccasin' involvement is seen. Recurrent vesicles also occur, sometimes with pompholyx

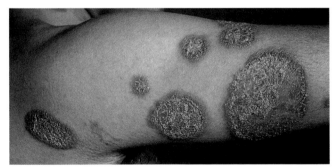

Fig. 1 **Tinea corporis.** The infection is due to animal ringworm (*T. verrucosum*) and shows intense inflammation.

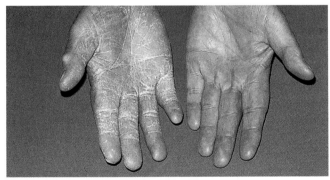

Fig. 3 **Unilateral tinea manuum caused by *T. rubrum*.**

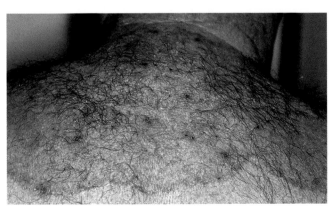

Fig. 2 **Tinea corporis showing a well-defined edge.**

Table 1 **Superficial mycoses: causative organisms and differential diagnosis**

Area	Commonest organism	Differential diagnosis
Body/limbs (corporis)	*T. verrucosum, M. canis, T. rubrum*	Discoid eczema, psoriasis, pityriasis rosea
Feet (pedis)	*T. rubrum, T. interdigitale, E. floccosum*	Contact dermatitis, psoriasis, pompholyx, erythrasma
Groin (cruris)	*T. rubrum, E. floccosum, T. interdigitale*	Intertrigo, candidiasis, erythrasma
Hand (manuum)	*T. rubrum*	Chronic eczema, psoriasis, granuloma annulare
Nail (unguium)	*T. rubrum, T. interdigitale*	Psoriasis, trauma, candidiasis
Scalp (capitis)	*M. canis, M. audouinii, T. tonsurans, T. schoenleinii*	Alopecia areata, psoriasis, seborrhoeic eczema, furunculosis

as an id reaction. The commonest organisms are *T. rubrum*, *T. mentagrophytes* var. *interdigitale* and *Epidermophyton floccosum*.

The differential diagnoses of superficial mycoses are shown Table 1. Microscopy and culture of skin scrapings are often helpful. Wood's ultraviolet light examination is used for tinea capitis, especially for screening during outbreaks. Hair infected by *Microsporum audouinii* and *M. canis* fluoresces green, but *Trichophyton tonsurans* does not fluoresce.

Management

Humid and sweaty conditions, including occlusive footwear, should be minimized, and dusting powder may help to keep the feet or body folds dry. Minor fungal infections respond to topical treatments, but widespread involvement or diseases of the nails or scalp requires systemic therapy.

Topical therapy

Whitfield's ointment (containing benzoic acid) and Magenta paint have been replaced by the imidazoles, e.g. clotrimazole (Canesten) and miconazole (Daktarin). Tinea corporis, tinea pedis and tinea cruris respond to topical creams, sprays or powders. Terbinafine (Lamisil) cream once daily is often effective. Amorolfine (Loceryl) nail lacquer, applied once weekly, produces a 40–50% cure for tinea unguium of one or two nails. Before antifungal agents, scalp ringworm sometimes required X-irradiation.

Systemic therapy

Tinea capitis, tinea manuum, tinea unguium and extensive tinea corporis often require systemic treatment. Griseofulvin is still the treatment of choice for tinea capitis in children (10 mg/kg/day for 1–2 months) but, for other indications, it has largely been superseded by the newer antifungals, terbinafine (Lamisil) and itraconazole (Sporanox), which show greater efficacy, have fewer side-effects and require shorter treatments.

Terbinafine 250 mg daily or itraconazole 100 mg daily may be used for tinea capitis, corporis, cruris, manuum and pedis, given for 2–4 weeks. In tinea unguium, terbinafine (250 mg daily for 6–12 weeks) is the drug of choice; itraconazole (200 mg daily for 12 weeks or as 'pulsed' courses) is an alternative. In the elderly, uncomplicated fungal toenail infection may not require any therapy. Itraconazole can potentially cause hepatotoxicity and requires cautious use in heart failure.

Ketoconazole (Nizoral) by mouth, although effective, is limited in use by hepatotoxicity.

Candida albicans infection

Candida albicans is a ubiquitous commensal of the mouth and gastrointestinal tract that can produce opportunistic infection. Predisposing factors include:

- moist and opposing skin folds
- obesity or diabetes mellitus
- immunosuppression (p. 55)
- pregnancy
- poor hygiene
- humid environment
- wet work occupation
- use of broad-spectrum antibiotic.

Clinical presentation

In infection, hyphal forms of *C. albicans* are seen in the stratum corneum. Infection may present as:

- **Genital.** Thrush commonly appears as an itchy, sore vulvovaginitis. White plaques adhere to inflamed mucous membranes, and a white vaginal discharge may occur. Males develop similar changes on the penis. It can be spread by sexual intercourse.
- **Intertrigo.** Superinfection with *C. albicans*, and often also with bacteria, gives a moist, glazed and macerated appearance to the submammary, axillary or inguinal body folds. The interdigital clefts are involved (Fig. 4) in wet workers who do not dry their hands properly.
- **Mucocutaneous candidiasis.** This rare, sometimes inherited disorder of immune deficiency starts in infancy. Chronic *C. albicans* intertrigo with nail and mouth infections is seen.
- **Oral.** White plaques adhere to an erythematous buccal mucosa. Broad-spectrum antibiotics, false teeth and poor oral hygiene predispose. Angular stomatitis may coexist.
- **Paronychia.** See page 66.
- **Systemic.** Systemic candidiasis can occur in immunosuppressed patients. Red nodules are seen in the skin.

Management

Candida albicans infections must be differentiated from other conditions (Table 2). General measures are important. Body folds are separated and kept dry with dusting powder. Hands are dried carefully (p. 36) and oral hygiene improved. Systemic antibiotics may need to be stopped. Specific agents

against *Candida* are used topically and systemically.

Topical therapy

Imidazoles are effective and available as creams, powders, pessaries and lotions. For oral candida, use amphotericin, nystatin or miconazole as lozenges, suspension or gels.

Systemic therapy

Bowel carriage may be reduced in recurrent candidiasis by oral nystatin. Itraconazole 100 mg daily or fluconazole (Diflucan) 50 mg daily, but not griseofulvin, can be given as a short course for persistent *C. albicans* infections and in the long term for mucocutaneous candidiasis. Vaginal candidiasis is treated by a single dose of 500 mg of clotrimazole (Canesten) or 150 mg of econazole (Gyno-Pevaryl) as a pessary, or with itraconazole or fluconazole by mouth.

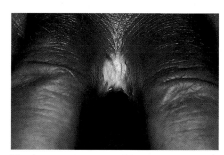

Fig. 4 **Intertrigo of the interdigital cleft due to *C. albicans*.**

Table 2 **Differential diagnosis: *C. albicans* infections**

Variant	Differential diagnosis
Genital	Psoriasis, lichen planus, lichen sclerosus
Intertrigo	Psoriasis, seborrhoeic dermatitis, bacterial secondary infection
Oral	Lichen planus, epithelial dysplasia
Paronychia	Bacterial infection, chronic eczema

Fungal infections

- Dermatophytes infect the feet, groin, body, nails, hands and scalp. The commonest dermatophyte pathogens are *Trichophyton rubrum*, *T. mentagrophytes* var. *interdigitale* and *Epidermophyton floccosum*.

- Topical imidazoles and oral terbinafine or itraconazole are effective for most dermatophyte infections.

- *C. albicans* produces opportunistic infection of the body folds, mouth, genitals and nail fold. These are predisposed to by humidity, obesity, diabetes and oral antibiotic therapy.

- Topical imidazoles are usually effective for candidiasis.

http://www.cdc.gov/az.do#C   http://www.nlm.nih.gov/medlineplus/fungalinfections.html

Tropical infections and infestations

Infections constitute one of the biggest problems in dermatology in tropical countries of the developing world. Leprosy, for example, despite being a treatable disease, continues to ravage in many parts of the globe.

However, tropical infections may also be seen in countries in which they are non-endemic – among visitors and immigrants, or when acquired abroad by the indigenous population.

Leprosy

Leprosy is a chronic disease caused by *Mycobacterium leprae*. This is an acid- and alcohol-fast bacillus that cannot be cultured in the laboratory. Nasal droplets spread the infection, and the incubation period is several years. The disease is usually acquired in childhood, as the risk to exposed adults is about 5%. Leprosy is no longer endemic in northern Europe, but it does occur in tropical and subtropical areas throughout the world. The manifestation of the disease depends on the degree of the delayed (type IV) hypersensitivity response in the infected individual. Those with strong cell-mediated immunity develop the tuberculoid type, whereas those in whom the cell-mediated reactivity is poor develop lepromatous leprosy. Borderline lesions are seen in those whose immune state is in between.

M. *leprae* has a predilection for nerves and the dermis but, in the lepromatous type, infection may be much more widespread. Tuberculoid leprosy is characterized by a granulomatous reaction in the nerves and dermis with no acid-fast bacilli demonstrated with the Ziehl–Neelsen stain. In contrast, bacilli are plentiful in the dermis of the lepromatous type, and large numbers of macrophages are seen on microscopy.

Clinical presentation

Tuberculoid leprosy affects the nerves and the skin. Nerves may be thickened, and anaesthesia or muscle atrophy is found. Skin lesions often occur on the face, and as few as one or two may be seen. They usually take the form of raised red plaques with a hypopigmented centre, which is typically dry and hairless (Fig. 1). Sensation may be impaired within the plaque.

The skin lesions of *lepromatous leprosy* are multiple and take the form of macules, papules, nodules and plaques. They are symmetrical and tend to involve the face, arms, legs and buttocks. Sensation is not impaired. Untreated, the condition is infectious from the nasal involvement. Progression gives a thickened furrowed appearance to the face (leonine facies) with loss of eyebrows (Fig. 2). *Borderline leprosy* shows features intermediate between lepromatous and tuberculoid.

Leprosy must be distinguished from a variety of other dermatological conditions (Table 1).

Complications

Tuberculoid leprosy may result in bone damage to a hand or foot from repeated trauma to an insensitive area. In lepromatous leprosy, nasal damage may progress to a saddle nose defect. Ichthyosis, testicular atrophy and leg ulcers are seen. A peripheral neuropathy leads to shortening of the toes and fingers from repeated trauma. Lepra reactions, which result from an upgrading or a downgrading of the immune response, can produce nerve destruction or acute skin lesions.

Management

Lepromatous (multibacillary) leprosy is treated with rifampicin, dapsone and clofazimine. Treatment is for at least 2 years, continued until skin smears are negative. Tuberculoid (paucibacillary) leprosy responds to rifampicin and dapsone, given for 6 months. The complications of leprosy may require the skills of rehabilitation specialists and orthopaedic and plastic surgeons.

In countries where leprosy is endemic, the education of the public about the disease is important in reducing the stigma attached to sufferers. Public health programmes aimed at leprosy control are active in several countries.

Leishmaniasis

Leishmaniasis is a disease caused by *Leishmania* protozoa, which are transmitted by sand fly bites. It exists in tropical and subtropical areas in a cutaneous, mucocutaneous or visceral form. Three protozoa cause disease:

- *Leishmania tropica* causes the cutaneous 'oriental sore' and is seen around the Mediterranean coast, in the Middle East and in Asia.
- *L. braziliensis*, endemic in central and South America, leads to cutaneous and mucosal disease.

Table 1 **Differential diagnosis of leprosy**	
Type of leprosy	**Differential diagnosis**
Tuberculoid	Vitiligo, pityriasis versicolor, pityriasis alba, sarcoidosis, lupus vulgaris, granuloma annulare, post-inflammatory hypopigmentation
Lepromatous	Disseminated cutaneous leishmaniasis, yaws, guttate psoriasis, discoid lupus erythematosus, mycosis fungoides

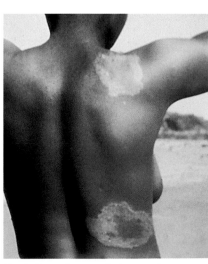

Fig. 1 **Hypopigmented plaques of tuberculoid leprosy.**

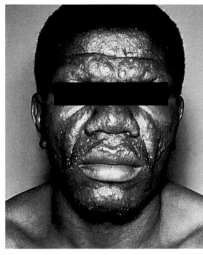

Fig. 2 **The leonine facies of lepromatous leprosy.**

- *L. donovani* is widely distributed in Asia, Africa and South America, and causes visceral disease (kala-azar) with associated skin lesions.

Clinical presentation

Oriental sore is a common infection in endemic areas normally affecting children, who subsequently develop immunity. In non-endemic regions, it is not infrequently seen in travellers after a Mediterranean holiday. The face, neck or arms are usually affected. At the site of inoculation, a red or brown nodule appears, which either ulcerates or spreads slowly to form a crust-topped plaque (Fig. 3). Untreated, the lesion will heal in 6–12 months, although a chronic form is seen. In *mucocutaneous leishmaniasis*, the skin lesion resembles an oriental sore but, subsequently, necrotic ulcers affect the nose, lips and palate with deformity. *Kala-azar* principally affects children and has a significant mortality. It causes hepatomegaly, splenomegaly, anaemia and debility. The cutaneous signs are patchy pigmentation on the face, hands and abdomen.

Leishmaniasis must be distinguished from some other disorders (Table 2).

Management

Cutaneous leishmaniasis may heal spontaneously, and small areas respond to cryotherapy. When specific treatment

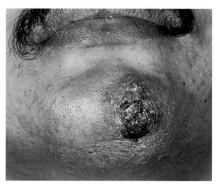

Fig. 3 **The oriental sore of cutaneous leishmaniasis.** Small lesions may respond to cryotherapy. Otherwise, intravenous sodium stibogluconate may be given.

is needed, it is usual to give sodium stibogluconate (Pentostam) intravenously for 10–21 days. The treatment for the mucocutaneous and visceral forms is similar.

Larva migrans

Larva migrans is a 'creeping' eruption due to penetration of the skin by the larval stage of animal hookworms. Larva migrans is often acquired from tropical beaches where ova from the hookworms of dogs and cats have hatched into larvae that are able to penetrate the human skin. Penetration usually occurs on the feet. The larvae advance at the rate of a few millimetres a day in a serpiginous route causing red intensely itchy tracks to appear (Fig. 4). They eventually die spontaneously after a few weeks, as they cannot complete their life cycle in humans.

Topical 10% thiabendazole cream or a single oral dose of ivermectin (200 μg/kg) is usually effective.

Deep mycoses

Deep mycoses are defined as the invasion of living tissue by fungi, causing

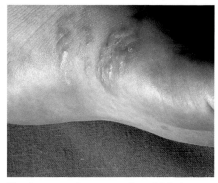

Fig. 4 **Larva migrans seen in a child who had just visited the beaches of the West Indies.** Treatment is with oral ivermectin or topical thiabendazole.

systemic disease. Brief details are given in Table 3.

Filariasis

Filariasis is seen in the tropics and is often due to the nematode worm *Wuchereria bancrofti*. Lymphatic damage ultimately results in gross oedema of the legs and scrotum ('elephantiasis'). Treatment is with diethylcarbamazine.

Onchocerciasis

Onchocerciasis is a disease affecting the eyes and skin, caused by the worm *Onchocerca volvulus*. It is endemic in Africa and Central America and is an important cause of blindness. A gnat transmits the worm to humans. Dermal nodules with lichenification and pigmentary change follow an itchy papular eruption. Microfilariae invade the eye and result in blindness.

Ivermectin, as a single dose, is the drug of choice for onchocerciasis. Retreatment at 6- or 12-monthly intervals may be needed until the worms die out.

Table 2 **Differential diagnosis of leishmaniasis**	
Variant	**Differential diagnosis**
Cutaneous	Lupus vulgaris, leprosy, discoid lupus erythematosus
Mucocutaneous	Syphilis, yaws, leprosy, blastomycosis
Kala-azar	Leprosy

Table 3 **The deep mycoses**		
Mycosis	**Clinical features**	**Management**
Actinomycosis (filamentous bacteria)	A chronic suppurating granulomatous infection with multiple sinuses discharging yellow granules, particularly around the jaw, chest and abdomen	Long-term, high-dose penicillin, surgical excision
Blastomycosis	Ulcerated discharging nodules that show central clearing with scarring; may spread from pulmonary infection	Oral itraconazole, systemic amphotericin B or ketoconazole
Histoplasmosis	Seen in immunosuppressed patients who develop lung disease with granulomatous skin lesions	Oral itraconazole or ketoconazole
Mycetoma	A chronic granulomatous infection usually of the foot, involving skin, subcutaneous tissue and bones, due to several types of fungi or actinomycetes; nodules with abscesses, sinuses, ulceration and tissue necrosis result	Depends on the organism; surgical excision, dapsone with co-trimoxazole, and itraconazole may help
Sporotrichosis	An abscess forms with nodules subsequently occurring proximally along the line of lymphatic drainage	Potassium iodide, itraconazole or terbinafine

> *Tropical infections*
>
> - **Leprosy:** tuberculoid and lepromatous forms mainly affect the skin and nerves; treatment is with dapsone, rifampicin and clofazimine.
> - **Leishmaniasis:** cutaneous, mucocutaneous and visceral types; treatment is with sodium stibogluconate.
> - **Larva migrans:** creeping eruption due to animal hookworms; responds to thiabendazole cream or oral ivermectin.
> - **Deep mycoses:** serious infections that may be difficult to eradicate.
> - **Onchocerciasis:** an important cause of blindness; skin shows lichenified nodules and pigmentary changes. Treatment is with oral ivermectin.

http://www.who.int/lep/ ■ http://www.cdc.gov/C

Infestations

Infestation is defined as the harbouring of insect or worm parasites in or on the body. Worms – on or in the skin – are infrequent except in tropical countries. Insect life on the skin is usually transient in temperate climes, although a mite (*Demodex folliculorum*) may live harmlessly in facial hair follicles.

Insects cause a variety of skin reactions (Table 1). Contact with an insect or an insect bite can produce a chemical effect, such as a bee sting, or an irritant effect, such as dermatitis from contact with a caterpillar or blistering due to cantharadin released from a crushed beetle. Contact may also cause an immune-mediated response.

Insects also act as vectors of skin disease, as in Lyme disease (p. 49), when animal ticks transmit *Borrelia burgdorferi*. They may involve the skin directly by burrowing (e.g. scabies) or by laying eggs in the skin (myiasis).

Insect bites
The cutaneous reaction following the bite of an insect is due to a pharmacological, irritant or allergic response to the introduced foreign material.

Clinical presentation
The lesions of insect bites vary from itchy wheals (Fig. 1) through papules

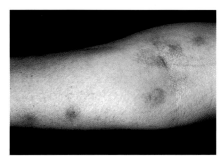

Fig. 1 **Papular urticaria, showing grouped and linear lesions.**

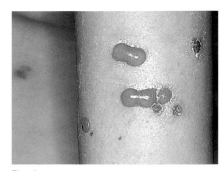

Fig. 2 **Grouped blisters due to insect bites.**

Table 1 **Insect effects on the skin**	
Insect	**Effect**
Animal ticks	Bites, disease vector
Ants, bedbugs, fleas	Bites
Bees, wasps	Stings
Caterpillars	Dermatitis
Cheyletiella	Papular urticaria
Demodex folliculorum	Normal inhabitant
Food and harvest mites	Bites
Lice	Infestation (bites), disease vector
Mosquitoes	Bites, myiasis, disease vector
Sarcoptes scabei	Scabies

to quite large bullae (Fig. 2). The morphology will depend on the insect (Table 1) and the type of response elicited. Insect bites are usually grouped or track up a limb. Papular urticaria defines recurrent itchy urticated papules on the limbs or trunk, quite often in a child. The culprits, which may be difficult to trace, include garden insects, fleas or mites on household pets. Bedbugs cause bites on the face, neck and hands. They lie inactive in crevices in furniture during the day and emerge at night. Secondary bacterial infection of excoriated insect bites is common.

Differential diagnosis
The linear or grouped nature of the lesions is usually suggestive, but sometimes urticaria, scabies, atopic eczema or dermatitis herpetiformis may need to be considered.

Management
Elimination of the cause is often not easy, as the insects are difficult to trace. Household pets must be inspected and treated if necessary. Cat fleas exist for months on carpets without a cat being present. Birds nesting or perching by a window can introduce *Cheyletiella* into a house. An individual with insect bites can be helped by Eurax hydrocortisone cream or calamine lotion.

Lice infestation (pediculosis)
Lice are flat, wingless, blood-sucking insects (Fig. 3). Their eggs (nits) are laid on hairs or clothing. There are two anthropophilic species:

- pubic louse
- body louse (the head louse is a variant).

Head lice are common among schoolchildren and spread by head-to-head contact. The nits are often easier to see than the lice (p. 20). The body louse is mainly seen in vagrants who live in unhygienic or poor social conditions. Spread is by infested bedding or clothing. The pubic louse is sexually transmitted and is mostly found in young adults. Lice induce intense itching which, through scratching, results in excoriation and secondary infection.

Clinical presentation
The itching of head lice usually starts at the sides and back of the scalp. Scratching results in secondary infection that may cause matted hair. Body lice result in excoriations on the trunk and, in chronic infestation, lichenification and pigmentation. The lice are found in the seams of clothes. Pubic lice, known colloquially as 'crabs', result in severe pruritus with secondary eczema and infection. They may involve the eyelashes. Lice infestation should not be confused with other conditions (Table 2).

Management
Head lice are treated with malathion or carbaryl lotion, applied to the scalp for 12 h, washed out and repeated in 7 days. Permethrin or phenothrin are alternatives. Nits are removed with a comb. Contacts are also treated. Body lice are eradicated by treating the

Table 2 **Differential diagnosis of pediculosis**	
Louse infestation	**Differential diagnosis**
Body louse	Scabies, chronic eczema
Head louse	Impetigo, eczema
Pubic louse	Scabies, eczema

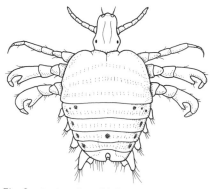

Fig. 3 **The female pubic louse.**

clothing with tumble drying, laundering or dry cleaning. Malathion or phenothrin lotions may be used on the skin. Infestation with pubic lice requires the application of malathion or carbaryl aqueous lotions to all the body. Sexual partners should be treated.

Scabies

The scabies mite, *Sarcoptes scabei* var. *hominis*, is 0.4 mm in length (Fig. 4) and is spread by direct physical transfer, including sexual contact. The fertilized female mite burrows through the stratum corneum at the rate of 2 mm/day, laying two or three eggs each day. The eggs hatch after 3 days into larvae, which form shallow pockets in the stratum corneum where they moult and mature within about 2 weeks. The mites mate in the pockets; the male dies, but the fertilized female burrows and continues the cycle. After first being infested, it takes 3–4 weeks for the hypersensitivity reaction to the mite, and the intense itching that it causes, to develop. On average, about 12 mites are present at the itching stage, but it can be many more.

Clinical presentation

The irregular, tortuous and slightly scaly burrows measure up to 1 cm long. They are commonest on the sides of fingers (Fig. 5), wrists, ankles and nipples, and on the genitalia where they form rubbery nodules. Small vesicles are often seen. Itching induces excoriations (Fig. 6). In infants, the feet are frequently involved and the face can be affected. The mite is occasionally visible as a white dot at the end of a burrow. If extracted with a needle and viewed under a microscope, the diagnosis is irrefutable.

Scabies is often accompanied by an ill-defined eczematous urticated papular hypersensitivity reaction on the trunk. Untreated, scabies becomes chronic.

Differential diagnosis

Other intensely itchy eruptions, such as lichen planus, dermatitis herpetiformis, papular urticaria and eczema, may need to be considered, but only scabies shows burrows. Animal scabies, due to animal mites, causes an itchy eruption, but burrows are absent.

Complications

Scabies commonly becomes secondarily infected. In institutionalized or immunosuppressed patients, very large numbers of mites proliferate to produce an extensive crusted eruption known as 'Norwegian' scabies (p. 114).

Patients commonly feel itchy for some days even after adequate treatment, and pruritic non-infested 'post-scabetic' nodules may persist for weeks. Scabicides often cause an irritant dermatitis, and care must be taken to distinguish this from persistent or recurrent infestation.

Management

An adequate application technique and the treatment of all contacts are most important in the treatment of scabies. If either is lacking, persistence or re-infestation may result. An instruction leaflet for patients is helpful. The aqueous preparations of permethrin (Lyclear) and malathion (Prioderm) are effective. Crotamiton (Eurax), benzyl benzoate (Ascabiol) and 10% sulphur ointment are alternatives. A single dose of ivermectin (200 μg/kg) may be used when topical therapy alone is ineffective, e.g. in crusted scabies. For topical treatment, the suggested technique is as follows:

- apply the lotion or cream to the entire body surface including scalp, face, neck and ears
- pay special attention to fingerweb and toeweb spaces, and under the nails
- leave the lotion on for 12–24 h and then wash off in the bath or shower
- if the hands are washed during this period, reapply the lotion or cream
- repeat the treatment after 1 week.

Recently infested individuals do not itch, and close contacts (such as the whole family) and sexual partners need treatment. Scabies often breaks out in old people's homes or geriatric wards and presents the problem of how far to extend the therapeutic net. The safe rule is to treat all members of a ward or home, including nurses, who have contact with the index case. Clothing and bedding is laundered. The mite dies within a few days away from the skin.

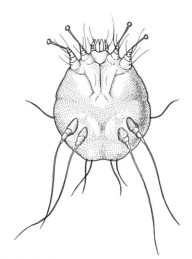

Fig. 4 **The female scabies mite.**

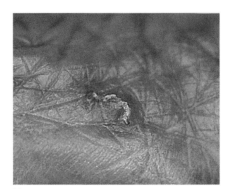

Fig. 5 **A scabetic burrow on the side of the finger in an elderly patient.**

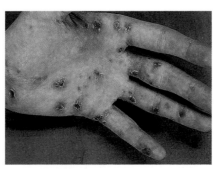

Fig. 6 **Multiple excoriations on the hand due to scabies infestation.**

Infestations

- **Insect bites** present on the trunk and limbs as groups of itchy, often blistering, papules; secondary infection is common.

- **Head lice** infestation is transmitted between schoolchildren by head contact. Secondary infection is common. Repeated treatment is often necessary.

- **Body lice** occur in those living in poor social conditions and produce excoriation and lichenification.

- **Pubic lice** are sexually transmitted and present with pruritus and secondary infection.

- **Scabies** is spread by direct transfer and is intensely itchy. All contacts need treatment. Outbreaks are frequently seen in nursing homes where there is quite often an 'index' case with crusted scabies.

Sebaceous and sweat glands – Acne, rosacea and other disorders

Acne

Acne is a chronic inflammation of the pilosebaceous units, producing comedones, papules, pustules, cysts and scars. It affects nearly every adolescent. Acne has an equal sex incidence and tends to affect women earlier than men, although the peak age for clinical acne is 18 years in both sexes. Acne results from:

- increased sebum excretion – seborrhoea (greasy skin)
- pilosebaceous duct hyperkeratosis and comedone formation
- colonization of the duct with *Propionibacterium acnes*
- release of inflammatory mediators (including cytokines).

In acne, the androgen-sensitive pilosebaceous unit (p. 4) shows a hyper-responsiveness that results in increased sebum excretion. Factors in sebum induce comedones, and *P. acnes* initiates inflammation through chemical mediators inducing enzymes (e.g. lipase) and prostaglandins (Fig. 1).

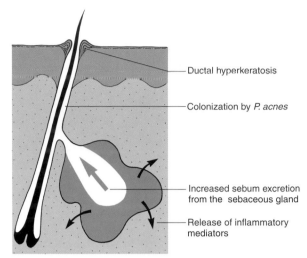

Ductal hyperkeratosis

Colonization by *P. acnes*

Increased sebum excretion from the sebaceous gland

Release of inflammatory mediators

Fig. 1 **Aetiopathogenesis of acne.**

Clinical presentation

Comedones are either open (blackheads: dilated pores with black plugs of melanin-containing keratin) or closed (whiteheads: small cream-coloured, dome-shaped papules). They appear at about the age of 12 years and evolve into inflammatory papules (Fig. 2), pustules or cysts (Fig. 3). The sites of predilection – the face, shoulders, back and upper chest – have many sebaceous glands. The severity of acne depends on its extent and the type of lesion, with cysts being the most destructive.

Acne usually persists until the early twenties, although in a few patients, particularly women, the disease continues into the fifth decade. Scars may follow healing, especially of cysts or abscesses. Scars may be 'ice-pick', atrophic (Fig. 4) or keloidal.

Some variants of acne are seen:

- *Acne excoriée*: due to squeezing, affects depressed or obsessional young women.
- *Chloracne*: caused by systemic toxicity of certain aromatic halogenated industrial chemicals.
- *Conglobate*: a mass of burrowing abscesses and sinuses with scarring.
- *Cosmetic*: pomade and cosmetic-induced comedonal and papular acne (mainly seen in the USA).
- *Drug-induced*: by systemic steroids, androgens and topical steroids.
- *Infantile*: mostly found on the faces of male infants; cause unknown.
- *Physical*: occlusion by the back of a wheelchair or on a violinist's chin.

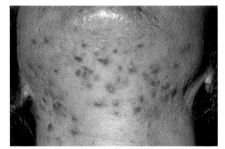

Fig. 2 **Papular–pustular acne of the chin, with some whiteheads.**

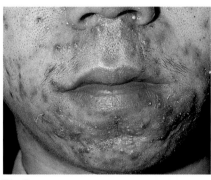

Fig. 3 **Pustulocystic acne on the face.**

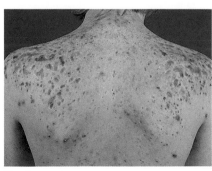

Fig. 4 **Scarring acne on the back.**

Complications and differential diagnosis

Embarrassment, social withdrawal and depression are important sequelae of acne. These can improve with effective treatment. The rare and severe acne fulminans, seen in adolescent males, is associated with fever, arthritis and vasculitis. Long-term antibiotic treatment may induce a Gram-negative folliculitis.

Rosacea can usually be differentiated from acne (see below). Bacterial folliculitis is more acute than acne, but the two may coexist.

Management

Treatment depends on the type and extent of acne and the patient's psychological state. 'Over-the-counter' creams have often already been used.

Local treatment is adequate for mild acne and is used with systemic drugs for more severe cases.

- *Benzoyl peroxide* (PanOxyl, Brevoxyl) cream or gel, applied twice a day, works by reducing the number of *P. acnes*. It may cause irritation, contact allergy and bleach clothing.
- *Tretinoin* (Retin A cream or gel) is good at reducing the number of comedones, but may be irritant.
- *Antibiotics*, e.g. clindamycin (Dalacin T), erythromycin alone (Stiemycin) or with zinc (Zineryt) or benzoyl peroxide (Benzamycin), can be used for mild or moderately severe acne.
- *Other topical agents*, e.g. azelaic acid, isotretinoin and adapalene.

Oral treatment with antibiotics, retinoid or hormones is prescribed for moderate or severe acne, acne excoriée and in depressed patients.

Antibiotics
The first-line systemic antibiotic drug is tetracycline, 500 mg twice daily (taken half an hour before food with water), given for a minimum of 4 months. Tetracyclines are contraindicated in children and in pregnancy, and may cause *Candida albicans* infection or photosensitivity. Minocycline (Minocin, Aknemin, 100 mg daily) and doxycycline (Vibramycin, 100 mg once daily) are alternative tetracyclines that are better absorbed.

Erythromycin (500 mg twice daily) and trimethoprim are second-choice antibiotics. Women on oral contraceptives who take an antibiotic are advised that, if diarrhoea develops, additional contraception is needed for the rest of the menstrual cycle.

Antiandrogen
The combination of an antiandrogen and an oestrogen (co-cyprindiol–cyproterone acetate, 2 mg, and ethinylestradiol, 35 µg: Dianette) is used in females (not males) with moderate to severe acne that is resistant to conventional therapy. The antiandrogen suppresses sebum production. Co-cyprindiol is given for 6–12 months and is also a contraceptive.

Retinoid
Isotretinoin (Roaccutane), which reduces sebum excretion, inhibits *P. acnes* and is anti-inflammatory, is a very effective treatment for acne. It is used if acne is severe or unresponsive to conventional treatment, or if acne relapses quickly once antibiotics are stopped. A course lasts 4 months and requires the monitoring of liver function and fasting lipids. Isotretinoin is teratogenic. Women given the drug must not be pregnant and need to take the oral contraceptive throughout treatment and for the month before and after. Common side-effects include cracked lips, dry skin, nose bleeds, hair loss and muscle aches.

Other therapies
Acne cysts may require injection with triamcinolone acetonide (a steroid), or sometimes excision or cryotherapy. Comedones can be removed using an extractor. Diet has no effect on acne.

Rosacea

Rosacea is a chronic inflammatory facial dermatosis characterized by erythema and pustules. The cause of rosacea is unknown. Histologically, dilated dermal blood vessels, sebaceous gland hyperplasia and an inflammatory cell infiltrate are seen. Sebum excretion is normal.

Clinical presentation
Rosacea has an equal sex incidence. Although commonest in middle age, it also affects young adults and the elderly. The earliest symptom is flushing. Erythema, telangiectasia, papules, pustules (Fig. 5) and, occasionally, lymphoedema involve the cheeks, nose, forehead and chin. Rhinophyma, hyperplasia of the sebaceous glands and connective tissue of the nose (Fig. 5), and eye involvement by blepharitis and conjunctivitis are complications. Sunlight and topical steroids exacerbate the condition. Rosacea persists for years, but usually responds well to treatment. Rosacea lacks the comedones of acne

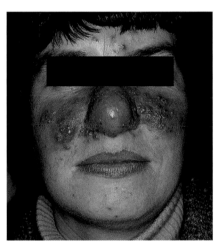

Fig. 5 **Rosacea with rhinophyma in a woman.** Rhinophyma usually affects men.

and occurs in an older age group. Contact dermatitis, photosensitive eruptions, seborrhoeic dermatitis and lupus erythematosus often involve the face but are more acute or scaly, or lack pustules.

Management
Topically, metronidazole 0.75% cream (Rozex) twice daily may be helpful. If this is ineffective, the usual oral treatment is tetracycline, initially 1 g daily, reducing to 250 mg daily after a few weeks and continued for 2–3 months. Erythromycin is an alternative. Repeated treatment is often needed. Isotretinoin can be used but is less effective than in acne. Plastic surgery is required for rhinophyma.

Other disorders

Perioral dermatitis is characterized by papules and pustules that may occur around the mouth and chin of a woman who has used topical steroids. They will clear with steroid cessation and oral tetracycline therapy.

Hidradenitis suppurativa is an unpleasant chronic inflammatory condition of the infundibulum of hair follicles (p. 4) in the apocrine sweat gland areas of the axillae, groin and perineum. Nodules, abscesses, cysts and sinuses form and scarring results (p. 110). Treatment is with topical antiseptics, a prolonged course of a systemic antibiotic or retinoid and surgical excision. Conglobate acne may coexist.

Hyperhidrosis (excess sweating) due to eccrine gland overactivity is usually emotional in origin. Treatment with 20% aluminium chloride in alcohol (Anhydrol Forte, Driclor) is often effective. Botox injection is a new treatment (p. 110).

Sebaceous/apocrine disorders

Acne
- *Due to* increased sebum excretion, comedone formation, *P. acnes* and inflammation.
- *Presentation*: comedones, pustules, cysts and scars seen over the face, chest and trunk.
- *Treatment*: topical treatments include benzoyl peroxide and tretinoin; systemic treatments include antibiotics, e.g. tetracyclines or erythromycin, co-cyprindiol and isotretinoin.

Rosacea
- *Affects* the middle-aged or elderly. Often starts with facial flushing.
- *Presentation*: facial erythema, telangiectasia and pustules; rhinophyma and conjunctivitis.
- *Treatment*: topical metronidazole 0.75% cream, oral tetracycline.

Hidradenitis suppurativa
- *Presentation*: chronic nodules or abscesses of axillae and groin, resulting in scarring.
- *Treatment*: local antiseptics, prolonged course of oral antibiotic or retinoid, excision.

Disorders of hair

Hair loss (Alopecia)

The division of alopecia into diffuse localized and scarring or non-scarring helps in diagnosis (Table 1).

Diffuse non-scarring

With diffuse, non-scarring alopecia, patients usually notice excessive numbers of hairs on the pillow, brush or comb, and after washing their hair. The scalp shows a diffuse reduction in hair density. The causes are described below.

Male pattern (androgenetic alopecia)

Male pattern baldness is inherited (the exact mode is unclear) and androgen dependent. Over several cycles, the androgen-sensitive follicles miniaturize from terminal to vellus hairs. Males are affected from the second decade and, by the seventh decade, 80% have involvement. Patterned balding also occurs in females, the majority of whom are hormonally normal. It becomes more pronounced after the menopause and is present in 70% of 80-year-old

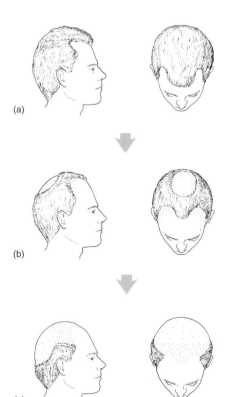

Fig. 1 **Male pattern baldness.** Hair loss may progress from bitemporal recession **(a)** to vertex involvement **(b)** to the most severe form **(c)**, where only a horseshoe of hair runs from the ears to the occiput.

Table 1 **Causes of hair loss**	
Type of hair loss	**Causes**
Diffuse non-scarring	Male pattern/androgenetic, hypothyroid, hypopituitary, hypoadrenal, drug induced, iron deficiency, telogen and anagen effluvium, diffuse alopecia areata
Localized/non-scarring	Alopecia areata, ringworm, traumatic, hair pulling, traction, secondary syphilis
Localized/diffuse scarring	Burns, radiation, shingles, kerion, tertiary syphilis, lupus erythematosus, morphoea, pseudopelade, lichen planus

women. In men, bitemporal recession followed by a bald crown is the usual pattern (Fig. 1); women may show this but more commonly exhibit a diffuse thinning. Mostly, no treatment is required but, if indicated, topical minoxidil (Regaine) produces some response in a third of cases, and finasteride can help.

Endocrine and nutrition related

Endocrine disorders often present with hair loss. Underactivity of the thyroid, pituitary or adrenals can cause diffuse alopecia, as may hyperthyroidism. Androgen-secreting tumours in women produce male pattern baldness with virilization. Malnutrition induces dry brittle hair that becomes pale or red in kwashiorkor (protein deficiency). Diffuse hair loss is also seen with iron or zinc deficiency.

Telogen effluvium

Hair follicles are not usually in phase but, if synchronized into the telogen-resting mode, they will be shed in unison about 3 months later. Such an *effluvium* can be a response to high fever, childbirth, surgery, drug reaction or other stress.

Drug induced

Abrupt cessation of growth (*anagen effluvium*) may follow ingestion of a poison such as thallium, but is more commonly drug induced, e.g. with cytotoxics (especially cyclophosphamide), heparin, warfarin, carbimazole, colchicine and vitamin A.

Localized non-scarring

Patchy hair loss results from a variety of causes, as described below.

Alopecia areata

Alopecia areata is a common condition, associated with autoimmune disorders, in which anagen is prematurely arrested. It generally starts in the second or third decade and presents with sharply defined non-inflamed bald patches on

the scalp. Pathognomonic exclamation mark hairs, which taper as they approach the scalp, are seen. The eyebrows and beard can also be affected, and nails may show pitting.

The course is unpredictable: bald patches may enlarge progressively but, for a first attack, regrowth (often initially with white hairs) is usual (Fig. 2). Prepubertal onset, extensive involvement (especially of the posterior scalp) and atopy signal a poor prognosis. Complete scalp alopecia (*totalis*) or loss of all bodily hair (*universalis*) is seen occasionally and, rarely, diffuse scalp alopecia occurs.

Treatment depends on the extent: if localized, spontaneous regrowth is probable, and intralesional steroid (e.g. triamcinolone acetonide) may accelerate this. If extensive, therapy is less successful. Contact immunotherapy by the application of the sensitizer diphencyprone is effective but not widely available. Wigs are often necessary.

Infections

Scalp ringworm infection can result in patchy hair loss and is described below. Secondary syphilis causes a patchy alopecia.

Trauma and traction

Constantly rubbing or pulling the hair can result in its loss. Traction from tight rollers or pulling hair into a bun causes

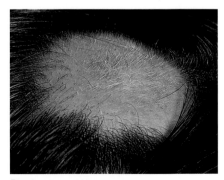

Fig. 2 **Alopecia areata showing some exclamation mark (!) hairs and growth of white hair.**

alopecia at the scalp margins. Hair straightening, bleaching and permanent waving produces a damaged hair shaft that is easily broken.

Localized/diffuse scarring alopecia

In scarring (cicatricial) alopecia, hair follicles are destroyed. This condition can result from:

- *Burns or irradiation*. Chemical or thermal burns will scar the scalp, as may X-irradiation, which was used in the past to induce epilation in the treatment of scalp ringworm.
- *Infection*. Shingles of the first trigeminal dermatome (p. 52), kerion (see below) and tertiary syphilis may leave a scarred scalp.
- *Lichen planus/lupus erythematosus*. Scarring alopecia, with erythema, scaling and follicular changes, is seen when these conditions affect the scalp (Fig. 3). Lesions may exist elsewhere. Topical or intralesional steroids or systemic therapies are prescribed.
- *Pseudopelade*. Pseudopelade describes a scarring alopecia, which represents the endstage of an idiopathic or unidentified destructive inflammatory process in the scalp.

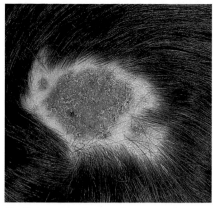

Fig. 3 **Scarring alopecia due to discoid lupus erythematosus, which involves the scalp with erythema and scaling.**

Excess hair (Hirsutism and Hypertrichosis)

Hirsutism is the growth of terminal hair in a male pattern in a female. *Hypertrichosis* is excessive terminal hair growth in a non-androgenic distribution. Often, hirsutism is racial or idiopathic and represents increased end-organ sensitivity to androgens (Table 2). Only a few cases are due to increased androgen secretion, although it is important to identify these. Hypertrichosis is less common and is usually caused by a systemic effect (Table 3).

Idiopathic hirsutism is quite common and presents with hair growth in the beard area, around the nipples and in the male pubic pattern. It frequently causes a lot of anxiety, even if mild. Virilizing features such as cliteromegaly, male pattern baldness and a deep voice must be excluded. In hypertrichosis, fine terminal hair appears on the face, limbs and trunk (Fig. 4). It is mostly drug induced.

Women with a normal menstrual cycle and no signs of virilization are unlikely to have a significant endocrine

Table 2	**Causes of hirsutism**
Type	**Example**
Pituitary	Acromegaly
Adrenal	Cushing syndrome, virilizing tumours, congenital adrenal hyperplasia
Ovarian	Polycystic ovaries, virilizing tumours
Iatrogenic	Androgens, progestogens
Idiopathic	End-organ hypersensitivity to androgens

Table 3	**Causes of hypertrichosis**
Type	**Example**
Localized	Melanocytic naevi, faun tail (associated with spina bifida occulta), chronic scarring or inflammation
Generalized	Malnutrition in children, anorexia nervosa, porphyria cutanea tarda, underlying malignancy, drugs, e.g. minoxidil, phenytoin, ciclosporin

cause for their hirsutism. However, investigation is needed if these symptoms are present.

Treatment is often unsatisfactory. Electrolysis is time consuming for large areas. Waxing, shaving and bleaching are other approaches. Laser hair

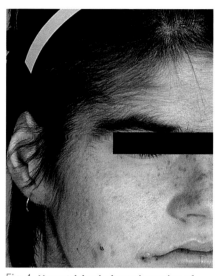

Fig. 4 **Hypertrichosis due to ingestion of minoxidil.**

removal is now widely available. Treatment with an antiandrogen (cyproterone acetate), usually with ethinylestradiol, is occasionally helpful. Eflornithine cream is effective for facial hair. The onset of hypertrichosis requires investigation to find the underlying cause.

Other disorders

Hair shaft defects are rare, usually inherited, conditions of the hair shaft (e.g. monilethrix) that result in broken hairs that are brittle, beaded and look abnormal.

Dandruff is an exaggerated physiological exfoliation of fine scales from an otherwise normal scalp. More severe forms merge with seborrhoeic dermatitis of the scalp (p. 36). Psoriasis (p. 31) produces scaling and may give localized alopecia.

Tinea capitis usually affects children. Common causative organisms and recommended treatments are shown on page 56. Anthropophilic species cause defined scaly areas with slight inflammation and alopecia with broken hair shafts. Zoophilic infection with *Trichophyton verrucosum* produces an inflamed boggy, pustular swelling known as a kerion (p. 110). Scarring may result. Infection with *T. schoenleinii* causes favus – a chronic crusted scarring alopecia.

> ### Common hair disorders
>
> - **Male pattern baldness:** the commonest cause of hair loss; if treatment is required, topical minoxidil or oral finasteride may help.
> - **Alopecia areata:** common; discrete bald patches may show exclamation mark (!) hairs. Early cases recover spontaneously.
> - **Scarring alopecia:** needs investigation to establish the underlying cause.
> - **Hirsutism:** often 'idiopathic' but investigation for androgen secretion is indicated if there are irregular menstrual periods or signs of virilization.

http://www.keratin.com/ ■ http://hirsutism.homestead.com/

Disorders of nails

Congenital disease

A number of usually rare congenital conditions can affect the nails. In the *nail–patella syndrome*, the nails (and patellae) are absent or rudimentary. The nails in *pachyonychia congenita* are thickened and discoloured from birth. Nail dystrophy is a feature of *dystrophic epidermolysis bullosa* (p. 88). *Racket nails*, characterized by a broad short thumbnail, is the commonest congenital nail defect. It is dominantly inherited and more common in women.

Trauma

Trauma, especially from sport, commonly causes nail abnormalities. *Subungual haematomas* usually occur when a fingernail has been trapped or a toenail stood on or stubbed, but the possibility of a subungual malignant melanoma must always be considered. *Splinter haemorrhages* are induced by trauma, although they also occur with infective endocarditis. Ill-fitting shoes contribute to *ingrowing toenails*, and chronic trauma predisposes to *onychogryphosis* – in which the big toenails become thickened and grow like a horn. Trauma may also induce onycholysis (separation of the nail from the nail bed). Constant picking of the thumbnail will produce *a habit-tic dystrophy* with transverse ridges and grooves. *Brittle nails* are a common complaint, usually due to repeated exposure to detergents and water, although iron deficiency, hypothyroidism and digital ischaemia are other causes.

Dermatoses

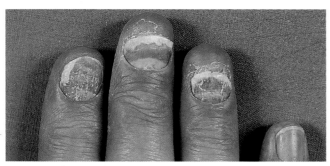

Fig. 1 **Psoriasis of the nails.** Pitting, onycholysis and brownish discoloration are apparent.

Table 1 **Nail involvement in common dermatoses**

Dermatosis	Nail changes
Alopecia areata	Fine pitting, roughness of nail surface
Darier's disease	Longitudinal ridges, triangular nicks at distal nail edge
Eczema	Coarse pitting, transverse ridging, dystrophy, shiny nails due to rubbing
Lichen planus	Thinned nail plate, longitudinal grooves, adhesion between distal nail fold and nail bed (pterygium), complete nail loss
Psoriasis	Pitting, nail thickening, onycholysis (separation of nail from nail bed), brown discoloration, subungual hyperkeratosis

The nails are commonly involved in skin disease (Figs 1 and 2), and are routinely assessed in a dermatological examination. Details are given in Table 1, and a differential diagnosis of the changes is shown in Table 2. Treatment is aimed at the associated dermatosis; care of the hands (p. 36) is especially important.

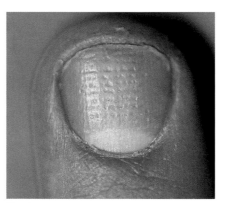

Fig. 2 **Alopecia areata.** Thimble pitting of the nail is seen.

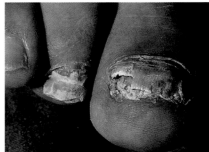

Fig. 3 **Fungal infection of toenails.** The nails are thickened, crumbly and discoloured. An adjacent nail is not affected. Dermatophytes, *C. albicans* and, occasionally, moulds such as *Fusarium* or *Scopulariopsis brevicaulis* are causative.

Infections

Bacterial or fungal infection may involve the nail fold (paronychia) or the nail itself.

Onychomycosis (tinea unguium)

Fungal infection of the nails (onychomycosis) increases with age – children are seldom affected. Toenails, especially the big toenails (Fig. 3), are involved more than fingernails. The process usually begins at the distal nail edge and extends proximally to involve the whole nail. The nail separates from the nail bed (onycholysis), the nail plate becomes thickened crumbly and yellow, and subungual hyperkeratosis occurs. Several – but almost never all – the toenails may be involved. Tinea pedis often coexists and, if the fingernails are diseased, *Trichophyton rubrum* infection of the hand is usually seen. Treatment is with oral terbinafine (Lamisil) or itraconazole (Sporanox).

Chronic paronychia

Chronic paronychia of the fingernails due to *Candida albicans* is often seen in wet workers. The cuticle is lost, the proximal nail fold becomes boggy and swollen (Fig. 4), and light pressure may extrude pus. The nail plate becomes irregular and discoloured. Gram-negative bacteria may be co-pathogens and turn the nail a blue–green colour. Management is directed towards keeping the hands dry, applying an imidazole lotion or cream to the nail fold twice daily, or oral itraconazole for 14 days.

Acute paronychia

Acute paronychia is usually bacterial, and staphylococci are often the cause. Oral flucloxacillin or erythromycin is required.

Table 2 Differential diagnosis of nail changes in dermatoses and systemic disease

Change	Description of nail	Differential diagnosis
Beau's lines	Transverse grooves	Any severe systemic illness that affects growth of the nail matrix
Brittle nails	Nails break easily, usually at distal margin	Effect of water and detergent, iron deficiency, hypothyroidism, digital ischaemia
Colour change	Black transverse bands	Cytotoxic drugs
	Blue	Cyanosis, antimalarials, haematoma
	Blue–green	*Pseudomonas* infection
	Brown	Fungal infection, stain from cigarette smoke, chlorpromazine, gold, Addison's disease
	Brown 'oil stain' patches	Psoriasis
	Brown longitudinal streak	Melanocytic naevus, malignant melanoma, Addison's disease, racial variant
	Red streaks ('splinter haemorrhages')	Infective endocarditis, trauma
	White spots	Trauma to nail matrix (not calcium deficiency)
	White transverse bands	Heavy metal poisoning
	White/brown 'half and half' nails	Chronic renal failure
	White (leuconychia)	Hypoalbuminaemia (e.g. associated with cirrhosis)
	Yellow	Psoriasis, fungal infection, jaundice, tetracycline
	Yellow nail syndrome (Fig. 5)	Defective lymphatic drainage – pleural effusions may occur
Clubbing	Loss of angle between nail fold and nail plate, bulbous finger tip, nail matrix feels spongy	*Respiratory*: bronchial carcinoma, chronic infection, fibrosing alveolitis, asbestosis *Cardiac*: infective endocarditis, congenital cyanotic defects *Other*: Inflammatory bowel disease, thyrotoxicosis, biliary cirrhosis, congenital
Koilonychia	Spoon-shaped depression of nail plate	Iron deficiency anaemia; also lichen planus and repeated exposure to detergents
Nail fold telangiectasia	Dilated capillaries and erythema at nail fold	Connective tissue disorders including systemic sclerosis, systemic lupus erythematosus, dermatomyositis
Onycholysis	Separation of nail from nail bed	Psoriasis, fungal infection, trauma, thyrotoxicosis, tetracyclines (*photo-onycholysis*)
Pitting	Fine or coarse pits may be seen in nail bed	Psoriasis, eczema, alopecia areata, lichen planus
Ridging	Transverse (across nail)	Beau's lines (see above), eczema, psoriasis, tic-dystrophy, chronic paronychia
	Longitudinal (up/down)	Lichen planus, Darier's disease

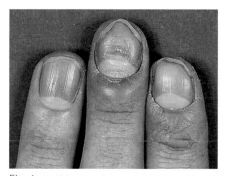

Fig. 4 **C. albicans is the commonest pathogen in chronic paronychia.** The nail fold is inflamed and swollen, and the nail is ridged transversely.

Systemic disease

Nail changes not infrequently indicate an underlying internal medical disorder. Table 2 shows some systemic associations.

Tumours

Tumours of the nail and nail bed are rare, but it is not uncommon to see benign tumours around the nail fold. Examples of both include:

- *Viral warts*. Periungual warts are common. Treatment is similar to that for warts elsewhere (p. 51).
- *Periungual fibromas*. These are seen in patients with tuberous sclerosis (p. 90) and appear at or after puberty.
- *Myxoid (mucous) cysts*. The cysts appear adjacent to the proximal nail fold, usually on the fingers. They are fluctuant, semitranslucent papules that contain a clear gel and may arise from folds of synovium. Treatment is by cryotherapy, injection with triamcinolone acetonide (a steroid) or excision.
- *Malignant melanoma*. A subungual malignant melanoma should be excluded by biopsy if a pigmented longitudinal streak appears and progresses in a nail. An acral malignant melanoma may be amelanotic and can resemble a pyogenic granuloma or even chronic paronychia. Any atypical or ulcerating lesion around the nail fold requires a biopsy to exclude a malignant melanoma.

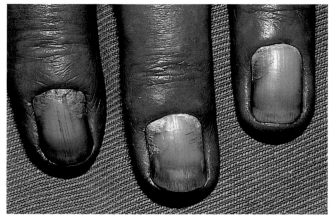

Fig. 5 **Yellow nail syndrome.** The nails grow very slowly, lymphatic drainage is abnormal, and pleural effusions may occur.

Disorders of nails

- **Congenital nail problems** are uncommon except for racket nails.
- **Sports trauma** often results in subungual haematoma, onychogryphosis or onycholysis.
- **Common dermatoses,** e.g. psoriasis, lichen planus and eczema, have distinctive nail changes.
- **Fungal infection** of the big toenails is common, especially in the elderly. Oral terbinafine or itraconazole are prescribed if needed.
- **Chronic paronychia** of fingernails is due to *C. albicans*. Improved skin care, topical imidazole or oral itraconazole are suggested.
- **Acute paronychia** is usually bacterial: antibiotics are given.
- **Systemic diseases** may cause nail changes that help in diagnosis.
- **Malignant melanoma** of the nail bed must be considered with any subungual pigmentation or nail destruction.

http://www.fortunecity.com/marina/victory/11/nail.htm ■ http://www.hooked-on-nails.com/naildisorders.html

Vascular and lymphatic diseases

Blood vessel disorders

Erythema

Erythema is redness of the skin, usually due to vasodilatation (Table 1). It may be localized, e.g. with pregnancy or liver disease (on palms), fixed drug eruption and infection (e.g. Lyme disease), or generalized, as with drug eruption, toxic erythema (e.g. viral exanthem) and connective tissue disease.

Flushing

Flushing is erythema due to vasodilatation. The causes are:

- physiological (autonomic response to emotion, heat or exercise)
- menopause (hormonal; often with associated sweating)
- foods (e.g. spices (gustatory), alcohol (aldehyde related))
- drugs (angiotensin-converting enzyme (ACE) inhibitors, 5-hydroxytryptamine (HT_3) antagonists, nifedipine)
- rosacea (mechanism unknown)
- carcinoid syndrome (serotonin (5-HT))
- phaeochromocytoma (catecholamine).

Flushing is common and affects the face, neck and upper trunk. It is usually benign. A sudden onset and systemic symptoms (e.g. diarrhoea or fainting) mean that carcinoid syndrome or phaeochromocytoma must be excluded. In treatment, first remove the cause, e.g. spices or alcohol. Embarrassing physiological flushing may improve with a small dose of propranolol.

Telangiectasia

Telangiectasia is a visible dilatation of dermal venules or, in spider naevi (Fig. 1), an arteriole. It results from:

Table 1 **Classification of blood vessel and lymphatic disorders**		
Vessel	**Process**	**Resulting lesion**
Small blood vessels	Dilatation (and/or increased flow)	Erythema, flushing, telangiectasia
	Release of extracellular fluid	Urticaria (p. 74), oedema
	Release of blood	Purpura, capillaritis
	Reduced flow	Livedo reticularis, chilblains, Raynaud's phenomenon
	Inflammation damage	Vasculitis, erythema ab igne
Arteries	Atherosclerosis, Buerger's disease	Ischaemia and ulceration
	Inflammation	Vasculitis (p. 80)
Veins	Inflammation, flow reduction, clotting abnormalities	Thrombosis, skin changes, ulceration (p. 70)
	Dilatation	Venous lake
Lymphatics	Congenital hypoplasia	Lymphoedema (primary)
	Blockage or inflammation	Lymphoedema (secondary)
	Infection	Lymphangitis

- *congenital* (e.g. hereditary haemorrhagic telangiectasia)
- *skin atrophy* (topical steroids, ageing skin, radiation dermatitis)
- *excess oestrogen* (e.g. liver disease, pregnancy, 'the pill')
- *connective tissue disease* (systemic sclerosis, lupus erythematosus, dermatomyositis)
- *rosacea* (on the face)
- *venous disease* (lower leg).

Isolated spider naevi are common and of little significance, but their number may increase with pregnancy and liver disease. A venous lake – acquired venous ectasia – is often seen on the lower lip of the elderly. Telangiectasia is treated by fine needle cautery, hyfrecation or laser (p. 109).

Purpura

Purpura is a blue–brown discoloration of the skin due to the extravasation of erythrocytes (Fig. 2). It results from a variety of mechanisms:

- *Vessel wall defects*
  –vasculitis (e.g. due to immune complexes), paraproteinaemia (e.g. cryoglobulinaemia)
  –infection (e.g. meningococcaemia)
  –raised vascular pressure (e.g. venous disease).

- *Defective dermal support*
  –dermal atrophy (ageing, steroids, disease, e.g. lichen sclerosus)
  –scurvy (vitamin C deficiency).
- *Clotting defects*
  –coagulation factor deficiency (e.g. disseminated intravascular coagulation) or inherited
  –anticoagulant (heparin, warfarin)
  –thrombocytopenia of any cause
  –abnormal platelet function.
- *Idiopathic pigmented purpuras.*

Petechiae are small dot-like purpura, whereas ecchymoses are more extensive. Purpura is often seen in the elderly or those on steroids, and develops spontaneously or after minor trauma. Idiopathic pigmented purpura is seen as brownish punctate lesions (capillaritis) on the legs.

Mostly, there is no specific therapy. Underlying causes, e.g. blood disorders or vasculitis, are treated as necessary.

Raynaud's phenomenon

Raynaud's phenomenon is characterized by a paroxysmal vasoconstriction of the digital arteries, usually provoked by cold, in which the fingers turn white (due to ischaemia), cyanotic blue (due to capillary dilatation with a stagnant blood flow) and then red (due to reactive hyperaemia). When no cause is found, it is known as 'Raynaud's disease'. Causes include:

- *arterial occlusion*: atherosclerosis, Buerger's disease
- *connective tissue disease*: systemic sclerosis (including CREST syndrome), systemic lupus erythematosus (p. 79)
- *hyperviscosity syndrome*: polycythaemia, cryoglobulinaemia
- *neurological defects*: syringomyelia, peripheral neuropathy

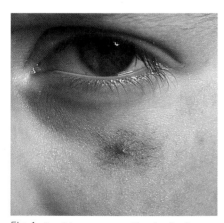

Fig. 1 **A spider naevus on the cheek of a child.**

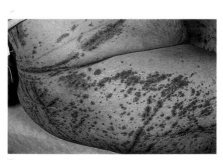

Fig. 2 **Purpura in a patient with thrombocytopenia.**

- *reflux vasoconstriction*: with use of vibration tools (p. 120)
- *toxins/drugs*: ergot, vinyl chloride, beta-blockers.

Raynaud's phenomenon mostly affects women. It may be the forerunner of a connective tissue disease. The hands should be kept warm and protected from the cold. Smoking must be stopped. A calcium channel blocker (e.g. nifedipine) or naftidrofuryl may help. In resistant cases, prostacyclin infusions are given.

Livedo reticularis

Livedo reticularis is a marble-patterned cyanosis of the skin, due to reduced arteriole blood flow, usually in women. The condition has the following causes:

- *physiological*, i.e. cold induced
- *vasculitis* due to connective tissue disease, e.g. systemic lupus erythematosus and polyarteritis nodosa
- *hyperviscosity* due to cryoglobulinaemia, polycythaemia
- *Sneddon syndrome*, which consists of livedo vasculitis with cerebrovascular disease and circulating antiphospholipid antibodies.

Cold-induced livedo reticularis gives a mottled meshwork pattern on the

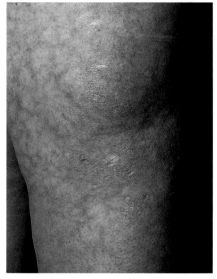

Fig. 3 **Livedo reticularis.** In this case, the condition was associated with systemic lupus erythematosus.

outer thighs of children and is reversible. Fixed livedo (Fig. 3) is due to vasculitis and requires investigation. Treatment is aimed at the underlying disease.

Erythema ab igne

Erythema ab igne is a reticulate pigmented erythema (Fig. 4) due to heat-induced damage. It is seen on the shins of elderly folk who sit before an open fire, or with the use of heat pads.

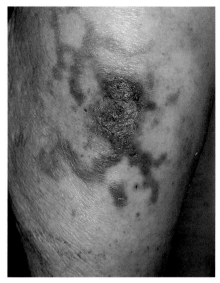

Fig. 4 **Erythema ab igne on the upper outer shin from sitting in front of a fire.**

Chilblains

Chilblains are inflamed and painful purple–pink swellings on the fingers, toes or ears that appear in response to cold. Chilblains result from an overcompensatory cold-induced vasoconstriction of cutaneous arterioles and venules. They occur in the winter and usually affect women. Warm housing and clothing are advised. Oral nifedipine may help.

Lymphatic disorders

Lymphoedema

Lymphoedema is oedema, often of a limb, due to inadequate lymphatic drainage. The condition may be primary or secondary. Primary lymphoedema is the result of a congenital developmental defect. Secondary causes include:

- *recurrent infection* – lymphangitis
- *blockage* – filariasis, tumour
- *destruction* – surgery, radiation.

Primary lymphoedema presents in adolescence and may follow infection. The lower legs are commonly affected. In chronic lymphoedema, the oedema is non-pitting and fibrotic, and the overlying epidermis hyperkeratotic (Fig. 5). Lymphangiography or radiolabelled lymphoscintigraphy shows the defect.

A lymphoedematous limb is at risk of repeated infection (particularly erysipelas), and long-term prophylaxis with oral phenoxymethylpenicillin is recommended. Exercise, compression support and massage can help. Surgical reconstruction is rarely possible.

Lymphangitis

Lymphangitis is defined as infection of the lymphatic vessels, usually due to streptococci. It presents as a tender red line extending proximally up a limb, usually from a focus of infection. Hospital admission is usually necessary. Therapy is with a suitable intravenous antibiotic (e.g. benzylpenicillin).

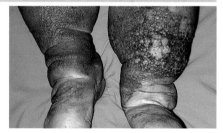

Fig. 5 **Chronic lymphoedema of the legs with papillomatosis.**

Vascular and lymphatic diseases

- **Erythema:** can be localized, e.g. liver palms, or generalized, e.g. toxic erythema.
- **Flushing:** usually emotional; rarely carcinoid syndrome or phaeochromocytoma.
- **Telangiectasia:** commonly seen with skin atrophy, but lesions can occur with oestrogen excess or connective tissue disease. Treatment is by hyfrecation or laser.
- **Purpura:** caused by defects of the vessel wall, supporting dermis or clotting mechanism, or 'idiopathic'. Treat the underlying disorder.
- **Livedo reticularis:** physiological or due to underlying hyperviscosity or connective tissue disorder.
- **Chilblains:** describes cold-induced perniosis of the fingers, toes and ears.
- **Raynaud's phenomenon:** vasoconstriction of the digital arteries with colour changes.
- **Lymphoedema:** results from absence of or damage to lymphatics. Long-term prophylaxis with antibiotics prevents recurrent infection in chronic cases.

Leg ulcers

Leg ulcers affect 1% of the adult population and account for 1% of dermatology referrals. They are twice as common in women as in men and are a major burden on the health service. One half is venous, a tenth arterial and a quarter 'mixed' – due to venous *and* arterial disease. The remainder are due to rare causes.

Venous disease

Damage to the venous system of the leg results in pigment change, eczema, oedema, fibrosis and ulceration.

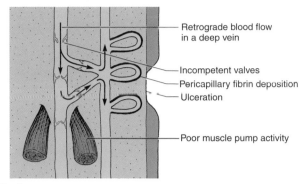

Fig. 1 **The aetiopathogenesis of venous ulceration.**

Aetiopathogenesis
The superficial low-pressure venous system of the leg is connected to the deep higher pressure veins by perforating veins. Blood flow relies on the pumping action of surrounding muscles and the integrity of valves. Valve incompetence, occasionally congenital but usually due to damage by thrombosis or infection, results in a rise in capillary hydrostatic pressure and permeability (Fig. 1). Fibrin is deposited as a pericapillary cuff, interfering with diffusion of nutrients and resulting in disease.

Clinical presentation
Venous disease usually starts in middle age and continues into later life. It is commoner in women and is predisposed to by obesity and venous thrombosis. Varicose veins are often present, but are not essential. The syndrome progresses through stages:

- *Heaviness and oedema*: early symptoms. The legs feel heavy and swell.
- *Discoloration*: brown haemosiderin deposits from extravasated red cells. Telangiectasia and white lacy scars (atrophie blanche) occur at the ankle (Fig. 2).
- *Eczema*: commonly occurs (p. 36), often complicated by allergic or irritant contact dermatitis.
- *Lipodermatosclerosis*: fibrosis of the dermis and subcutis around the ankle results in firm induration.
- *Ulceration*: often follows minor trauma, and typically affects the medial and, to a lesser extent, the lateral malleolus (Fig. 3). Neglected ulcers enlarge and may encircle the lower leg. Initially, venous ulcers are exudative but, under favourable conditions, they granulate and enter a healing phase in which the epidermis grows in from the sides

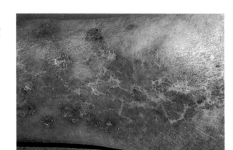

Fig. 2 **Atrophie blanche with white lace-like scarring and haemosiderin deposition.**

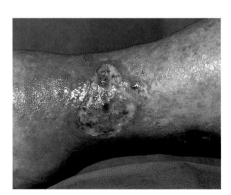

Fig. 3 **A venous ulcer at the lateral malleolus.**

and from small epithelial islands in the middle. Healing is invariably slow, often taking months. Some large ulcers never heal.
- *Post-ulcer leg*: fibrosis may lead to a slender sclerosed ankle.

Differential diagnosis and complications
Venous ulcers can be differentiated from other ulcers (Table 1) by history, position and additional signs. Arterial ulcers are deep, painful and gangrenous, and situated on the foot or mid-shin. Complications of venous ulcers are common and include:

Table 1 **Causes of leg ulceration**	
Division	**Condition**
Venous disease	Damaged valves (e.g. deep vein thrombosis), clotting disorder, congenital valve incompetence
Arterial disease	Atherosclerosis, Buerger's disease, polyarteritis nodosa
Small vessel disease	Diabetes mellitus, rheumatoid arthritis, vasculitis, sickle cell disease, hypertension
Infection	Tuberculosis, Buruli ulcer (p. 48), mycetoma (p. 58), syphilis (p. 116)
Neuropathy	Diabetes mellitus, leprosy, syphilis, syringomyelia
Neoplasia	Squamous cell carcinoma, Kaposi's sarcoma, malignant melanoma
Trauma	Direct injury, artefact
Unknown	Pyoderma gangrenosum (p. 87), necrobiosis lipoidica (p. 82)

- *Infections*. Bacteria invariably colonize ulcers. Systemic antibiotics are needed only for overt infection, as suggested by a purulent discharge, a rapidly advancing ulcer edge, cellulitis or septicaemia.
- *Lymphoedema*. Lymphatic drainage is impaired in legs with chronic venous ulcers, adding to the oedema.
- *Contact dermatitis*. Contact sensitivity to topical medicaments and bandages frequently develops, especially to lanolin, neomycin, rubber chemicals and preservatives. Allergic contact dermatitis can resemble an exacerbation of venous eczema and is suspected if there is generalized secondary spread. Some local therapies, and the ulcer exudate itself, are irritant.
- *Malignant change*. Rarely, squamous cell carcinoma develops in an ulcer.

Management
Treatment of a leg ulcer is long term and progress usually slow. The initial

Table 2   Topical therapy for venous ulcers

Type of wound	Role of dressing	Examples of dressing	Qualities of dressing
Dry, necrotic, black, yellow, sloughy	Moisture retention or rehydration, especially if dry; if moist, fluid absorption; removal of excess slough; possibly absorption of odour; possibly antimicrobial activity; infrequent changes so as not to disturb wound	Irrigation fluid, e.g physiological saline Hydrocolloid, e.g. Comfeel Granuflex, DuoDERM Extra Thin or Aquacel Odour-absorbing dressing, e.g. Actisorb Silver 200 Larval therapy may be considered in suitable cases (see p. 110)	Use of irritant cleansers may be harmful; debris and dressing remnants can be removed with saline irrigation Absorbent layer on vapour-permeable film. Occlusive; facilitates rehydration/autolytic debridement of dry slough or necrotic wounds; promote granulation; change daily or less Absorb odour; may bind bacteria; change daily or less frequently as dictated by clinical response
Clean, exudating, granulating	Fluid absorption; thermal insulation to give optimal temperature for healing; possibly odour absorption; possibly antimicrobial activity; optimal pH for wound healing	Alginate, e.g. Kaltostat, Sorbsan or SeaSorb Foam, e.g. Allevyn or Lyofoam Extra Low adherent tulle, e.g. Paratulle or Unitulle	Highly absorbent; suitable for moderate/heavily exudating wounds; not for dry wound or eschar; change daily or less Suitable for exudative wound; useful for overgranulation resulting from occlusive dressing; used as secondary dressing Used as interface layer under a secondary absorbent dressing; medicated tulle dressings are not generally recommended
Dry, low exudate, epithelializing	Moisture retention or rehydration; low adherence; thermal insulation	Hydrogel, e.g. Aquaform, Intrasite or Iodosorb	Amorphous cohesive material; takes shape of wound; needs secondary dressing; moisturizes/debrides dry wound

examination includes palpation of peripheral pulses and an assessment of contributing factors such as obesity, anaemia, cardiac failure and arthritis. Doppler studies, to exclude coexisting arterial disease, are essential when compression bandaging is proposed. Treatments are as follows:

- *Compression bandages*. These reduce oedema and promote venous return. Bandages are applied from the toes to the knee. Self-adhesive bandages (e.g. Coban) are preferred, and are left on for 2–7 days. A four-layer bandage technique uses a layer of orthopaedic wool (e.g. Softexe), a standard crepe (e.g. Setocrepe), an elasticated bandage (e.g. Elset) and an elasticated cohesive bandage (e.g. Coban). Arterial disease precludes compression bandaging. Once an ulcer has healed, a toe-to-knee compression stocking maintains venous return.
- *Elevation, exercise and diet*. Some doctors recommend rest with leg elevation. Walking is encouraged, as is dieting for obese individuals and ankle exercises to maintain joint mobility.
- *Topical therapy*. Table 2 shows what to use and when to use it. Venous eczema is treated with a mild to moderate potency steroid or an emollient.
- *Oral therapy*. Adequate analgesia is vital. Diuretics are given for cardiac oedema, and antibiotics for overt infection. An anabolic steroid, stanozolol (Stromba), may help lipodermatosclerosis, but side-effects (fluid retention, jaundice) limit its use. Oxerutins (Paroven) reduce capillary permeability, relieving oedema.

- *Surgery*. Vein surgery may prevent problems in younger patients, but is rarely applicable in the elderly. Split skin grafts or pinch grafts (from the thigh) are of limited use. However, experimental culturing of keratinocytes in a 'skin equivalent', to use as a graft, is promising and gives rapid pain relief (p. 110).

Arterial disease

Lower leg ischaemia and ulceration can result from arterial disease. Ischaemia presents with claudication, coldness of the foot, loss of hair, toenail dystrophy and dusky cyanosis. Deep, sharply defined ulcers occur on the foot or mid-shin (Fig. 4). Pulses in the legs are absent or reduced. Buerger's disease, seen in young male smokers, is a severe form of arterial disease.

Doppler studies and contrast angiography define the arterial lesions, which may be amenable to vascular reconstruction or angioplasty. Compression bandaging is contraindicated.

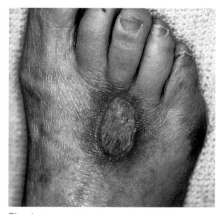

Fig. 4   **An arterial ulcer on the dorsal aspect of the foot.**

Other causes of leg ulceration

Vasculitic ulcers start as purpura, but become necrotic and punched out (Table 1). *Neuropathic ulcers* occur on the feet (Fig. 5) and are due to neurological disease. *Buruli ulcer* and deep mycoses are important in the tropics.

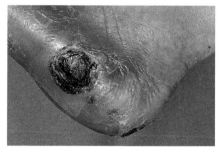

Fig. 5   **A necrotic neuropathic ulcer on the side of the foot.**

Leg ulcers

Venous ulcers
- Result from venous hypertension.
- Show associated skin discoloration, eczema and fibrosis.
- Occur at the medial or lateral malleolus.
- Require compression bandaging after checking Doppler pressures.
- May coexist with arterial disease.
- May be complicated by contact allergy.

Arterial ulcers
- Are associated with other symptoms and signs of leg ischaemia.
- Occur on the foot or mid-shin.
- Are usually deep and painful.
- Prohibit compression bandaging.

Other causes
- Vasculitis, trauma to a neuropathic limb and some types of infection can also cause leg ulceration.

http://www.legulcers.co.uk/   ■   http://www.sign.ac.uk/pdf/sign26.pdf

Pigmentation

Skin colour is due to a mixture of the pigments melanin (p. 8), oxyhaemoglobin (in blood) and carotene (in the stratum corneum and subcutaneous fat). Pigmentary diseases are common and particularly distressing to those with darker skin. Disorders of pigmentation mainly involve melanocytes, but other causes are mentioned where relevant.

Hypopigmentation

Pigment loss may be generalized or patchy. Generalized hypopigmentation occurs with albinism, phenylketonuria and hypopituitarism; patchy loss is seen in vitiligo, after inflammation, following exposure to some chemicals and with certain infections (Table 1).

Vitiligo

Vitiligo is an acquired idiopathic disorder showing white non-scaly macules. The association with pernicious anaemia, thyroid disease and Addison's disease suggests an autoimmune aetiology in some cases. About 30% of patients give a family history of the disorder. Melanocytes are absent from affected skin on histology.

Clinical presentation

Vitiligo affects 1% of the population, is seen in all races and is most troublesome in those with a dark skin. The sex incidence is equal, and the onset, usually between 10 and 30 years of age, may be precipitated by injury or sunburn. The sharply defined white macules are often symmetrical (Fig. 1). The hands, wrists, knees, neck and areas around orifices (e.g. the mouth) are frequently affected. Occasionally, vitiligo is segmental (e.g. down an arm), generalized or universal. The course is unpredictable; areas may remain static, spread or (infrequently) repigment. In light-skinned individuals, vitiligo may only be discernible in summer, when the non-vitiliginous areas become sun-tanned.

Differential diagnosis

Post-inflammatory hypopigmentation is often accompanied by other skin changes (Table 1). In chemical leucoderma, a history of exposure to phenolic chemicals should be sought. The hypopigmented macules of leprosy are normally anaesthetic.

Management

Treatment is unsatisfactory. Camouflage cosmetics require patience and skill to apply. Sunscreens help the lightly pigmented patient by reducing the tanning and contrast of the non-vitiligo areas. In patients with a darker skin, potent topical steroids occasionally induce repigmentation. Ultraviolet (UV)B, psoralen with UVA (PUVA) or the use of oral psoralens and natural UV radiation sometimes helps, although it may take months. Rarely, depigmentation using monobenzyl ether of hydroquinone is considered when vitiligo is near universal and other treatments have failed.

Albinism

Albinism is an autosomal recessive condition in which the melanocytes fail to synthesize pigment in the epidermis, hair bulb and eye.

There are several syndromes of albinism. All are autosomal recessive and show a lack of pigment in the skin, hair, iris and retina. Melanocyte numbers are normal, but melanosome production fails due to defective gene control of tyrosinase (p. 8).

Albinism is uncommon (the prevalence is 1/20 000), although the diagnosis is straightforward. The skin is white or pink, the hair white, and pigmentation is lacking in the eye (Fig. 2). Albinos have poor sight, photophobia and nystagmus. 'Tyrosinase-positive' albinos may pigment slightly with age, so that African skin becomes yellow and freckled. In the tropics, albinos risk premature skin photoageing and the early onset of skin tumours, especially squamous cell carcinomas.

Strict sun avoidance from childhood is essential. Opaque clothing, a wide-brimmed hat and sunscreens are needed. Prenatal diagnosis is possible.

Phenylketonuria

Phenylketonuria is an autosomal recessive inborn error of metabolism. Phenylalanine hydroxylase, which converts phenylalanine into tyrosine, is deficient. Phenylalanine and metabolites accumulate and damage the developing neonatal brain. The prevalence is 1/10 000 births.

Phenylketonuria is detected after birth by routine screening tests. Untreated, mental retardation and choreoathetosis develop. Patients have fair hair and skin, due to impaired melanin synthesis. Atopic eczema is common. A low phenylalanine diet, given early, prevents neurological damage.

Table 1 **Causes of hypopigmentation**	
Cause	**Example**
Chemical	Substituted phenols, hydroquinone
Endocrine	Hypopituitarism
Genetic	Albinism, phenylketonuria, tuberous sclerosis, piebaldism
Infection	Leprosy, yaws, pityriasis versicolor
Post-inflammatory	Cryotherapy, eczema, psoriasis, morphoea, pityriasis alba
Other	Vitiligo, lichen sclerosus, halo naevus, scarring

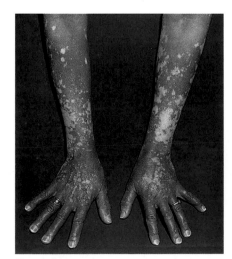

Fig. 1 **Vitiligo.** In this case, there is symmetrical involvement of the forearms in a patient with pigmented skin.

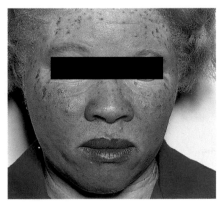

Fig. 2 **Albinism in an Afro-Caribbean patient.**

Hyperpigmentation

Hyperpigmentation is mostly hypermelanosis (Table 2), but sometimes other pigments colour the skin, e.g. iron deposition (with melanin) in haemochromatosis, and carotene (causing an orange discoloration) in carotenaemia, usually due to eating too many carrots.

Freckles and lentigines

Freckles are small, light-brown macules, typically facial, which darken on sun exposure. Lentigines are also brown macules but are scattered and do not darken in the sun. Freckles have normal basal layer melanocyte numbers but increased melanin. Lentigines have an *increased* number of melanocytes.

Freckles are common, especially in red-haired children. Lentigines may develop in childhood but are more common in sun-exposed elderly skin.

Table 2 Causes of hyperpigmentation

Cause	Example
Drugs	Photosensitizers, psoralens, oestrogens, phenothiazines, minocycline, amiodarone
Endocrine	Addison's disease, Cushing syndrome, Graves' disease
Genetic	Racial, freckles, neurofibromatosis, Peutz–Jeghers syndrome
Metabolic	Biliary cirrhosis, haemochromatosis, porphyria
Nutritional	Carotenaemia, malabsorption, malnutrition, pellagra
Post-inflammatory	Eczema, lichen planus, systemic sclerosis, lichen amyloidosis
Other	Acanthosis nigricans, naevi, malignant melanoma, argyria, chronic renal failure

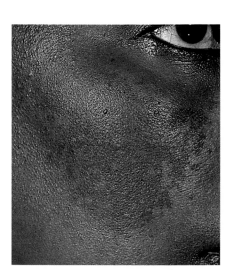

Fig. 3 **Melasma affecting the cheek and causing a cosmetic disability.**

Freckles require no treatment. Lentigines respond to cryotherapy.

Melasma (chloasma)

Melasma is a patterned macular facial pigmentation occurring with pregnancy and in women on oral contraceptives. The pigmentation is symmetrical and often involves the forehead (Fig. 3). Pregnancy stimulates melanocytes generally, and also increases pigmentation of the nipples and lower abdomen and in existing melanocytic naevi. Melasma may improve spontaneously. Topical tretinoin, azelaic acid or hydroquinone can reduce pigmentation. Sunscreens and camouflage cosmetics can help.

Peutz–Jeghers syndrome

Peutz–Jeghers syndrome is a rare autosomal dominant condition. Lentigines around the lips (Fig. 4), buccal mucosa and fingers are associated with small bowel polyps. The polyps may cause intussusception and rarely undergo malignant change.

Addison's disease

Addison's disease is characterized by hypoadrenalism with pituitary overproduction of adrenocorticotrophic hormone (ACTH). The skin signs are due to excess ACTH, which stimulates melanogenesis. Pigmentation may be

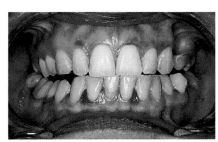

Fig. 4 **The Peutz–Jeghers syndrome showing perioral lentigines.**

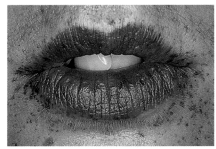

Fig. 5 **Addison's disease, with hyperpigmentation of the gingival and labial mucosa.**

Table 3 Drug-induced pigmentation

Drug	Effect
Amiodarone	Blue–grey pigmentation of exposed areas (p. 85)
Bleomycin	Diffuse pigmentation, often flexural
Busulfan	Diffuse brown pigment
Chloroquine	Blue–grey pigmentation of face and arms
Chlorpromazine	Slatey-grey pigment in sun-exposed sites
Clofazimine	Red and black pigment
Mepracrine	Yellow (drug deposited)
Minocycline	Blue–black pigment in scars and sun-exposed sites
Psoralens	Topical or systemic photosensitizers (cosmetics)

generalized or limited to the buccal mucosa (Fig. 5), palmar creases, scars, flexures or areas subjected to friction. Addisonian-like pigmentation is also seen in Cushing syndrome, hyperthyroidism and acromegaly.

Drug-induced pigmentation

Drug-induced pigmentation may be due to stimulation of melanogenesis or deposition of the drug in the skin, but the mechanism is often not well understood (Table 3, p. 84). Of the commonly used drugs, amiodarone, phenothiazines and minocycline not infrequently induce pigmentation.

Disorders of pigmentation

- **Vitiligo:** common, autoimmune; well-defined depigmented macules.
- **Albinism:** rare, autosomal recessive; lack of skin and eye pigment; need strict sun avoidance; risk of skin cancer.
- **Phenylketonuria:** autosomal recessive enzyme defect; fair skin and hair.
- **Freckles:** brown macules darken with sun; normal number of melanocytes.
- **Lentigines:** brown macules; melanocyte numbers are increased.
- **Peutz–Jeghers syndrome:** autosomal dominant disorder of perioral lentigines and intestinal polyps.
- **Melasma:** facial pigmentation; related to pregnancy and 'the pill'.
- **Addison's disease:** ACTH-stimulated melanogenesis of mucosae and flexures.
- **Drug-induced pigmentation:** due to deposition of pigment or stimulation of melanogenesis.

Urticaria and angioedema

Urticaria (hives) is a common eruption characterized by transient, usually pruritic, wheals due to acute dermal oedema from extravascular leakage of plasma. Angioedema signifies a larger area of oedema involving the dermis and subcutis. A classification is shown in Table 1.

Aetiopathogenesis

Urticaria is mediated through immune (allergic) or non-immune mechanisms. Lesions result from the release from mast cells of biologically active substances, particularly histamine, which produce vasodilatation and increased vascular permeability. Several pathways are recognized:

- *IgE-mediated (type I) hypersensitivity* (p. 11) is the best understood mechanism; antigen cross-links immunoglobulin (Ig)E molecules on the surface of mast cells, resulting in degranulation with release of vasoactive agents.
- *Complement activation* can produce dermal oedema, as in hereditary angioedema or urticaria associated with circulating immune complexes.
- *Direct release of histamine* from mast cells, in a non-immune manner, is caused by some drugs, e.g. opiates and contrast media.
- *Blocking of the prostaglandin pathway* from arachidonic acid, by some drugs such as aspirin and non-steroidal anti-inflammatory agents, promotes urticaria by accumulating vasoactive leukotrienes.
- *A serum histamine-releasing factor* has been suggested in 'chronic' urticaria, with IgG autoantibodies found in 60% of patients, although the mechanisms involved in this and in the physical urticarias are poorly understood.

Pathology

The dermis is oedematous with dilatation of vessels and mast cell degranulation. Vessel damage and a lymphocytic infiltrate may be seen with urticarial vasculitis.

Clinical presentation

Three-quarters of cases of urticaria fall into the 'chronic idiopathic' or acute categories. Another 20% are due to dermographism, cholinergic urticaria or physical factors. Other causes are rare.

Chronic idiopathic urticaria

Itchy pink wheals appear as papules or plaques anywhere on the skin surface (Fig. 1). Typically, they last for less than 24 h and disappear without a trace. Wheals may be round, annular or polycyclic, and vary in diameter from a few millimetres to several centimetres. Their number ranges from a few to many appearing each day, depending on the severity of the condition. Angioedema, usually with swelling of the tongue or lips, may occur (Fig. 2).

Pharmacological agents often act as provoking factors, but normally no underlying cause is found. The condition resolves spontaneously within 6 months in 50% of cases, although a minority are troubled for years.

Acute urticaria

The sudden onset of urticaria or angioedema may be due to an IgE-mediated type I reaction. The patient can often identify the offending allergen. Commonly, it is a food (e.g. egg, fish or peanuts), a drug (e.g. an antibiotic) or contact with latex (p. 121). Sometimes no cause is found.

Physical urticarias

Cold, heat, sun exposure, pressure and even water can all induce urticaria at the stimulated site. Dermographism, found in 5% of normal people, describes whealing induced by firm stroking of the skin (Fig. 3). In a few individuals, it is exaggerated and symptomatic. The wheals in cholinergic urticaria are small intensely itchy papules that appear in response to sweating, as induced by

exercise, heat, emotion or spicy food. The eruption lasts for a few minutes to an hour.

Hereditary angioedema

Hereditary angioedema is a rare and potentially fatal autosomal dominant

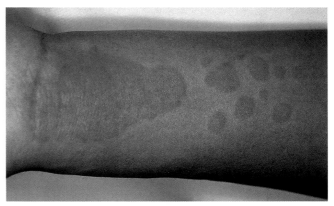

Table 1 **Classification of urticaria and angioedema**	
Group	**Example**
Chronic	Idiopathic (although 60% of patients show IgG autoantibodies)
Acute	IgE mediated, e.g. food allergy, drug reaction, latex
Physical	Dermographism, cholinergic, cold, solar, heat, delayed pressure
Contact	Immune, e.g. animal saliva, or non-immune, e.g. nettle sting
Pharmacological	Aspirin, opiates, non-steroidal drugs, food additives
Systemic cause	Systemic lupus erythematosus, lymphoma, thyrotoxicosis, infection, infestation
Inherited	Hereditary angioedema (C1 esterase inhibitor deficiency)
Other	Urticarial vasculitis, papular (insect bites, p. 60), mastocytosis (p. 112), pregnancy (Fig. 5)

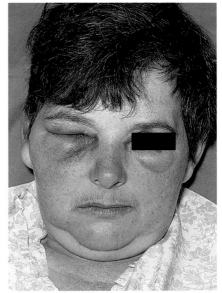

Fig. 1 **Chronic urticaria.** Typical wheals are seen on the forearm.

Fig. 2 **Angioedema involving the face.**

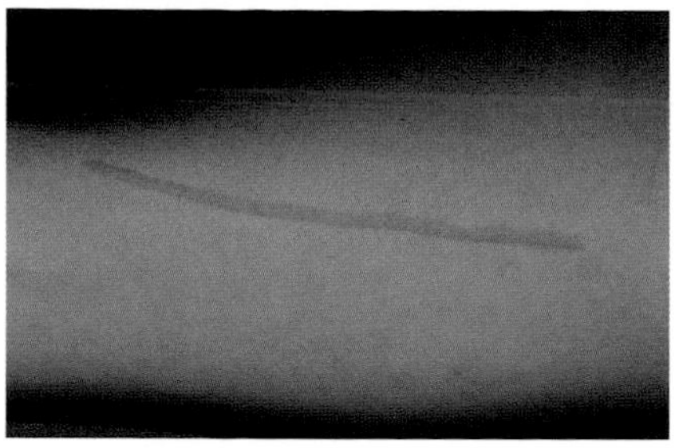

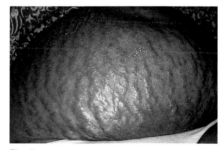

Fig. 3 **Dermographism.** This was induced by stroking the forearm.

condition. It usually presents in childhood, with episodes of angioedema sometimes involving the larynx (producing respiratory obstruction) and the gastrointestinal tract (causing vomiting and abdominal pain). A deficiency of C_1 esterase inhibitor allows complement activation (e.g. caused by trauma) to go unchecked, with an accumulation of vasoactive mediators. Acute attacks are treated with intravenous infusion of C_1 esterase inhibitor concentrate. In the long term, anabolic steroids such as danazol (Danol) are used to promote hepatic synthesis of C_1 esterase inhibitor.

Urticarial vasculitis

Urticarial vasculitis often has an acute onset with widespread urticarial lesions that are unusual as they persist for more than 24 h and fade leaving purpura (Fig. 4). Systemic abnormalities and low complement levels may be found.

Differential diagnosis

Urticaria is usually differentiated from other dermatoses, although pemphigoid (p. 76) or dermatitis herpetiformis (p. 77) occasionally present with an urticarial eruption. Toxic erythema and erythema multiforme (p. 80) may be urticated at first but, when the lesions persist for over 48 h, urticaria can be excluded. Facial erysipelas sometimes resembles angioedema but has a sharper margin and the patient is unwell with a fever.

Investigation

Underlying causes or provoking factors are better revealed by a careful history and examination than by laboratory tests. However, a full blood count, liver function tests, antinuclear antibody test and urinalysis are often done to exclude systemic conditions (Table 1). Dermographism is demonstrated by firmly stroking the skin, and cold urticaria induced by holding an ice cube on the arm for up to 20 min. If congenital angioedema is suspected, the serum C_1 esterase inhibitor level is assayed.

Management

Any underlying cause should be eliminated. Provoking factors, e.g. aspirin ingestion or swimming (for those with cold urticaria), are to be avoided. Desensitization may be possible for some physical urticarias; for example, individuals with cold urticaria can build up tolerance by gradual immersion of progressively more of the body in cold water. However, the mainstay of treatment is with antihistamines.

Antihistamines

Histamine type 1 receptor blockers (H_1 blockers) reduce the wheal size and the severity of the itch and, given regularly, provide relief. The newer, non-sedative antihistamines, such as cetirizine 10 mg daily, fexofenadine (Telfast) 180 mg once daily, desloratadine (Neoclarityn) 5 mg once daily or acrivastine (Semprex) 8 mg three times daily, are now preferred unless the sedative qualities of the older preparations are desired. The addition of an H_2 blocker has only a small summative effect if any.

Corticosteroids

Systemic steroids are very occasionally used to control severe acute urticaria or angioedema and urticarial vasculitis, but are not indicated for chronic urticaria.

Adrenaline (epinephrine)

Acute airways obstruction or anaphylactic shock is treated with adrenaline as an intramuscular injection (500 μg: 0.5 mL of 1/1000), repeated 5 min later if necessary. An antihistamine such as chlorphenamine (Piriton), 10–20 mg given by slow intravenous injection, is a useful adjunct. Intravenous steroids are often given, although their onset of action is delayed by several hours.

Diet

Salicylates in food aggravate chronic urticaria in up to a third of cases, and dietary azo dyes and benzoic acid preservatives produce an exacerbation in 10%. Diets low in these compounds are tried if routine measures are ineffective.

Fig. 5 **An urticated pregnancy-associated eruption.** Often starts in abdominal striae.

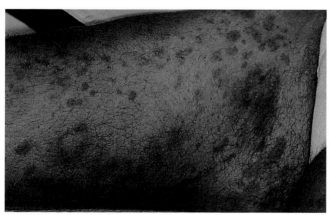

Fig. 4 **Urticarial vasculitis.** Resolving areas have left bruising.

Urticaria

- Urticaria is a common eruption of transient pruritic wheals that typically clear within 1 day.
- Associated dermal oedema is usually the result of mast cell degranulation and the release of vasoactive amines.
- No cause is usually found, but urticaria may result from histamine-releasing IgG autoantibodies, IgE-mediated allergy, physical stimuli, the pharmacological effect of drugs or food additives, or complement deficiencies.
- Causative or provoking factors should be eliminated, and non-sedating antihistamines prescribed.
- Systemic steroids are rarely used in treatment. Aspirin is avoided. Intramuscular adrenaline is given for an anaphylactic reaction.

Blistering disorders

Blistering is often seen with skin disease. It is found with common dermatoses such as acute contact dermatitis, pompholyx, herpes simplex, herpes zoster and bullous impetigo, and it also occurs after insect bites, burns and friction or cold injury. The type of blister depends on the level of cleavage: subcorneal or intraepidermal blisters rupture easily, but subepidermal ones are not so fragile (Fig. 1). The primary bullous disorders, dealt with here, are rare but important.

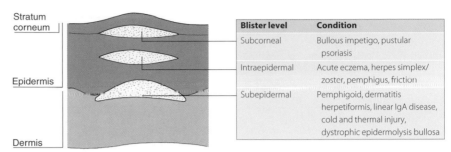

Blister level	Condition
Subcorneal	Bullous impetigo, pustular psoriasis
Intraepidermal	Acute eczema, herpes simplex/zoster, pemphigus, friction
Subepidermal	Pemphigoid, dermatitis herpetiformis, linear IgA disease, cold and thermal injury, dystrophic epidermolysis bullosa

Fig. 1 **The level of cleavage in blistering disorders.**

Pemphigus

Pemphigus is an uncommon, severe and potentially fatal autoimmune blistering disorder affecting the skin and mucous membranes.

Aetiopathogenesis

Over 80% of patients have circulating immunoglobulin (Ig)G autoantibodies detectable in the serum by indirect immunofluorescence (p. 123), which bind with desmoglein, a desmosomal cadherin involved in epidermal intercellular adhesion. The antibodies, possibly with complement activation and protease release, result in loss of adhesion and an intraepidermal split. Direct immunofluorescence shows the intercellular deposition of IgG in the suprabasal epidermis. Pemphigus is associated with other organ-specific autoimmune disorders such as myasthenia gravis.

Clinical presentation

In Europe, pemphigus is much less common than pemphigoid, and tends to affect middle-aged or young adults. Oral erosions signal the onset of *pemphigus vulgaris* in 50–70% of patients and often precede cutaneous blistering by months. Flaccid superficial blisters develop over the scalp, face, back, chest and flexures. The blistering is not always obvious, and lesions may consist of crusted erosions. Untreated, the blistering is progressive and, prior to the introduction of steroids, three out of four patients died within 4 years, usually from uncontrolled fluid and protein loss or secondary infection.

Less common variants include *pemphigus foliaceus*, in which shallow erosions appear on the scalp, face and chest (Fig. 2), and *pemphigus vegetans*, in which pustular and vegetating lesions affect the axillae and groins. In

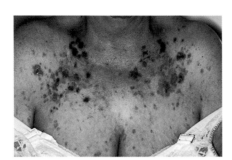

Fig. 2 **Pemphigus foliaceus showing blisters and erosions on the chest.**

Brazil, an endemic form of pemphigus foliaceus, *fogo selvagem*, seems to be induced by an infective agent. *Paraneoplastic pemphigus* describes a variant associated with underlying malignancy.

Differential diagnosis

Aphthous ulcers or Behçet's disease can simulate the oral erosions of pemphigus. Widespread skin erosions may suggest epidermolysis bullosa or pemphigoid. The diagnosis relies on the histological examination of a bulla and direct immunofluorescence.

Management

Systemic steroids and other immunosuppressive agents are required. Prednisolone is given initially in a high dose (1.0–1.5 mg/kg/day), often with azathioprine or cyclophosphamide. Once blistering is controlled, the steroid dosage can be lowered. Treatment usually needs to be continued for years, although remission occurs occasionally. Mortality and morbidity are now more likely to be due to side-effects of the steroid and immunosuppressive therapy than to the disease itself.

Pemphigoid

Pemphigoid is a chronic and not uncommon blistering eruption of the elderly.

Aetiopathogenesis

IgG autoantibodies to bullous pemphigoid antigens BP230 and BP180 in the hemidesmosomes at the basement membrane zone bind complement, which induces inflammation and protease release, leading to subepidermal bulla formation. The IgG and C_3 are detected by direct immunofluorescence (p. 123). Indirect methods demonstrate circulating autoantibodies in 75% of cases.

Clinical presentation

Bullous pemphigoid usually affects the elderly. Tense large blisters arise on red or normal-looking skin, often of the limbs, trunk and flexures (Fig. 3). Oral lesions occur in only 10% of cases. A pruritic urticarial eruption may precede the onset of blistering. Pemphigoid is sometimes localized to one site, often the lower leg. The differential diagnosis of pemphigoid may include dermatitis herpetiformis, linear IgA disease or pemphigus. Immunofluorescence and histology reveal the diagnosis.

Cicatricial pemphigoid mainly affects the ocular and oral mucous membranes. Scarring results, and this can cause serious eye problems. *Pemphigoid (herpes) gestationis* is a rare but characteristic intensely itchy bullous eruption associated with pregnancy, which remits after the delivery but can recur during subsequent pregnancies.

Management

Pemphigoid responds to a lower dose of steroids than pemphigus: 30–60 mg daily

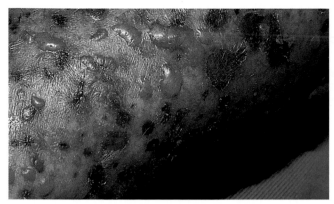

Fig. 3 **Bullous pemphigoid.** Tense blisters on an arm.

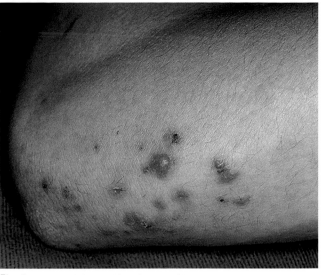

Fig. 4 **Dermatitis herpetiformis.** Itchy blisters on an elbow.

of oral prednisolone is usually sufficient, and this can normally be reduced to below 15 mg within weeks. Azathioprine is sometimes also prescribed. The disease is self limiting in many cases, and steroids can often be stopped after 2–3 years. Cicatricial pemphigoid does not respond so well, but pemphigoid gestationis is controlled by standard doses. Steroid-induced side-effects may be a problem, especially in the elderly.

Dermatitis herpetiformis

Dermatitis herpetiformis (DH) is an uncommon eruption of symmetrical itchy blisters on the extensor surfaces. Jejunal villus atrophy is an associated finding in most cases.

Aetiopathogenesis

DH is characterized by the finding of granular IgA at the dermal papillae on immunofluorescence, and by the response of the skin lesions (and the villus atrophy seen in over 75% of patients) to a gluten-free diet. Despite this, the cause of the eruption – and its relationship to the undoubted gluten sensitivity of both the gut and the skin – remains unclear. It is doubtful whether the IgA induces the itch, as it is present in asymptomatic patients.

Clinical presentation

DH usually presents in the third or fourth decade and is twice as common in males as in females. The classical onset is with groups of small intensely itchy vesicles on the elbows, knees, buttocks and scalp (Fig. 4). The blisters are often broken by scratching to leave excoriations. Although most patients have small bowel villus atrophy, symptoms of gastrointestinal disturbance and malabsorption are uncommon.

Differential diagnosis

Distinction from scabies, eczema and linear IgA disease is important. Biopsy shows a subepidermal bulla, and direct immunofluorescence of normal-looking skin demonstrates granular IgA at the dermal papilla (p. 123). The small bowel can be investigated by jejunal biopsy. Serum folate, vitamin B12 and ferritin estimates detect any biochemical malabsorption. Antiendomysial antibodies are present.

Management

A gluten-free diet is the treatment of choice, as this corrects both the bowel and the skin lesions. Dapsone (50–200 mg daily) will control the eruption and is often given until the gluten-free diet has its beneficial effect. A haemolytic anaemia may occur with dapsone. Regular blood counts are necessary.

Linear IgA disease

Linear IgA disease is a rare heterogeneous condition of blisters and urticarial lesions on the back or extensor surfaces (Fig. 5). The disorder responds to dapsone and may resemble DH or pemphigoid. Direct immunofluorescence reveals linear IgA at the basement membrane. In the childhood variant, blisters occur around the genitalia.

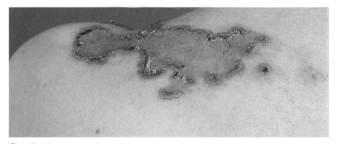

Fig. 5 **Linear IgA disease.** A figurate lesion with peripheral blisters.

Blistering disorders

Disorder	Clinical details	Direct (and indirect) immunofluorescence	Treatment
Bullous pemphigoid (BP)	Not uncommon, seen in elderly, limbs > trunk, oral lesions rare, tense blisters often seen	Linear IgG at basement membrane zone (to hemidesmosome BP antigens), indirect 75% positive	Modest dose of oral prednisolone with or without azathioprine
Pemphigus vulgaris	Rare, middle-aged affected, trunk > limbs, often starts with oral lesions, flaccid blisters may be seen	Intercellular epidermal IgG (to desmoglein in desmosomes), indirect 80% are positive	High dose of oral prednisolone and azathioprine or other immunosuppressive
Dermatitis herpetiformis	Young adults (M > F), extensor surfaces show itchy blisters, villus atrophy is usual	Granular IgA at dermal papilla (exact antigen is unknown), indirect test is negative	Gluten-free diet with or without dapsone

Connective tissue diseases

The inflammatory disorders of connective tissue often affect several organs, as in systemic lupus erythematosus (LE), but they may also involve the skin alone (e.g. discoid LE). Autoantibodies and cell-mediated immunity against normal cellular components (e.g. nuclei) are a feature of these diseases, which can thus be regarded as 'autoimmune'.

Lupus erythematosus

Systemic LE is a serious multisystem disease that involves vascular and connective tissues. *Discoid LE* is a chronic indolent cutaneous disorder of scaly atrophic plaques in sun-exposed sites.

Aetiopathogenesis

Autoantibodies to nuclear, nucleolar and cytoplasmic antigens are found in LE. Over 80% of systemic LE patients have circulating antinuclear antibodies compared with 35% of those with discoid LE. Subjects with systemic LE have impaired T-cell immunity. Ultraviolet (UV) radiation often brings out the eruption, perhaps by generating nuclear products in the skin. Systemic LE is associated with human leucocyte antigen (HLA) phenotypes -B8, -DR3, -A1 and -DR2, and certain drugs may trigger it.

Pathology

Discoid lesions show epidermal atrophy, hyperkeratosis and basal layer degeneration. Systemic lesions have similar changes with dermal oedema and fibrinoid change, inflammatory infiltrate and sometimes vasculitis. Direct immunofluorescence shows a 'lupus band' of immunoglobulins and complement at the dermoepidermal junction of the lesional and normal sun-exposed skin in systemic LE, and of lesional skin in discoid LE.

Clinical presentation

Systemic lupus erythematosus

Skin signs are found in 80%. The facial butterfly eruption (Fig. 1) is well known, but photosensitivity, discoid lesions, diffuse alopecia, mouth lesions and vasculitis also occur. Multisystem involvement with serological or haematological abnormalities must be demonstrated to diagnose systemic LE (Table 1). The female:male ratio is 8:1.

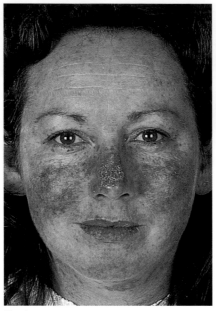

Fig. 1 **Systemic LE.** The typical butterfly eruption is present on the face.

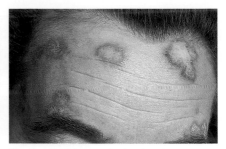

Fig. 2 **Discoid LE on the forehead.**

Table 1	**Organ involvement in systemic LE**
Organ	**Involvement**
Skin	Photosensitivity, facial rash, vasculitis, hair loss, Raynaud's phenomenon
Blood	Anaemia, thrombocytopenia
Joints	Arthritis, tenosynovitis, calcification
Kidney	Glomerulonephritis, nephrotic syndrome
Heart	Pericarditis, endocarditis, hypertension
Central nervous system	Psychosis, infarction, neuropathy
Lungs	Pneumonitis, effusion

Discoid lupus erythematosus

One or more round or oval plaques appear on the face, scalp or hands (Fig. 2). The lesions are well demarcated, red, atrophic, scaly and show keratin plugs in dilated follicles. Scarring leaves alopecia on the scalp and hypopigmentation in those with a pigmented skin. Remission occurs in over 50%. Internal involvement is not a feature, and only 6% develop systemic LE. Women outnumber men by 2:1.

Other forms

Subacute cutaneous LE is characterized by widespread symmetrical scaly plaques on sun-exposed sites of the face and forearms. Internal disease may occur, and anti-Ro antibodies are found. *Neonatal LE* is due to the placental transfer of anti-Ro antibodies from affected mothers to their neonates, who develop an annular atrophic eruption, sometimes with heart block.

Differential diagnosis

Discoid LE can usually be differentiated from other facial rashes such as rosacea, seborrhoeic dermatitis, lupus vulgaris or psoriasis. A biopsy should be performed. The photosensitive eruption of systemic LE may resemble polymorphic light eruption, dermatomyositis or drug reaction. Skin biopsy, with immunofluorescence, is helpful.

Management

Discoid LE usually responds to potent or very potent topical steroids which, in this instance, can be applied to the face. Sunblock creams are helpful. Widespread disease may need systemic therapy with hydroxychloroquine: the small risk of retinopathy demands regular tests of visual acuity. The treatment of systemic LE depends on the type of involvement. Sunscreens reduce photosensitivity but, if there is internal disease, systemic steroids are required, often with immunosuppressive agents.

Systemic sclerosis

Systemic sclerosis is an uncommon, progressive multisystem disease in which collagen deposition and fibrosis occur in several organs.

Aetiopathogenesis

Most patients have circulating antibodies to nuclear, nucleolar or cytoplasmic antigens, but their importance is unclear. Endothelial cell damage is central and leads to inflammation and fibrosis. T-cell factors may be involved. Immunofluorescence of telangiectatic skin shows immunoglobulin and complement at the dermoepidermal junction.

Clinical presentation

Raynaud's phenomenon (p. 68) is frequently the presenting sign. The skin of the fingers, forearms and lower legs becomes tight, waxy and stiff, and the finger pulps are resorbed (Fig. 3). Facial signs include perioral furrowing, telangiectasia (p. 111) and restricted mouth opening. Internal organ involvement, e.g. renal failure, may prove fatal (Table 2). Women are affected more than men (F:M 4:1). The diagnosis is rarely in doubt, although chronic graft-versus-host disease shows similar changes. In the CREST syndrome, a variant with a better prognosis, involvement is confined to *C*alcinosis, *R*aynaud's phenomenon, o*E*sophageal dysmotility, *S*clerodactyly and *T*elangiectasia.

Management

Treatment is mainly supportive. Nifedipine can help Raynaud's phenomenon. Hypertension is controlled. Systemic steroids, penicillamine and immunosuppressives have been used with little benefit. Photophoresis may be tried (p. 111).

Morphoea (localized scleroderma)

Morphoea consists of localized indurated plaques or bands of sclerosis on the skin. Internal disease is not found. The cause is unknown, although it may follow trauma. Histology shows bands of collagen with loss of appendages.

Morphoea presents with round or oval plaques of induration and erythema, often with a purplish edge (Fig. 4). These become shiny and white, eventually leaving atrophic hairless pigmented patches. The trunk or proximal limbs are affected. Morphoea is more common in women (F:M 3:1). *Linear morphoea* may involve the face or a limb and, when seen in a child, can retard growth of the underlying tissues, including bone. A rare, *generalized form* may encase the trunk but avoids the hands and feet.

There is no well established treatment (p. 111), although topical steroids are often given. The disease usually resolves spontaneously within months to years.

Dermatomyositis

Dermatomyositis is an uncommon disorder in which inflammation of skin, muscle and blood vessels gives a distinctive eruption, with muscle weakness of varying severity.

Clinical presentation

In dermatomyositis/polymyositis, skin changes or muscle weakness may predominate, and underlying malignancy is found in a subgroup. The cause is unknown, but autoimmune mechanisms with vascular damage are proposed. The typical eruption is a lilac–blue discoloration around the eyelids, cheeks and forehead, often with oedema. Bluish-red papules or streaks on the dorsal aspects of the hands (Fig. 5), elbows and knees are seen, sometimes with pigmentation and nail fold telangiectasia. Photosensitivity is common. An association with malignancy exists in patients over 40 years, 40% of whom have an underlying tumour, usually of the lung, breast or stomach. A childhood variant mainly affects the muscles and causes calcinosis and contractures.

Management

Investigations must define the degree of myositis and, in the middle-aged or elderly, exclude the possibility of underlying neoplasia. Treatment is with systemic steroids in moderate to high dosage, often with an immunosuppressive such as azathioprine. Immunoglobulin infusion and possibly photophoresis (p. 111) may help.

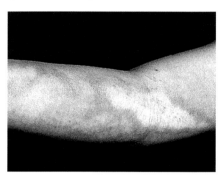

Fig. 4 **Morphoea.** Seen here on the arm of a child. The white indurated plaque has an erythematous edge.

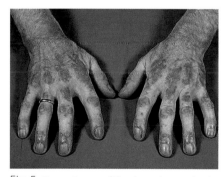

Fig. 5 **Dermatomyositis.** A streaky eruption is seen on the dorsal aspects of the hands.

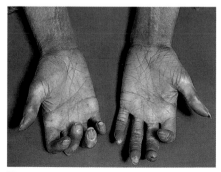

Fig. 3 **Systemic sclerosis.** Note the tightly bound waxy skin on the fingers (sclerodactyly) and resorption of the finger pulps.

Table 2 **Organ involvement in systemic sclerosis**	
Organ	**Involvement**
Skin	Raynaud's phenomenon, calcinosis, sclerodactyly, telangiectasia
Gut	Oesophageal dysmotility, malabsorption, dilated bowel
Lung	Fibrosis, pulmonary hypertension
Heart	Pericarditis, myocardial fibrosis
Kidney	Renal failure, hypertension
Muscle	Myositis, tendon involvement

Connective tissue diseases

- **Systemic LE** is an autoimmune, multisystem disease in which a butterfly rash, photosensitivity, vasculitis and alopecia may be seen. Treatment depends on the type and degree of involvement and often includes systemic steroids and immunosuppressive agents.

- **Discoid LE** is confined to the skin. Scaly atrophic plaques and scarring alopecia are found. Topical steroids and sunscreens are helpful. Sometimes, systemic therapy, e.g. with hydroxychloroquine, is used.

- **Systemic sclerosis** is a serious multisystem disorder. Sclerodactyly, Raynaud's phenomenon, telangiectasia and calcinosis are seen.

- **Morphoea** is characterized by white indurated plaques, usually on the trunk and proximal limbs. In children, it may retard growth of underlying tissues, producing atrophy. In adults, the condition is generally self-limiting.

- **Dermatomyositis** is an autoimmune inflammation of skin and muscle. The skin signs are a lilac–blue discoloration around the eyelids and red streaks on the dorsa of the hands. Exclude underlying malignancy in those over 40 years of age.

Vasculitis and the reactive erythemas

Vasculitis and the reactive erythemas are characterized by inflammation within or around blood vessels. This may result from a type III hypersensitivity response, with circulating immune complexes, but other mechanisms are also possible.

Vasculitis

Vasculitis is a disease process usually centred on small or medium-sized blood vessels. It is often due to circulating immune complexes (CIC).

Aetiopathogenesis

The CIC, which may be associated with several conditions (Table 1), lodge in the vessel wall where they activate complement and cytokine release, attract polymorphs and damage tissue. Inflammatory cells infiltrate vessels. Endothelial cells may show swelling, fibrinoid change or necrosis.

Clinical presentation

This depends on the size and site of the vessels involved. Vasculitis may be confined to the skin, or may be systemic and involve the joints, kidneys, lungs, heart, gut and nervous system. The skin signs are of palpable purpura, often painful and usually on the lower legs or buttocks (Fig. 1). Specific types are as follows:

■ *Henoch–Schönlein purpura* describes these signs, with arthritis, abdominal pain and haematuria. It is a small vessel immunoglobulin (Ig)A–CIC vasculitis that mainly affects children and often follows a streptococcal infection.
■ *Nodular vasculitis*, characterized by tender subcutaneous nodules on the lower legs, results when deeper dermal vessels are involved.
■ *Polyarteritis nodosa* is characterized by a necrotizing vasculitis in medium-sized arteries. It is uncommon and afflicts middle-aged men who, in addition to tender subcutaneous nodules along the line of arteries, may develop hypertension, renal failure and neuropathy.
■ *Wegener's granulomatosis* is a rare but potentially fatal granulomatous vasculitis of unknown cause. Malaise, upper and lower respiratory tract necrosis, glomerulonephritis and, in 40% of cases, a cutaneous vasculitis

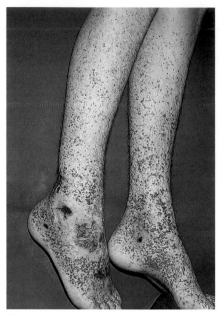

Fig. 1 **Vasculitis with purpura and impending skin necrosis.**

Table 1	**Causes of vasculitis**
Group	**Example**
Idiopathic	50% of cases (no cause found)
Blood disease	Cryoglobulinaemia
Connective tissue disease	Systemic lupus erythematosus, rheumatoid arthritis
Drugs	Antibiotics, diuretics, non-steroidals, anticonvulsants, allopurinol, cocaine
Infections	Hepatitis B, streptococci, *Mycobacterium leprae*, *Rickettsia*
Neoplasia	Lymphoma, leukaemia
Other	Wegener's granulomatosis, giant cell arteritis, polyarteritis nodosa

are found. Antineutrophil cytoplasm antibodies are present.
■ *Giant cell arteritis* affects medium-sized arteries in the elderly. Visual loss may result if prednisolone is withheld. Patients present with scalp tenderness due to temporal artery involvement that can progress to scalp necrosis.

In vasculitis, a skin biopsy is helpful along with tests to look for internal organ involvement. Other causes of purpura need exclusion.

Management

The cause is identified and remedied if possible. Some idiopathic cases settle with bedrest but, if lesions continue to develop and if internal organs are involved, treatment is indicated.

Dapsone, 100 mg daily, is often effective for cutaneous vasculitis. Otherwise, prednisolone (sometimes with an immunosuppressive) is prescribed. Giant cell arteritis, polyarteritis nodosa and Wegener's granulomatosis nearly always require oral steroids and immunosuppression.

Erythema multiforme

Erythema multiforme is an immune-mediated disease, characterized by target lesions on the hands and feet. It has a variety of causes (Table 2).

Aetiopathogenesis

Cell-mediated immunity seems to be involved. CIC are also present and can be demonstrated in blood vessels. No provoking factor is found in 50% of cases. On histology, the epidermis is necrotic and the dermis shows oedema, an inflammatory infiltrate and vasodilatation.

Clinical presentation

Typical target lesions, seen on the hands and feet, consist of red rings with central pale or purple areas, which may blister (Fig. 2). Involvement of the oral, conjunctival and genital mucosae is not uncommon and, if extreme, is known as the *Stevens–Johnson syndrome*. Crops of new lesions appear for 2–3 weeks. The

Table 2	**Causes of erythema multiforme**
Group	**Cause**
Idiopathic	50% of cases (no cause found)
Viral	Herpes simplex, hepatitis B, orf, adenovirus, mumps, *Mycoplasma*
Bacterial	Streptococci, *Rickettsia*
Fungal	Coccidioidomycosis, histoplasmosis
Drugs	Antibiotics, phenytoin, non-steroidals
Other	Lupus erythematosus, pregnancy, malignancy

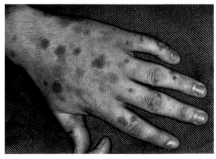

Fig. 2 **Erythema multiforme.** Target lesions are seen here on the dorsal aspect of the hand.

differential diagnosis includes toxic erythema (p. 84), toxic epidermal necrolysis, Sweet's disease, urticaria or pemphigoid. A biopsy is often helpful. *Toxic epidermal necrolysis* (p. 85) may sometimes represent erythema multiforme in a severe form.

Management
Identification and treatment of the underlying cause is the ideal. Mild cases resolve spontaneously and require symptomatic measures only. Extensive involvement necessitates hospital admission for supportive therapy. Systemic steroids are often prescribed to moderate the acute symptoms, although it is debatable whether they affect the outcome.

Erythema nodosum
Erythema nodosum is a panniculitis (i.e. an inflammation of the subcutaneous fat) that usually presents as painful red nodules on the lower legs. It is believed to result from CIC deposition in vessels of the subcutis. Infection, drugs and some systemic diseases are underlying causes (Table 3).

Clinical presentation
Deep, firm and tender reddish-blue nodules, 1–5 cm in diameter, develop on the calves (Fig. 3), shins and occasionally on the forearms. Joint pains and fever are common. Spontaneous resolution usually occurs within 8 weeks. Women are affected more than men (F:M 3:1). Other causes of panniculitis (e.g. pancreatic disease, cold, trauma and lupus erythematosus), cellulitis and phlebitis need to be excluded. A skin biopsy is helpful. If tuberculosis or sarcoidosis is suspected, a chest radiograph and Mantoux test are indicated.

Management
As spontaneous remission is usual, active therapy is rarely needed, although

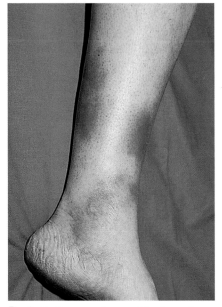

Fig. 3 **Erythema nodosum of the lower leg.**

a non-steroidal anti-inflammatory, potassium iodide or dapsone may help.

Sweet's disease
Sweet's disease (*acute febrile neutrophilic dermatosis*) occurs as raised plum-coloured plaques on the face or limbs (Fig. 4), typically with fever and a raised neutrophil count. It is not a true vasculitis but results from polymorph infiltration of the dermis. Leukaemia, ulcerative colitis and other disorders

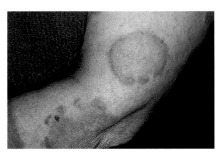

Fig. 4 **Sweet's disease.** A variant associated with rheumatoid arthritis is shown. Infiltrated annular plaques are seen on the arm.

may be associated and must be excluded. Drugs are another cause. Treatment with prednisolone is usually required.

Graft-versus-host (GVH) disease
GVH disease occurs when immunologically competent donor lymphocytes react against host tissues, principally the skin and gut. It is mostly associated with bone marrow transplantation, e.g. given for leukaemia or aplastic anaemia. Fever, malaise and a morbilliform eruption (Fig. 5), which may progress to toxic epidermal necrolysis, typify the acute GVH reaction. The acute type may be difficult to differentiate from a drug eruption, a viral infection or a cutaneous reaction to radiation therapy. Chronic GVH disease may resemble lichen planus or systemic sclerosis. A skin biopsy often helps, and treatment with systemic steroids is usually needed.

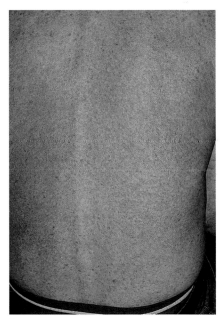

Fig. 5 **Graft-versus-host disease.** An acute eruption is shown in a patient following bone marrow transplant.

Table 3	**Causes of erythema nodosum**
Group	**Cause**
Idiopathic	About 20% of cases
Bacterial	Streptococci, TB, leprosy, *Yersinia*, *Mycoplasma*, *Salmonella*
Fungal	Coccidioidomycosis, *Trichophyton*
Viral	Cat-scratch fever, chlamydiae
Drugs	Sulphonamides, oral contraceptives
Systemic diseases	Inflammatory bowel disease, sarcoidosis, Behçet's disease, malignancy (rare)

Vasculitis *and the reactive erythemas*

- **Vasculitis** is a circulating immune complex (CIC) disorder showing palpable purpura, sometimes with internal organ involvement. Investigations may reveal the underlying cause. Treatment with dapsone, prednisolone or other immunosuppressive drugs is often indicated.

- **Erythema multiforme** is an immune-mediated reaction with target and mucosal lesions, often due to infection, commonly *Herpes simplex*, or drugs. The underlying cause should be sought.

- **Erythema nodosum** presents as painful red nodules on the lower legs and is regarded as a CIC response to infection (e.g. streptococcal), drugs or internal disease (e.g. sarcoidosis).

- **Sweet's disease** is characterized by plum-coloured plaques on the face and limbs. Leukaemia or a systemic disorder may be associated. A course of prednisolone is often required.

Skin changes in internal conditions

Skin signs are seen with many internal disorders and are not uncommonly their presenting feature. The astute dermatologist can therefore recognize hitherto undiagnosed systemic disease.

Skin signs of endocrine and metabolic disease

Almost all endocrine diseases (and several metabolic defects) have cutaneous signs that depend on the over- or underproduction of a hormone or metabolite (Table 1).

Diabetes mellitus

Candida albicans or bacterial infection is more common with untreated or poorly controlled diabetes. The neuropathy or arteriopathy of diabetes may result in *ulcers* on the feet (p. 71), and an associated secondary hyperlipidaemia can produce *eruptive xanthomas* (Fig. 4). *Diabetic dermopathy* describes depressed pigmented scars on the shins, associated with diabetic microangiopathy. *Necrobiosis lipoidica* (Fig. 1), characterized by shiny atrophic yellowish-red plaques on the shins, was associated with diabetes in 65% of cases in one series, although others find a much lower figure. It affects less than 1% of all diabetics. Histologically, degenerate dermal collagen is seen with epithelioid cells and giant cells. The condition is chronic and may ulcerate. It is unresponsive to treatment. In contrast, *granuloma annulare* – recognized as palpable annular lesions on the hands, feet or face (Fig. 2) – is only rarely associated with diabetes and usually fades in 2 years. It must be differentiated from tinea corporis.

Thyroid disease

Both over and underproduction of thyroxine result in skin and hair changes (Table 1). *Pretibial myxoedema* (Fig. 3), seen in 1–10% of patients with hyperthyroidism, presents on the shins as raised erythematous plaques due to the deposition of mucin in the dermis. Topical steroids may be of benefit.

Hyperlipidaemia

Both primary (genetic metabolic defects) and secondary (associated with diabetes, hypothyroidism or the nephrotic syndrome) lipid abnormalities may produce a variety of xanthomatous deposits. These may be:

- *eruptive* – red–yellow papules on shoulders and buttocks (Fig. 4)
- *tendinous* – subcutaneous nodules; hand, foot or Achilles tendons
- *plane* – yellow–orange macules in palmar creases
- *tuberous* – yellow–orange nodules on knees and elbows.

Xanthelasma, seen as yellowish plaques on the eyelids, are not always due to a lipid abnormality. Treatment of xanthomas is usually aimed at the underlying hyperlipidaemia.

Table 1 **Skin signs of endocrine and metabolic disorders**	
Disorders	**Skin signs**
Diabetes mellitus	Necrobiosis lipoidica, granuloma annulare, xanthomas, *Candida albicans* infection, 'dermopathy', neuropathic ulcers
Thyrotoxicosis	Pink soft skin, hyperhidrosis, alopecia, pigmentation, vitiligo, onycholysis, clubbing, pretibial myxoedema, palmar erythema
Myxoedema	Alopecia (including eyebrows), coarse hair, dry puffy yellowish skin (e.g. hands, face), asteatotic eczema, xanthomas
Addison's disease	Pigmentation (p. 73), vitiligo, loss of axillary and pubic hair
Cushing's disease	Pigmentation, hirsutism, striae, acne, obesity, buffalo 'hump'
Acromegaly	Thickened moist greasy skin, pigmentation, skin tags
Phenylketonuria	Fair hair and skin, atopic eczema (p. 34), photosensitivity
Hyperlipidaemia	Xanthomas (tuberous, tendinous, eruptive, plane), xanthelasma
Cutaneous porphyrias	Photosensitivity, blistering, skin fragility, atrophic scarring, thickening of skin, hypertrichosis, pigmentation (p. 44)

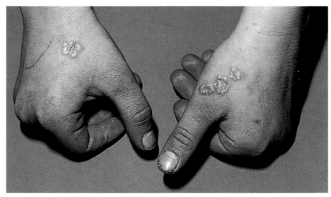

Fig. 2 **Granuloma annulare, seen on the dorsal aspects of the hands.**

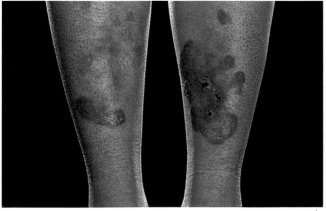

Fig. 1 **Necrobiosis lipoidica.** Yellowish-red atrophic areas are seen on the shins of a diabetic patient.

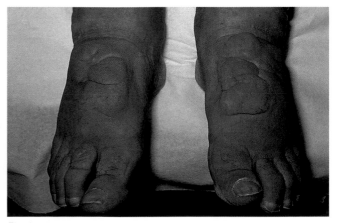

Fig. 3 **Pretibial myxoedema.** The patient had been thyrotoxic.

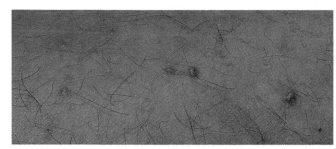

Fig. 4 **Eruptive xanthomas.** The patient had recently presented with diabetes mellitus.

Skin signs of nutritional and other internal disorders

Skin changes are common with nutritional deficiency and are not infrequent with gastrointestinal, hepatic and renal disease.

Nutritional deficiency

Protein malnutrition results in retarded growth, wasted muscles, oedema and skin changes of altered pigmentation, desquamation and ulcers with, in Black Africans, dry and pale-brown/red hair. *Vitamin C deficiency* (scurvy) and *niacin deficiency* (pellagra) produce distinct lesions. In Europe, scurvy is mainly seen in elderly men who do not eat fresh fruit or vegetables. Deficiencies of other B vitamins and of iron also produce cutaneous changes (Table 2). *Acrodermatitis enteropathica* is a rare inherited defect of zinc absorption seen in weaned infants and cured by zinc supplements.

Gastrointestinal disease

Malabsorption and its deficiency states have accompanying skin problems that include dryness, eczema, ichthyosis, pigmentation and defects of the hair and nails. Some gut disorders show specific skin changes (Table 2). *Coeliac disease* is associated with an eczema (in addition to the link of dermatitis herpetiformis with gluten enteropathy, p. 77). and both *Crohn's disease* and *ulcerative colitis* induce various eruptions. *Peutz–Jeghers syndrome* (p. 73) and *pseudoxanthoma*

elasticum (p. 91) affect both the skin and the gut. *Bowel bypass surgery* induces a vesiculopustular eruption.

Other internal disorders

Hepatic and *renal diseases* often produce troublesome itching and pigmentation. Lesions may also be related to the underlying disease process, e.g. primary biliary cirrhosis (associated with systemic sclerosis) or vasculitis.

Sarcoidosis, a disorder of unknown aetiology in which granulomas commonly develop in the lungs, lymph nodes, bone and nervous tissue, affects the skin in a third of cases. Cutaneous changes are variable and include brownish-red papules (typically on the face), nodules, plaques (on the limbs and shoulders, Fig. 5) and scar involvement. *Lupus pernio* is a particular pattern of sarcoidosis that appears as dusky-red infiltrated plaques on the nose or, occasionally, the fingers. *Erythema nodosum* may also result. Topical steroids have little effect. Resistant lesions may improve with intralesional steroid injection, but oral prednisolone or methotrexate is sometimes prescribed, particularly when there is progressive internal disease.

Skin changes in pregnancy

Skin changes are common in pregnancy. Pigmentation generally increases (p. 72), melanocytic naevi become more prominent, and spider naevi and abdominal striae develop. Telogen effluvium may occur in the postpartum period (p. 64). Pruritus and an urticated papular eruption (p. 74) are not uncommon, although pemphigoid gestationis (p. 76) is rare. The effect on common dermatoses is variable and unpredictable: psoriasis tends to improve, but eczema may get worse.

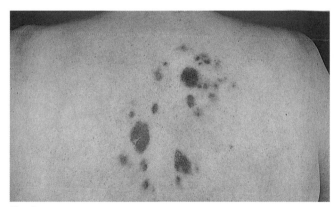

Fig. 5 **Sarcoidosis.** Plum-coloured plaques are seen on the upper back.

Table 2 **Skin signs of nutritional and internal disorders**	
Disorder	**Skin signs**
Protein malnutrition	Pigmentation, dry skin, oedema, pale-brown/orange hair
Iron deficiency	Alopecia, koilonychia, itching, angular cheilitis
Scurvy	Perifollicular purpura, bleeding gums, woody oedema
Pellagra	Light-exposed dermatitis and pigmentation
Acrodermatitis enteropathica	Perianal/perioral red scaly pustular eruption in infants, failure to thrive, diarrhoea, poor wound healing
Malabsorption	Dry itchy skin, ichthyosis, eczema, oedema
Liver disease	Pruritus, jaundice, spider naevi, palmar erythema, white nails, pigmentation, xanthomas, porphyria cutanea tarda, zinc deficiency, striae, gynaecomastia, lichen planus (p. 38)
Renal failure	Pruritus, pigmentation, white/red nails, dry skin with fine scaling
Pancreatic disease	Panniculitis, thrombophlebitis, glucagonoma syndrome
Crohn's disease	Perianal abscesses, sinuses, fistulae, erythema nodosum, Sweet's disease, necrotizing vasculitis, aphthous stomatitis, glossitis
Ulcerative colitis	Pyoderma gangrenosum, erythema nodosum, Sweet's disease
Sarcoidosis	Nodules, plaques, erythema nodosum, dactylitis, lupus pernio, scar granulomas, small papules, nail involvement

Skin changes in internal conditions

- Endocrine and metabolic disorders, nutritional deficiencies and malabsorption are frequently associated with skin changes.

- Hyperlipidaemias are associated with a variety of xanthomata and xanthelasma, although the latter can occur with normal lipid levels.

- Liver and kidney failure, in particular, are complicated by pruritus and pigmentation. Treatment is often difficult.

- Inflammatory bowel disease and sarcoidosis have specific skin manifestations, often granulomatous or with cellular infiltration.

- Pregnancy can be associated with increased pigmentation (e. g. melasma), an urticated papular eruption and, rarely, with the blistering eruption pemphigoid gestationis.

Drug eruptions

Reactions to drugs are common and often produce an eruption. Almost any drug can result in any reaction, although some patterns are more common with certain drugs. Not all reactions are 'allergic' in nature.

Aetiopathogenesis

Drug-induced skin reactions have several possible mechanisms:

- *excessive therapeutic effect*, e.g. purpura resulting from accidental overdosage with anticoagulants
- *pharmacological side-effects*, e.g. dry lips and nasal mucosa with isotretinoin or bone marrow suppression by cytotoxics
- *modulation of the immune response*, e.g. a type IV skin reaction in leprosy when cell-mediated immunity improves following drug therapy
- *deposition* of the drug (or metabolites) in the skin, e.g. gold
- *idiosyncratic reaction* peculiar to that individual
- *facilitative effect*, e.g. when antibiotics suppress the normal skin flora or drugs exacerbate psoriasis
- *immune hypersensitivity* in any of the four types (p. 11).

Clinical presentation

Drug eruptions present in many guises and come into the differential diagnosis of several rashes. When suspected, it is vital to obtain a detailed history of all the drugs taken over the preceding 2 or 3 weeks. This must include 'over-the-counter' preparations (e.g. for headaches or constipation) not normally regarded as 'drugs' by the patient. In subjects taking several preparations, a drug introduced during a 2-week period before the eruption starts must be viewed as the most likely culprit, although a reaction may occur to a drug taken safely for years. The majority of drug eruptions fit into a defined category (Table 1). The most common and characteristic ones are outlined below. Other patterns, e.g. lichenoid, photosensitive, pigmentation and erythroderma, have been mentioned previously.

Toxic erythema

Toxic erythema, the commonest type of drug eruption may be *morbilliform* (measles-like) or *urticarial*, or may resemble *erythema multiforme*. It usually affects the trunk more than the extremities (Fig. 1), and may be accompanied by fever or followed by peeling of the skin. Drugs commonly implicated include amoxicillin, proton pump inhibitors and carbamazepine. It is also caused by scarlet fever (group A streptococci) or viral infections. The eruption clears 1–2 weeks after stopping the offending drug.

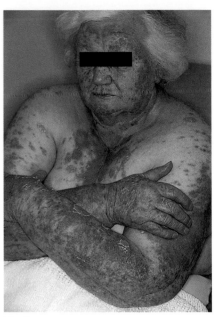

Fig. 1 **Toxic erythema.** This morbilliform variant was due to chlorpropamide.

Fixed drug eruption

This specific but uncommon eruption is characterized by round red or purplish plaques (Fig. 2) that recur at the same site each time the causative agent is taken. The lesions may blister and leave pigmentation on clearing. Non-steroidals, paracetamol, antibacterials and oral antifungals are often responsible.

Table 1 **Patterns of drug eruptions**		
Drug eruption	**Description**	**Drugs commonly responsible**
Acneiform	Like acne: papulopustules, no comedones	Androgens, bromides, dantrolene, isoniazid, lithium, phenobarbital, quinidine, steroids
Bullous	Various types; some phototoxic, some 'fixed'	Barbiturates (overdose), furosemide, nalidixic acid (phototoxic), penicillamine (pemphigus-like)
Eczematous	Not common; seen when topical sensitization is followed by systemic treatment	Neomycin, penicillin, sulphonamide, ethylenediamine (cross-reacts with aminophylline), benzocaine (cross-reacts with chlorpropamide), parabens, allopurinol
Erythema multiforme	Target lesions (p. 80)	Antibiotics, anticonvulsants, ACE inhibitors, calcium channel blockers, non-steroidals
Erythroderma	Exfoliative dermatitis (p. 42)	Allopurinol, captopril, carbamazepine, diltiazem, gold, isoniazid, omeprazole, phenytoin
Fixed drug eruption	Round red–purple plaques recur at same site	Antibiotics, tranquillizers, non-steroidals, phenolphthalein, paracetamol, quinine
Hair loss	Telogen effluvium (p. 64)	Anticoagulants, bezafibrate, carbimazole, oral contraceptive pill, propranolol, albendazole
	Anagen effluvium (p. 64)	Cytotoxic drugs, acitretin
Hypertrichosis	Excess vellus hair growth (p. 64)	Minoxidil, ciclosporin, phenytoin, penicillamine, corticosteroids, androgens
Lupus erythematosus	LE-like syndrome (p. 78)	Hydralazine, isoniazid, penicillamine, anticonvulsants, beta-blockers, etanercept
Lichenoid	Like lichen planus (p. 38)	Chloroquine, beta-blockers, anti-TB drugs, penicillamine, diuretics, gold, captopril
Photosensitive	Sun-exposed sites, may blister or pigment (Fig. 4)	Non-steroidals, ACE inhibitors, amiodarone, thiazides, tetracyclines, phenothiazines
Pigmentation	Melanin or drug deposition (Fig. 5)	Amiodarone, bleomycin, psoralens, chlorpromazine, minocycline, antimalarials
Psoriasiform	Psoriasis-like appearance (see text)	Beta-blockers, gold, methyl dopa; lithium and antimalarials exacerbate psoriasis
Toxic epidermal necrolysis	Scalded skin appearance (see text)	Antibiotics, anticonvulsants, non-steroidals, omeprazole, allopurinol, barbiturate
Toxic erythema	Commonest pattern (see text)	Antibiotics (e.g. amoxicillin), proton pump inhibitors, gold, thiazides, allopurinol, carbamazepine
Urticaria	Many mechanisms (p. 74)	ACE inhibitors, penicillins, opiates, non-steroidals, X-ray contrast media, vaccines
Vasculitis	Immune complex reaction	Allopurinol, captopril, penicillins, phenytoin, sulphonamides, thiazides

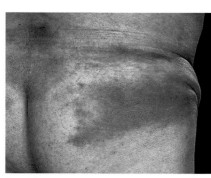

Fig. 2 **Fixed drug eruption.** The typical dusky erythematous lesion followed the ingestion of penicillin.

Toxic epidermal necrolysis

Toxic epidermal necrolysis, a serious and life-threatening eruption, is a drug-induced adult disorder similar to *staphylococcal scalded skin syndrome* of childhood (p. 47). The skin is red, swollen and separates as in a scald (Fig. 3). The split is intraepidermal. Mucosal lesions are usual, and the condition may on occasions be a severe form of erythema multiforme. The extensive skin loss results in problems of fluid and electrolyte balance, as seen with extensive burns, and the patient must be managed in an intensive care unit. Overall mortality is 30%. Drugs that commonly cause this condition include non-steroidals, anticonvulsants, antibiotics and allopurinol.

Psoriasiform and bullous eruptions

Drugs including non-steroidals or angiotensin-converting enzyme (ACE) inhibitors, but especially lithium and chloroquine, can exacerbate existing psoriasis. Other agents, e.g. beta-blockers and gold, may provoke a psoriasis-like eruption.

Fixed drug eruption, phototoxic reaction, drug-induced pemphigus and barbiturate overdosage (at pressure sites) may all blister (Table 1).

Differential diagnosis

The exact differential diagnosis depends on the type of drug eruption. A typical morbilliform rash occurring a few days after antibiotic therapy usually presents no diagnostic difficulties, but could be confused with a toxic erythema associated with the infection for which the antibiotic was prescribed. The situation is more complicated when an eruption occurs in an ill patient treated with a multiplicity of drugs. The determination of which drug is responsible depends on accurate prescribing records and a knowledge

of the potential of each drug to cause a reaction. Table 2 shows the types of eruption seen with some commonly prescribed drugs. Allergen-specific immunoglobulin (Ig)E tests are often not helpful, but patch or intradermal tests may be of use in diagnosing a drug eruption.

Management

Withdrawal of the offending drug usually leads to clearance of the eruption within 2 weeks or so. Simple emollients or topical steroids can help to ease the eruption until it resolves. Patients should be given advice about which drugs they must avoid. Provocation tests to confirm that a drug has been culpable are not recommended because of the possibility of inducing a severe reaction.

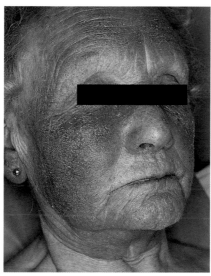

Fig. 4 **Photosensitivity.** This was caused by taking a thiazide diuretic, associated with being out of doors on a sunny day.

Table 2 **Eruptions seen with some commonly prescribed drugs**

Drug	Eruption
ACE inhibitors	Pruritus, urticaria, toxic erythema
Antibiotics	Toxic erythema, urticaria, fixed drug eruption, erythema multiforme
Beta-blockers	Psoriasiform, Raynaud's phenomenon, lichenoid eruption
Non-steroidal anti-inflammatories	Toxic erythema, erythroderma, toxic epidermal necrolysis
Oral contraceptive	Melasma, alopecia, acne, candidiasis
Phenothiazines	Photosensitivity, pigmentation
Thiazides	Toxic erythema, photosensitivity, lichenoid eruption, vasculitis

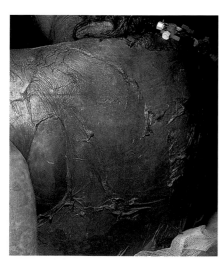

Fig. 3 **Toxic epidermal necrolysis.** The damaged epidermis has sheared off to leave extensive areas of eroded skin.

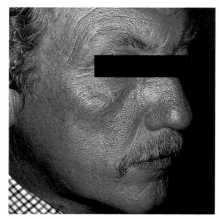

Fig. 5 **Pigmentation.** This was due to treatment with amiodarone for a cardiac arrhythmia. An erythematous eruption occurring within 2 h of sun exposure is more common.

Drug eruptions

- Drug reactions may be pharmacological or idiosyncratic, as well as immune mediated.

- Drugs that commonly cause drug eruptions are *amoxicillin, ACE inhibitors, sulphonamides, thiazides* and *non-steroidal anti-inflammatory drugs*.

- The commonest pattern is *toxic erythema*, often morbilliform.

- The most severe involvement is *toxic epidermal necrolysis*, which may be fatal.

- A drug eruption typically begins within 3 days of starting a drug (if it has been taken before) and clears about 2 weeks after stopping it.

- Withdrawal of the drug and avoidance of related compounds are necessary.

- Provocation tests are not recommended because of the possibility of a severe reaction.

Associations with malignancy

Internal malignancy causes a variety of skin changes (Table 1). Apart from direct infiltration, the mechanisms of these effects are often poorly understood.

Conditions associated with malignancy

The following rare skin eruptions are characteristic and strongly indicate an underlying malignancy:

- acanthosis nigricans
- erythema gyratum repens
- necrolytic migratory erythema
- Paget's disease of the nipple
- extramammary Paget's disease
- skin secondaries.

Acanthosis nigricans

True acanthosis nigricans is uncommon. The flexures and neck typically show epidermal thickening and pigmentation (Fig. 1), and the skin is velvety or papillomatous. Warty lesions are seen around the mouth and on the palms and soles. *Benign acquired acanthosis nigricans* is more frequent and describes similar milder changes, seen with obesity or endocrine disorders such as insulin-resistant diabetes or acromegaly. Very rarely, acanthosis nigricans is *inherited* and appears in childhood or at puberty. In the malignancy-associated type, usually found in a middle-aged or elderly patient, the cancer is most commonly of the gastrointestinal tract.

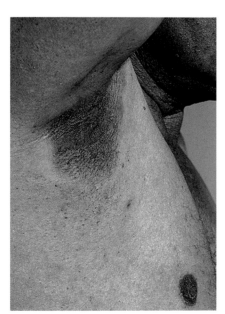

Fig. 1 **Acanthosis nigricans.** Pigmented velvety papillomatosis at the axilla and nipples is shown.

Growth factors, released from the tumour or associated with the endocrine disorder, cause the skin changes. The underlying disease must be identified and treated.

Erythema gyratum repens

Erythema gyratum repens is an exceptionally rare pattern of concentric scaly rings of erythema that shift visibly from day to day (Fig. 2). The appearance resembles wood grain. An underlying neoplasm, frequently a carcinoma of the lung, is almost invariably detected.

Necrolytic migratory erythema

Necrolytic migratory erythema is a rare paraneoplastic eruption of serpiginous erythematous plaques, with a migratory eroded edge. It typically starts in the perineum. The eruption indicates a tumour, or occasionally a hyperplasia, of the glucagon-secreting alpha cells of the pancreas (a *glucagonoma*). Weight loss, anaemia, mild diabetes, diarrhoea and glossitis are associated. Liver metastases are often present at diagnosis.

Paget's disease and extramammary Paget's disease

Paget's disease presents as a unilateral eczema-like plaque of the nipple areola and represents the intraepidermal spread of an intraductal breast carcinoma. Extramammary Paget's disease is seen as an eczema-like eruption around the perineum or axilla. It usually results from intraepidermal spread of a ductal apocrine carcinoma. A skin biopsy confirms the diagnosis prior to surgical excision.

Secondary deposits

Cutaneous metastases are not uncommon. They occur late, indicate a poor prognosis and may be the presenting sign of an internal tumour. Skin secondaries are multiple or solitary and appear as firm asymptomatic pink nodules (Fig. 3). The scalp, umbilicus and upper trunk are favoured sites. They occur most commonly with tumours of the breast, gastrointestinal

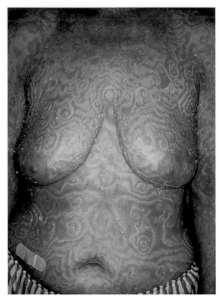

Fig. 2 **Erythema gyratum repens.** Note the 'wood grain' pattern.

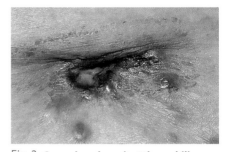

Fig. 3 **Secondary deposit at the umbilicus from a carcinoma of the breast.**

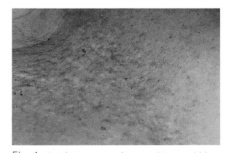

Fig. 4 **Carcinoma en cuirasse.** Direct pebbly infiltration of the skin of the chest wall from a carcinoma of the breast.

tract, ovary and lung, and with malignant melanoma (p. 96). Leukaemias and lymphomas often show skin involvement (p. 100). Direct infiltration of the skin – carcinoma en cuirasse – is sometimes found with carcinoma of the breast (Fig. 4).

Conditions occasionally associated with malignancy

Conditions occasionally associated with underlying neoplasia but also seen with benign disease include:

- acquired ichthyosis
- dermatomyositis (p. 79)
- erythroderma (p. 42)
- flushing (p. 68)
- generalized pruritus
- hyperpigmentation
- hypertrichosis (p. 65)
- pyoderma gangrenosum
- superficial thrombophlebitis
- tylosis (keratoderma; p. 88).

Acquired ichthyosis
Ichthyosis is usually inherited and starts in infancy (p. 88), but it may be acquired in adult life due to an underlying malignancy (e.g. Hodgkin's disease), essential fatty acid deficiency (e.g. caused by intestinal bypass malabsorption) or drug therapy with nicotinic acid, allopurinol and clofazimine.

Generalized pruritus
Generalized pruritus not associated with an eruption has several causes:

- idiopathic ('senile'): see page 114
- iron deficiency
- liver disease (cholestasis)
- malignancy, e.g. Hodgkin's disease
- neurological disorders
- polycythaemia
- renal failure (chronic)
- thyroid dysfunction.

Patients with generalized pruritus need careful examination and investigation to exclude liver disease (e.g. biliary obstruction), iron deficiency, polycythaemia, hypothyroidism, hyperthyroidism and renal failure. Pruritus may occur with multiple sclerosis and neurofibromatosis. Sometimes, especially in the elderly, no cause is found, and the itching is labelled *idiopathic*. The commonest malignant causes of pruritus are Hodgkin's disease (one-third of patients with this disease itch) and polycythaemia rubra vera. The aetiology of the itching is poorly understood. Treatment, once any underlying disorder has been dealt with, is symptomatic. Sedative antihistamines, calamine lotion and topical antipruritics (e.g. 0.5% menthol or 1% phenol in aqueous cream) are used.

Hyperpigmentation
Malignancy-associated pigmentation may result from ectopic adrenocorticotrophic hormone (ACTH) or melanocyte-stimulating hormone (MSH)-like hormone production by the tumour. It is also seen in patients with malignant cachexia. The axillae, groins and nipples are involved.

Pyoderma gangrenosum
Pyoderma gangrenosum starts as a pustule or inflamed nodule, which breaks down to produce an ulcer with an undermined purplish margin and a surrounding erythema (Fig. 5). The ulcer may extend rapidly. Lesions may be multiple. A bacterial gangrene (e.g. necrotizing fasciitis, p. 46) is sometimes misdiagnosed. Pyoderma gangrenosum often occurs on the trunk or lower limbs. An immune-mediated process is suggested. The following diseases are associated:

- ulcerative colitis, Crohn's disease
- chronic autoimmune liver disease
- rheumatoid arthritis
- Behçet's syndrome (p. 117)
- multiple myeloma and monoclonal gammopathy
- leukaemia (a bullous form is seen).

Treatment is with systemic steroids, ciclosporin or infliximab. Minocycline helps mild disease. Cases associated with bowel disease can improve as this is controlled.

Superficial thrombophlebitis
Migratory superficial thrombophlebitis, mainly associated with carcinoma of the pancreas or lung, also occurs with Behçet's syndrome.

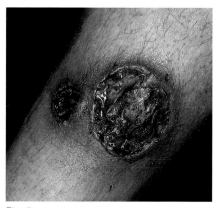

Fig. 5 **Pyoderma gangrenosum.** Necrotic ulcers shown on the lower leg.

Table 1 **Cutaneous manifestations of malignancy**	
Condition associated	**Commonest malignancies**
Almost always	
Acanthosis nigricans	Gastrointestinal tract
Erythema gyratum repens	Lung, breast
Extramammary Paget's disease	Apocrine glands
Necrolytic migratory erythema	Pancreas (alpha cells)
Paget's disease of the nipple	Breast
Skin secondaries	Breast, gastrointestinal, ovary, lung, kidney
Occasionally	
Acquired ichthyosis	Lymphoma (Hodgkin's disease)
Dermatomyositis	Lung, breast, stomach
Erythroderma	T-cell lymphoma
Flushing	Carcinoid syndrome
Generalized pruritus	Hodgkin's disease, polycythaemia rubra vera
Hyperpigmentation	Cachectic malignancy
Hypertrichosis	Various tumours
Migratory thrombophlebitis	Pancreas, lung, stomach
Paraneoplastic pemphigus	B-cell lymphoma, thymoma
Pyoderma gangrenosum	Leukaemia, myeloma
Tylosis	Oesophagus

Associations with malignancy

- **Acanthosis nigricans,** characterized by pigmentation and epidermal thickening of the flexures, neck, palms and soles, is seen with gastrointestinal cancers.
- **Benign acanthosis nigricans** is more common and occurs with obesity or endocrine disorders.
- **Erythema gyratum repens** is a migratory erythema almost invariably associated with a neoplasm.
- **Paget's disease,** an eczema-like plaque at the nipple, is due to epidermal spread of an intraductal carcinoma. The *extramammary* form comes from an apocrine carcinoma.
- **Secondary deposits** are not uncommon and may present as single or multiple pink firm nodules often on the scalp or upper trunk. They occur with tumours of the breast, gastrointestinal tract, ovary and lung and with malignant melanoma.
- **Acquired ichthyosis** is associated with Hodgkin's disease, fatty acid deficiency (e.g. intestinal bypass malabsorption) and as a side-effect of some drugs.
- **Generalized pruritus** may occur with malignancy (e.g. Hodgkin's disease), liver disease, renal failure, iron deficiency and thyroid dysfunction.
- **Pyoderma gangrenosum** is a necrotic ulceration seen with ulcerative colitis, Crohn's disease, rheumatoid arthritis, multiple myeloma or leukaemia.

Keratinization and blistering syndromes

Common skin disorders, e.g. atopic eczema or psoriasis, have a genetic component that is often subject to environmental influences. The *genodermatoses* differ in being single gene defects and include keratinization, blistering and neurocutaneous syndromes.

The ichthyoses

The ichthyoses are inherited disorders of keratinization and epidermal differentiation. They are characterized by dry scaly skin and vary from mild and asymptomatic to severe and incompatible with life (Table 1). Keratinization is abnormal. Some of the biochemical defects have been identified, e.g. steroid sulphatase is deficient in X-linked ichthyosis.

Clinical presentation

Ichthyosis vulgaris is common and unrecognized if mild. Small branny scales are seen on the extensor aspects of the limbs and the back (Fig. 1). The flexures are often spared.

The other types of ichthyosis are uncommon or rare and can usually be identified by their clinical features, onset and inheritance. Autosomal dominant conditions tend to improve with age, whereas recessive ichthyoses may worsen. *Collodion baby* describes a newborn infant with a tight shiny skin that causes feeding problems and ectropion. It is mainly due to non-bullous ichthyosiform erythroderma. *Acquired ichthyosis* (p. 86) usually starts in adulthood.

Table 1 **A classification of the ichthyoses**		
Disorder	**Inheritance**	**Clinical features**
Ichthyosis vulgaris	Autosomal dominant	Common (1 in 250). Onset 1–4 years. It occurs with atopic eczema. Often mild. Small bran-like scale seen. Flexures spared. Defect in filaggrin, needed for keratin assembly
X-linked ichthyosis	X-linked recessive	1 in 2000 males. Generalized involvement with large brown scale. Onset in first week of life. Improves in summer. Due to a deficiency of steroid sulphatase
Non-bullous ichthyosiform erythroderma*	Autosomal recessive	Rare (1 in 300 000). At birth may present as collodion baby. Red scaly skin and ectropion may follow. Erythema improves with age
Bullous ichthyosiform erythroderma†	Autosomal dominant	Rare (< 1 in 100 000). Redness and blisters occur after birth but fade. Warty rippled hyperkeratosis appears in childhood

*Lamellar ichthyosis is similar but rarer.
†Also called epidermolytic hyperkeratosis.

Management

Emollient ointments, creams and bath additives (p. 22) are essential and adequate for mild ichthyosis. Urea-containing creams (e.g. Aquadrate or Calmurid) help, but severe forms may need oral acitretin (p. 30).

Keratoderma

Keratoderma describes gross hyperkeratosis of the palms and soles, and may be acquired or inherited.

Clinical presentation

The degrees of involvement and modes of inheritance vary. A common pattern, *tylosis*, shows diffuse hyperkeratosis of the palms and soles (Fig. 2) and is usually of autosomal dominant inheritance. In a few families, tylosis is associated with carcinoma of the oesophagus. Other keratodermas may give punctate papular lesions on the palms and soles or, in 'mutilating' types, fibrous bands that strangulate digits.

Acquired palmoplantar keratoderma is seen in pityriasis rubra pilaris (p. 42) and lichen planus, and may develop in women at the menopause, particularly around the heels. Corns and callosities are different from keratoderma.

Callosities are painless localized thickenings of the keratin layer and are seen as a protective response, induced by friction or pressure, which is often occupational in origin. *Corns* are painful and develop at areas of high local pressure on the feet, where shoes squeeze against bony points.

Management

Treatment is with keratolytics, e.g. 5–10% salicylic acid ointment or 10% urea cream. Topical calcipotriol can be helpful. Sometimes the use of oral acitretin is justified.

Keratosis pilaris

Keratosis pilaris is a common, sometimes inherited condition in which multiple small horny follicular plugs affect the upper thigh, upper arm and face (Fig. 3). It is occasionally associated with ichthyosis vulgaris. Application of 5% salicylic acid ointment or 10% urea cream lessens, but does not cure, the problem.

Darier's disease

Darier's disease (keratosis follicularis) is a rare autosomal dominant condition characterized by brownish scaly papules.

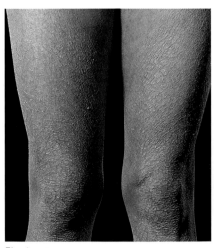

Fig. 1 **Ichthyosis vulgaris showing bran-like scaling.**

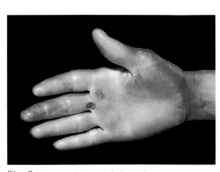

Fig. 2 **Keratoderma of the palm.**

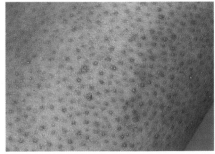

Fig. 3 **Keratosis pilaris on the upper arm.**

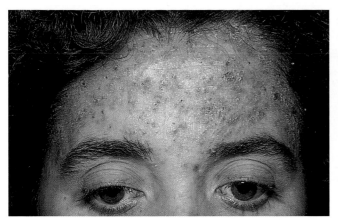

Fig. 4 **Darier's disease affecting the forehead.**

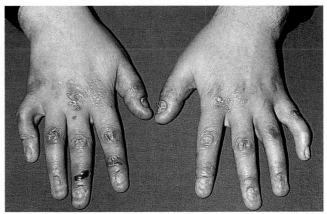

Fig. 5 **Epidermolysis bullosa.** The dystrophic dominant type is shown.

The abnormal gene is sited on chromosome 12q and encodes for calcium adenosine triphosphatase. Keratinocyte tonofilaments and desmosomes are dissociated on electron microscopy.

Clinical presentation
The disease presents in teenagers or young adults, with small brown greasy scaled papules, typically on the flexures, upper back, chest and forehead (Fig. 4). Its onset may follow sunburn. The severity varies from being mild and almost unnoticed to being extensive and severe. Nail changes (p. 66) and palmar pits or keratoses are found. Bacterial infection or eczema herpeticum (p. 34) may occur.

Management
Mild Darier's disease requires topical keratolytics only (e.g. 5% salicylic acid ointment) and advice on sun avoidance. More severe cases are greatly helped by oral acitretin (p. 31).

Flegel's disease
Flegel's disease (hyperkeratosis lenticularis perstans) is a rare, dominantly inherited disorder, characterized by keratotic plugs on the legs and arms. It starts in middle age. When larger plugs are seen, it is called *Kyrle's disease*, but the two types may coexist.

Epidermolysis bullosa
Epidermolysis bullosa (EB) defines a group of genetically inherited diseases characterized by skin fragility and blistering on minimal trauma. They range from being mild and trivial to being incompatible with life (Table 2).

Aetiopathogenesis
Keratin synthesis is defective in simple EB (genes mapped to chromosomes 12

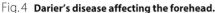

Table 2 **The main types of epidermolysis bullosa (EB)**

Disease	Inheritance	Clinical features
Simple EB	Autosomal dominant	Commonest type. Often mild and limited to hands and feet. Blisters caused by friction. Nails and mouth unaffected
Junctional EB	Autosomal recessive	Rare and often lethal. At birth, large erosions seen around mouth and anus. Slow to heal. No effective treatment
Dystrophic EB	Autosomal dominant	Hands, knees and elbows are affected. Scarring with milia is found. Deformity of the nails may occur
Dystrophic EB	Autosomal recessive	Starts in infancy. Severe blistering results in fusion of fingers and toes, with mucosal lesions and oesophageal stricture

and 17). Collagen VII is abnormal in dystrophic EB (gene sited on chromosome 3). Anchoring fibrils (p. 2) are defective in certain types of EB.

Clinical presentation and management
Simple EB is fairly common and requires avoidance of trauma. The more severe forms (Table 2; Fig. 5) need to be managed in specialized centres. Avoidance of trauma, supportive measures and the control of infection are important. Treatment with various drugs has given disappointing results. *Acquired EB*, with an onset in adult life, shows trauma-induced blistering and resembles pemphigoid on immunofluorescent studies.

Prenatal diagnosis of inherited disorders
DNA-based prenatal diagnosis is now possible for junctional and recessive dystrophic EB, bullous ichthyosiform erythroderma and oculocutaneous albinism. DNA is obtained in the first trimester from chorionic villus samples or amniotic cells. Mid-second trimester fetal skin biopsy is still used for diseases where the gene is unknown but biopsy changes are specific.

Inherited keratinization and blistering disorders

- The **ichthyoses** are inherited disorders of keratinization. The skin is dry and scaly. Emollient therapy is helpful. Certain ichthyoses may present at birth as a collodion baby.
- **Darier's disease** is a rare autosomal dominant condition. Greasy scaly papules are seen on the chest, back and in the flexures. Severe cases are treated with acitretin.
- **Keratoderma** is typified by hyperkeratosis of the palms and soles and is treated by keratolytics.
- **Keratosis pilaris** is a common condition in which horny follicular plugs are seen on the limbs and face. Treatment is difficult; emollients may help.
- **Flegel's disease** is a rare dominantly inherited disorder characterized by keratotic plugs on the legs and arms.
- **Epidermolysis bullosa** describes inherited bullous diseases ranging from mild blistering induced by ill-fitting shoes to severe and lethal blistering present at birth.
- **Prenatal diagnosis** of several rare severe inherited skin diseases is now possible using DNA technology.

http://www.scalyskin.org/   ■   http://www.dermatlas.com/derm/result.cfm?Diagnosis=62

Neurocutaneous disorders and other syndromes

Certain inherited skin disorders also have significant involvement of internal organs. The neurocutaneous disorders, the inherited diseases of connective tissue and the premature ageing syndromes are included.

Neurofibromatosis

von Recklinghausen's neurofibromatosis (NF1) is relatively common, affecting about 1 in 3000 births. Café-au-lait spots, cutaneous neurofibromas and other bony or neurological abnormalities characterize NF1. The disease shows autosomal dominant inheritance, although 50% of cases are new mutations.

Aetiopathogenesis

The *NF1* gene is a tumour suppressor gene, mapped to chromosome 17. This finding offers the prospect of devising a prenatal DNA screening test.

Clinical presentation

The two main cutaneous features are:

- *Café-au-lait spots*: round or oval coffee-coloured macules, due to increased melanin pigment. They often appear in the first year of life. One or two café-au-lait spots are seen in 10% of normal people but, in neurofibromatosis, six or more are usually present. Freckling of the axilla is also found (Fig. 1).
- *Dermal neurofibromas*: small nodules that appear during childhood and increase in number at the time of puberty (Fig. 2). Their number varies from a few to several hundred.

A proportion of patients with NF1 have short stature and macrocephaly. Rare variants of the disease are occasionally seen. The commonest is NF2 (*central neurofibromatosis*) in which patients have bilateral acoustic neuromas but few if any café-au-lait spots or dermal nodules. NF2 also shows autosomal dominant inheritance. The *NF2* gene is on chromosome 22.

Complications

Complications develop in many cases and include the following:

- *Plexiform neurofibromas* are larger than their dermal counterparts and measure up to several centimetres in size. They are associated with

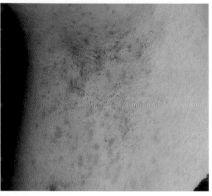

Fig. 1 **Neurofibromatosis showing axillary freckling.**

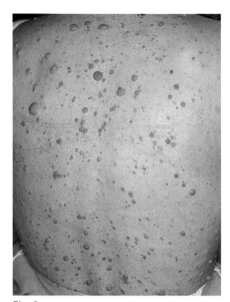

Fig. 2 **Neurofibromatosis.** Multiple neurofibromas are present on the back.

pigmentation and hypertrophy of the overlying skin or underlying bone, and present a cosmetic problem.
- *Benign tumours of the nervous system* may develop. These include optic gliomas, acoustic neuromas and spinal neurofibromas that arise from nerve roots of the spinal cord.
- *Sarcomatous change* in a neurofibroma, typically non-cutaneous, occurs in 1.5–15% of cases.
- *Kyphoscoliosis* (in 2%) or bowing of the tibia and fibula may occur.
- *Other problems* include iris hamartomas, hypertension, epilepsy and learning difficulties.

Management

Once the diagnosis has been made, genetic counselling and the exclusion of any complicating factors are important. Troublesome nodules can be excised,

and larger disfiguring neurofibromas removed by plastic surgery. Patients are often helped by contact with a patient support group (p. 128).

Tuberous sclerosis complex

Tuberous sclerosis complex is a not infrequent autosomal dominant condition of variable expression. About 60–70% of patients are new mutations. Hamartomas occur in several organs. The abnormal genes have been mapped to chromosomes 9 and 16.

Clinical manifestations

The features may not appear until puberty. Patients typically show:

- *Adenoma sebaceum*: red–brown angiofibromatous papules that are usually found around the nose (Fig. 3). They appear in childhood.
- *Periungual fibromas*: pink fibrous projections are seen under the nail folds (Fig. 4).

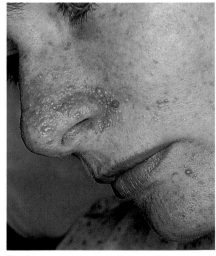

Fig. 3 **Tuberous sclerosis.** Angiofibromas are seen at the sides of the nose.

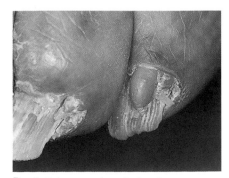

Fig. 4 **Tuberous sclerosis showing periungual fibromas.**

- *Shagreen patches*: connective tissue naevi, soft, yellowish with a cobblestone surface, are found on the lumbosacral region.
- *Ash-leaf macules*: small (1–3 cm long) white oval macules, sometimes present at birth, and best seen with a Wood's light.
- *Neurological involvement*: mental retardation and epilepsy affect more than 70% of cases. Intracranial calcification is seen.
- *Other features*: retinal phacomas, cardiac rhabdomyomas and renal tumours are found.

Management

An affected individual should have a full clinical examination, often with radiographs and magnetic resonance imaging (MRI) scan of the head. Children are screened for ash-leaf macules using a Wood's light. The angiofibromas may be improved by hyfrecation or laser, but tend to recur. Genetic counselling is given once the diagnosis is made. The support group is helpful (p. 128).

Incontinentia pigmenti

Incontinentia pigmenti is a rare X-linked dominant condition that is usually lethal *in utero* in males. In females, it presents within a few days of birth as a widespread blistering eruption (p. 13). Warty papules follow, but are replaced by hyperpigmentation, which appears in a whorled pattern. Skeletal, ocular, neurological and dental abnormalities are associated.

Xeroderma pigmentosum

Xeroderma pigmentosum is a group of rare autosomal recessive conditions characterized by defective repair of ultraviolet (UV)-damaged DNA. Photosensitivity begins in infancy, and freckles and keratoses appear on exposed skin in childhood. Squamous cell and basal cell carcinomas, keratoacanthomas and malignant melanomas subsequently develop in the UV-damaged skin (Fig. 5). Strict sunlight avoidance is necessary but, in its severe form, the disease can be fatal in the first or second decade. The gene loci are known (p. 12). Prenatal diagnosis is possible (p. 89) and is used when parents have already had one affected child.

Ehlers–Danlos syndrome

At least 10 inherited disorders of defective collagen structure and biochemistry are included in this group of conditions (gene loci: p. 12). The diseases may be dominant, recessive or X-linked, and present in varying degrees of severity. The features include:

- elasticity of the skin
- joint hyperextensibility
- skin fragility with bruising and scarring (Fig. 6).

In the more severe types, aneurysms and rupture of large arteries may be found.

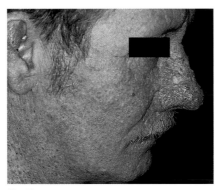

Fig. 5 **Xeroderma pigmentosum.** This patient shows severely sun-damaged skin with freckling, keratoses and scars from excision of tumours.

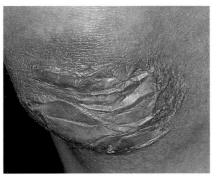

Fig. 6 **Ehlers–Danlos syndrome.** Ugly scarring has resulted from fragile skin and poor wound healing.

Pseudoxanthoma elasticum

Pseudoxanthoma elasticum describes a group of at least five disorders. The inheritance is autosomal recessive. The affected gene controls transmembrane peptide transport and results in calcified elastic fibres. The skin is loose, wrinkled and yellow and contains small papules (resembling xanthomas), giving a 'chicken skin' appearance. These changes are most obvious at the neck and flexures. Angioid streaks in the retina are seen in more than 50% of cases. Arterial involvement may result in gastrointestinal or cerebral haemorrhage.

The premature ageing syndromes

The features of ageing include an increased susceptibility to neoplasia, dementia, diabetes, autoimmune disease, cataracts, premature alopecia and hair greying, osteoporosis and degenerative vascular disease. *Down syndrome* shows several of these stigmata and is the most common condition in which premature ageing occurs. Many of the other disorders of premature ageing, such as *Werner syndrome* or *progeria*, are very rare and often show autosomal recessive inheritance.

Aged skin is dry, wrinkled, atrophic, shows loss of elasticity and uneven pigmentation and is susceptible to develop benign and malignant tumours. Photoageing from chronic sun exposure (p. 102) can produce similar changes, although certain of the features are more prominent. Some conditions, such as pseudoxanthoma elasticum or xeroderma pigmentosum, have the signs of aged skin without necessarily showing more generalized features of ageing.

Neurocutaneous disorders and other syndromes

- **NF1 neurofibromatosis** is a relatively common autosomal dominant condition characterized by café-au-lait spots, dermal neurofibromas and often skeletal or neurological anomalies. The abnormal gene is on chromosome 17.

- **Tuberous sclerosis complex** is a not infrequent autosomal dominant disorder with prominent skin signs (e.g. facial angiofibromas and periungual fibromas), neurological problems (mental retardation and epilepsy) and ocular, cardiac and renal tumours.

- **Incontinentia pigmenti** is a rare X-linked dominant disease, present at birth, which evolves through vesicular and warty stages to leave whorled patterns of pigmentation. Skeletal, ocular and neurological defects are associated.

- **Xeroderma pigmentosum** represents a group of rare recessive conditions showing defects of DNA repair, characterized by skin tumours and premature death.

- **Ehlers–Danlos syndrome** is a group of at least 10 inherited collagen disorders in which skin elasticity and scarring and joint hypermobility are found.

- **Pseudoxanthoma elasticum** represents at least five disorders that result in calcification of elastin. The skin is wrinkled with yellowish papules. Retinal angioid streaks are seen.

Benign tumours

Skin tumours are common, and their incidence is rising in western countries (p. 24). The treatment of skin tumours makes up a large part of current dermatological practice (p. 24). Many skin tumours are benign, and these are described in this section. Viral warts, actinic keratoses and naevi are mentioned elsewhere.

Benign epidermal tumours

Seborrhoeic wart (basal cell papilloma)

A seborrhoeic wart (seborrhoeic keratosis) is a common, usually pigmented, benign tumour consisting of a proliferation of basal keratinocytes (Fig. 1). The cause is unknown, although they may be 'naevoid'. Seborrhoea is not a feature.

Clinical presentation

Seborrhoeic warts have the following features:

- often multiple (Fig. 2), sometimes solitary
- affect the elderly or middle-aged
- mostly found on the trunk and face
- generally round or oval in shape
- start as small papules, often lightly pigmented or yellow
- become darkly pigmented warty nodules 1–6 cm in diameter
- have a 'stuck-on' appearance, with keratin plugs and well-defined edges.

Differential diagnosis

The diagnosis is usually obvious from the physical findings and multiplicity of the lesions. Occasionally, a seborrhoeic wart can resemble an actinic keratosis, melanocytic naevus, pigmented basal cell carcinoma or malignant melanoma.

Management

Multiple lesions can be adequately dealt with using liquid nitrogen cryotherapy. Thicker seborrhoeic warts are best treated by curettage or shave biopsy, with cautery or hyfrecation. If there is doubt about the diagnosis, excision and histological examination are advised.

Skin tags

Skin tags are pedunculated benign fibroepithelial polyps, a few millimetres in length. They are common, mainly seen in the elderly or middle-aged, and show a predilection for the neck, axillae, groin and eyelids (Fig. 3). The cause is unknown, but they are often found in obese individuals. Occasionally, skin tags are confused with small melanocytic naevi or seborrhoeic warts. The

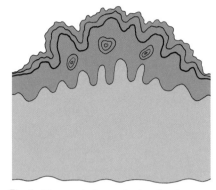

Fig. 1 **Histopathology of seborrhoeic wart.** The illustration shows a hyperkeratotic epidermis, thickened by basal cell proliferation, with keratin cysts.

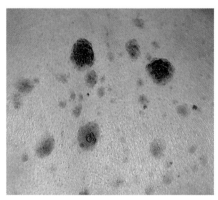

Fig. 2 **Seborrhoeic warts on the trunk, with a few small Campbell-de-Morgan spots.**

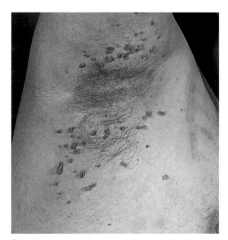

Fig. 3 **Skin tags in the axilla.**

treatment, usually for cosmetic reasons, is by snipping the stalk with scissors or cutting through it with a hyfrecator (under local anaesthetic if necessary), or using cryotherapy.

Epidermal (epidermoid) cyst

Epidermal cysts, usually seen on the scalp, face or trunk, are sometimes incorrectly called sebaceous cysts. They are keratin filled and derived from the epidermis or, in the case of the related pilar cyst, the outer root sheath of the hair follicle. The cysts are firm, skin coloured, mobile and normally 1–3 cm in diameter. Bacterial infection is a complication. Excision is curative.

Milium

Milia are mostly seen on the face, where they typically appear as small white keratin cysts (1–2 mm in size) around the eyelids and on the upper cheeks. They are often seen in children, but may appear at any age. Occasionally, milia may develop as part of healing after a subepidermal blister, e.g. with porphyria cutanea tarda. Milial cysts can normally be extracted using a sterile needle.

Benign dermal tumours

Dermatofibroma (fibrous histiocytoma)

Dermatofibromas are common dermal nodules, and are usually asymptomatic. Histologically, they show a proliferation of histiocytes and fibroblasts, with dermal fibrosis and sometimes epidermal hyperplasia. They may represent a reaction pattern to an insect bite or other trauma, although often no such history is obtained.

Clinical presentation

Dermatofibromas are usually seen in young adults, most commonly women, and mainly occur on the lower legs. They are firm, dermal nodules 5–10 mm in diameter and may be pigmented (Fig. 4). They enlarge slowly, if at all.

Management

A pigmented dermatofibroma may be confused with a melanocytic naevus or a malignant melanoma. Excision of symptomatic or diagnostically doubtful lesions is recommended.

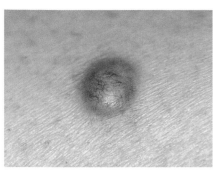

Fig. 4 **Dermatofibroma on the lower leg.**

Pyogenic granuloma

A pyogenic granuloma is a rapidly developing bright red or blood-crusted nodule that may be confused with a malignant melanoma. It is neither pyogenic nor granulomatous, but is an acquired haemangioma.

Clinical presentation

A pyogenic granuloma typically:

- develops at a site of trauma, e.g. a prick from a thorn
- presents as a bright red, sometimes pedunculated, nodule 5–10 mm in diameter that bleeds easily (Fig. 5)
- enlarges rapidly over 2–3 weeks
- is seen on a finger (also on lip, face and foot)
- occurs in young adults or children.

Management

Curettage and cautery, or excision, is needed. The specimen is sent for histological examination to exclude a malignant melanoma. Not infrequently, a pyogenic granuloma may recur after curettage.

Keloid

A keloid is an excessive proliferation of connective tissue in response to skin trauma and differs from a hypertrophic scar because it extends beyond the limit of the original injury. Keloids show the following characteristics:

- present as protuberant and firm smooth nodules or plaques (Fig. 6)
- occur mainly over the upper back, neck, chest and ear lobes
- develop more commonly in black Africans
- have their highest incidence in the second to fourth decades.

Treatment is with topical silicone gel or steroid injection (p. 21).

Campbell-de-Morgan spot (cherry angioma)

Campbell-de-Morgan spots are benign capillary proliferations, commonly seen as small bright-red papules on the trunk in elderly or middle-aged patients (see Fig. 2). If necessary, they can be removed by hyfrecation or cautery.

Tumours of the skin appendages

Tumours of the skin appendages, i. e. of the eccrine and apocrine sweat ducts, hair follicles and sebaceous glands, are relatively rare. Clinically, they often present as rather non-specific cutaneous nodules, and they are difficult to diagnose without histology following excision. Occasionally, these tumours are malignant.

Lipoma

Lipomas are benign tumours of fat, and present as soft masses in the subcutaneous tissue. They are often multiple and are mostly found on the trunk, neck and upper extremities. Sometimes they are painful. Removal is rarely needed.

Chondrodermatitis nodularis

Chondrodermatitis nodularis is not a neoplasm, but presents as a painful small nodule on the upper rim of the helix of the pinna, usually in elderly men (p. 114). It is due to inflammation in the cartilage that may be a response to degenerative changes in the dermis induced by chronic sun exposure. They are often confused with basal cell carcinomas. Excision is curative.

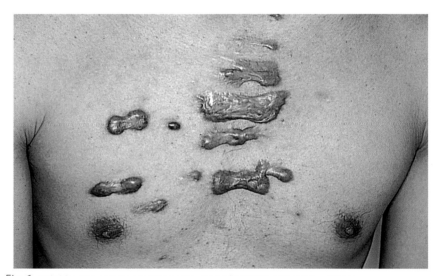

Fig. 6 **Keloids.** The nodules are seen on the chest of a patient with a history of acne.

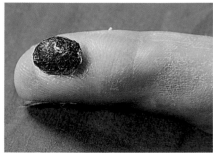

Fig. 5 **Pyogenic granuloma on the finger.**

Benign tumours		
Lesion	**Age at onset**	**Main features**
Epidermal		
Viral wart	Childhood mainly	Usually on hands or feet (p. 50)
Actinic keratosis	Old age	Sun-exposed areas (p. 102)
Seborrhoeic wart	Old/middle age	Keratosis, often on trunk or face
Milia	Childhood	White cysts, often on face
Epidermal cyst	After childhood	Mostly on face or scalp
Skin tags	Middle/old age	Seen on neck, axillae and groin
Dermal		
Dermatofibroma	Young adult, F > M	Nodule, often on leg
Melanocytic naevus	Teens/young adult	Brown macule or papule (p. 94)
Cherry angioma	Old/middle age	Small red papule on trunk
Pyogenic granuloma	Child/young adult	Red nodule, often on finger
Keloid	Second–fourth decades	Chest/neck, affects black Africans
Lipoma	Any age	Soft tumour on trunk or limbs
Chondrodermatitis nodularis	Old/middle age	Nodule on upper pinna, M > F

http://www.aafp.org/afp/20030215/729.html

Naevi

A naevus is a benign proliferation of one or more of the normal constituent cells of the skin. Naevi may be present at birth or may develop later. The commonest naevi are those containing benign collections of melanocytic naevus cells, but other types of naevi are found (Table 1).

Melanocytic naevi

Melanocytic naevi ('moles') are common. They are present in most caucasoids but are less prevalent in mongoloids and black Africans.

Aetiopathogenesis and pathology

The naevus cells in melanocytic naevi are thought to be derived from melanocytes that migrate to the epidermis from the neural crest during embryonic development (p. 3). The reason for the development of naevi is unknown, but they seem to be an inherited trait in many families.

The position of the naevus cells within the dermis determines the type of naevus (Fig. 1). The junctional type has clusters of naevus cells at the dermoepidermal junction, the intradermal type has nests of naevus cells in the dermis, and the compound naevus shows both components.

Naevus cells produce melanin and, if the pigment is deep in the dermis, an optical effect can give the lesion a blue colour, as in a blue naevus.

Clinical presentation

A congenital naevus, that is one present at or soon after birth, is seen in about 1–3% of infants, but most naevi develop during childhood or adolescence. Their number reaches a peak in the third decade, and they tend to become less numerous thereafter. However, it is not unusual to see a few new naevi appear after the third decade, especially if provoked by excessive sun exposure or pregnancy. The average young white adult has between 20 and 50 melanocytic naevi. The clinical features are as follows:

- *Congenital naevi.* Present at or shortly after birth, they are usually more than 1 cm in size, vary in colour from light brown to black and often become protuberant and hairy. They can be disfiguring, as in the rare bathing trunk naevus, and carry a lifetime risk of up to 5% for the development of malignant melanoma (p. 96).
- *Junctional naevi.* These are flat macules, varying in size from 2 to 10 mm and in colour from light to dark brown (Fig. 2). They are usually round or oval in shape and have a predilection for the palms, soles and genitalia.
- *Intradermal naevi.* The intradermal naevus is a dome-shaped papule or nodule that may be skin coloured or pigmented, and is most often seen on the face or neck.
- *Compound naevi.* Compound naevi are usually less than 10 mm in diameter, have a smooth surface and vary in their degree of pigmentation (Fig. 3). Larger lesions may develop a warty or cerebriform appearance. They may occur anywhere on the skin surface.
- *Spitz naevi.* A Spitz naevus is a firm, reddish-brown, rounded nodule seen typically on the face or leg of a child. The initial growth may be rapid. Histologically, the naevus cells are proliferative, and the dermal blood vessels are dilated.
- *Blue naevi.* This variant, so-called because of its steely-blue colour, is usually solitary and is most common on the extremities, particularly the hands and feet.
- *Halo naevi.* Halo (or Sutton's) naevi are mainly seen on the trunk in children or adolescents and represent the destruction, by the body's immune system, of naevus cells in a naevus. A white halo of depigmentation surrounds the pre-existing naevus that subsequently involutes (Fig. 4).

Table 1	**A classification of naevi**	
Group	**Example**
Melanocytic	Congenital (p. 96)
	Junctional
	Intradermal
	Compound
	Spitz
	Blue
	Halo
	Becker's
	Dysplastic (p. 96)
Vascular	Salmon patch (p. 112)
	Port wine stain (p. 112)
	Strawberry (p. 112)
	Cavernous haemangioma
Epidermal	Warty naevus
Connective tissue	Tuberous sclerosis (p. 90)

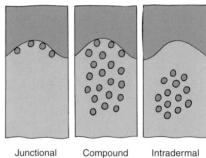

| Junctional | Compound | Intradermal |

Fig. 1 **Types of melanocytic naevi.** The site of the naevus cells, either at the dermoepidermal junction or in the dermis, or at both places, determines the type of melanocytic naevus.

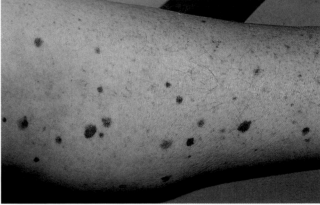

Fig. 2 **Multiple junctional (and compound) naevi on the lower leg.**

This may be due to antimelanocyte autoimmune attack. There is an association with vitiligo. Multiple halos often appear simultaneously.

- *Becker's naevi.* This rare variant usually develops in adolescent males as a unilateral lesion on the upper back or chest (Fig. 5). Hyperpigmented at first, it later becomes hairy and is prone to acne. It may represent mosaicism.
- *Dysplastic naevi.* Dysplastic naevi show some irregularity in outline and in pigmentation (p. 97).

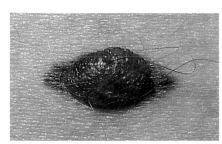

Fig. 3 **A compound melanocytic naevus.**

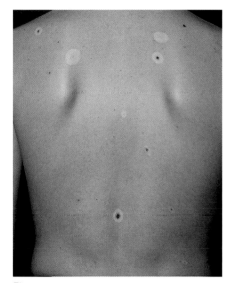

Fig. 4 **Multiple halo naevi on the back of an adolescent.**

Management

Over recent years, publicity in the media and in public health campaigns has promoted the early diagnosis of malignant melanoma. This has led to a greater public awareness about the significance of change in pigmented lesions, and many patients are now referred because of concern about their 'moles'. Any change merits serious attention (p. 96). The differential diagnosis of melanocytic naevi is shown in Table 2. Naevi are excised because of:

■ *concern about malignancy*, e.g. recent increase in size or itching
■ *an increased risk of malignant change*, e.g. in a large congenital naevus
■ *cosmetic reasons*, e.g. ugly naevi, usually on the face or neck
■ *repeated inflammation*, e.g. bacterial folliculitis, often in hairy facial naevi
■ *recurrent trauma*, e.g. naevi on the back that catch on bra straps.

All excised naevi should be sent for histology. Some clearly benign protuberant naevi, to be removed for cosmetic reasons, can be dealt with by shave biopsy (p. 106).

Epidermal naevi

Epidermal naevi are usually present at birth or develop in early childhood. They are warty, often pigmented and frequently linear (Fig. 6). Most are a few centimetres long, but they can be much larger and involve the length of a limb or the side of the trunk. They can be excised, but recurrence is common. A variant on the scalp, *naevus sebaceus*, carries a risk of malignant transformation and should be excised.

Connective tissue naevi

Connective tissue naevi are rare. They appear as smooth, skin-coloured papules or plaques and may be multiple. Coarse collagen bundles are seen in the dermis on histology. An example is the collagen-containing cobblestone naevus (shagreen patch) seen in tuberous sclerosis (p. 90).

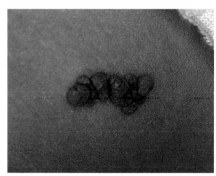

Fig. 6 **An epidermal naevus on the thigh.**

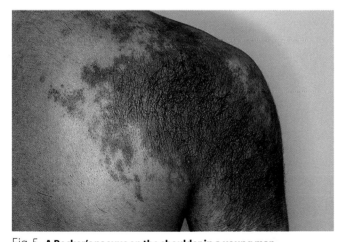

Fig. 5 **A Becker's naevus on the shoulder in a young man.**

Table 2 **Differential diagnosis of melanocytic naevi**	
Lesion	**Distinguishing features**
Freckle	Tan-coloured macules on sun-exposed sites (p. 73)
Lentigine	Usually multiple, onset in later life (p. 73)
Seborrhoeic wart	Stuck-on appearance, warty lesions, may show keratin plugs, but easily confused (p. 92)
Haemangioma	Vascular but may show pigmentation
Dermatofibroma	On legs, elevated nodule, firm and pigmented (p. 92)
Pigmented basal cell carcinoma	Often on face, pearly edge, increase in size, can ulcerate, other photodamage may coexist
Malignant melanoma	Variable colour and outline, may have increased in size, be inflamed, bled or be itchy (p. 96)

Naevi

■ **Melanocytic naevi** are very common, usually multiple, pigmented and benign. They appear during childhood or adolescence. Young white adults have 20–50. Variants include:

– *Congenital naevi* are present at birth, may be protuberant or hairy and have a small risk of malignant change.

– *Junctional naevi* are flat macules, often round or oval. Typically found on soles, palms or genitalia.

– *Intradermal naevi* are dome-shaped, usually skin-coloured papules. Typically seen on the face.

– *Compound naevi* are pigmented nodules or papules, sometimes warty or hairy. Histology shows junctional and dermal components.

– *Spitz naevi* are firm reddish-brown nodules typically seen on the face or legs in children.

– *Blue naevi* are steely-blue in colour due to melanin in the deep dermis. They are mainly solitary and found on the extremities.

– *Halo naevi* show depigmentation where a naevus has involuted due to autoimmune attack. Mostly seen on the trunk.

– *Becker's naevi* are pigmented hairy lesions on the upper back or chest, usually in males and appearing in adolescence.

■ **Epidermal naevi** are warty, pigmented and often linear. Usually small, they are sometimes extensive. A scalp variant, *naevus sebaceus*, should be excised as it has malignant potential.

■ **Connective tissue naevi** are skin-coloured papules composed of coarse collagen in the dermis. They can occur as cobblestone naevi (shagreen patches) in tuberous sclerosis.

Malignant melanoma

Malignant melanoma is a malignant tumour of melanocytes, usually arising in the epidermis. It is the most lethal of the main skin tumours and has increased in incidence over the last three decades. Malignant melanoma has received attention from public education campaigns, particularly because of its putative relationship to episodes of excessive ultraviolet radiation exposure. Genetics may be important, and up to 5% of patients have a family history of malignant melanoma.

Clinical presentation

Four main clinicopathological variants are recognized. These are described below.

Superficial spreading malignant melanoma

This type accounts for 50% of all British cases, shows a female preponderance and is commonest on the lower leg. The tumour is macular and shows variable pigmentation, often with regression (Fig. 1).

Lentigo malignant melanoma

Malignant melanoma developing in a longstanding lentigo maligna (Fig. 2) constitutes 15% of UK cases. A lentigo maligna arises in sun-damaged skin often on the face of an elderly person who has spent many years in an outdoor occupation.

Acral lentiginous malignant melanoma

The acral lentiginous type makes up 1 10 of British cases, but is the commone form in dark-skinned races. The tumou

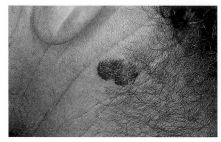

Fig. 1 **Superficial spreading malignant melanoma.**

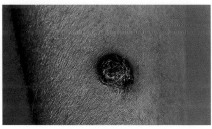

Fig. 4 **Nodular malignant melanoma.**

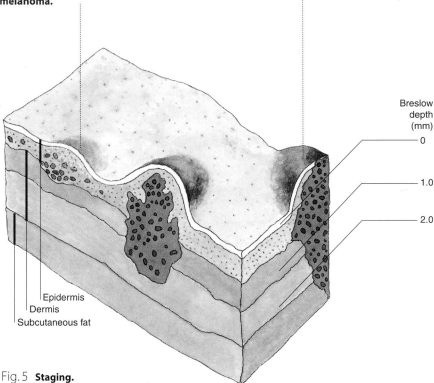

Breslow depth (mm)
0
1.0
2.0

Epidermis
Dermis
Subcutaneous fat

Fig. 5 **Staging.**

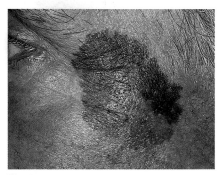

Fig. 2 **Lentigo maligna showing irregular outline and pigmentation.**

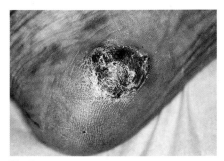

Fig. 3 **Acral lentiginous malignant melanoma.**

affects the palms, soles (Fig. 3) and nail beds, is often diagnosed late and has poor survival figures.

Nodular malignant melanoma

The nodular variant is seen in 25% of British patients; it shows a male preponderance and is commonest on the trunk. The pigmented nodule (Fig. 4) may grow rapidly and ulcerate.

Epidemiology

Malignant melanoma has an incidence in the UK of 15–20 per 100 000 population per year. The incidence has been rising at 7% each year and has trebled in the last two decades. It occurs in all races, but is particularly a problem in caucasoids, in whom it becomes much more common the closer the population lives to the equator. In the UK, women are affected twice as frequently as men. Superficial spreading and nodular melanomas tend to occur in those in the 20- to 60-year age group, whereas lentigo malignant melanomas mostly affect those over 60 years old. In males, the commonest site is the back; in females, it is the lower leg (about half occur here).

Staging

Malignant melanomas usually, although not invariably, progress through two stages (Fig. 5), horizontal and vertical. The *horizontal* phase of malignant melanocytic growth within the epidermis may evolve into a stage of dermal involvement and *vertical* growth.

Local invasion by the tumour is assessed using the *Breslow method*, which is the measurement in millimetres of the distance between the granular cell layer to the deepest identifiable melanoma cell. Metastasis is uncommon in tumours restricted to the epidermis.

Aetiopathogenesis

The cause of malignant melanoma is not known, but repeated short, intensive exposure to ultraviolet radiation, e.g. on sun-seeking holidays, may be involved. Major risk factors are shown in Figure 6. Histological evidence of a pre-existing melanocytic naevus is found in 30% of malignant melanomas but, with the exception of dysplastic or congenital naevi (Fig. 7), the risk of change in a common melanocytic naevus is small.

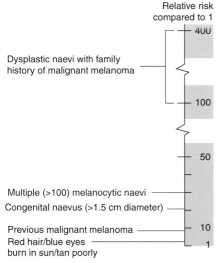

Fig. 6 **Major risk factors.** The major risk factors and their relative risk for the development of malignant melanoma are shown.

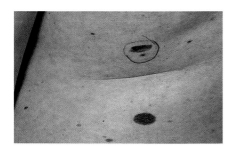

Fig. 7 **Dysplastic naevus syndrome.** This condition, which may be familial, is characterized by large numbers of atypical and 'dysplastic' naevi, which are often over 7 mm in diameter with an irregular edge and variable pigmentation. Affected individuals have a greatly increased risk of developing malignant melanoma. They should avoid the sun and be closely observed. Changing or suspicious pigmented lesions should be excised for histological examination.

Diagnosis

Any of the following changes in a naevus or pigmented lesion may suggest malignant melanoma:

- *size*: usually a recent increase
- *shape*: irregular in outline
- *colour*: variation, darker or lighter
- *inflammation*: may be at the edge
- *crusting*: some ooze or bleed
- *itch*: a common symptom.

The *differential diagnosis* of malignant melanoma includes:

- benign melanocytic naevus (p. 94)
- seborrhoeic wart (p. 92)
- haemangioma (p. 93)
- dermatofibroma (p. 92)
- pigmented basal cell carcinoma
- benign lentigo (p. 73).

Prognosis

The prognosis relates to the tumour depth. Tumours can be divided into three prognosis groups: good (thickness < 1 mm), intermediate (1–4 mm) and poor (> 4 mm). The approximate 5-year survival rates are:

- < 1 mm   95%
- 1–2 mm   90%
- 2.1–4 mm   77%
- > 4 mm   65%

Examples of thin and thick tumours are given in Figures 8 and 9.

Management

The primary treatment is surgical excision. Tumours up to 1 mm thick

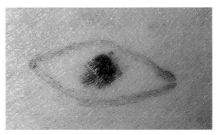

Fig. 8 **A thin (0.8-mm Breslow thickness) superficial spreading malignant melanoma with a good prognosis.**

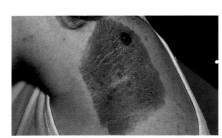

Fig. 9 **A thick (11-mm Breslow thickness) nodular malignant melanoma developing within a large congenital naevus.** Local lymph nodes were involved; the prognosis was poor.

require a 1-cm margin, those of 1–2 mm thickness need a 2-cm margin, and thicker tumours require a 3-cm clearance. A skin graft may be necessary to close the defect. Regular follow-up is needed to detect any recurrence, of which there are three main types:

- *local* (Fig. 10)
- *lymphatic* – either in the regional lymph nodes or in transit in the lymphatics draining from the tumour to the nodes
- *blood-borne* to distant sites.

Routine sentinel node biopsy (p. 111) or elective lymph node dissection is not recommended as a standard procedure at present. Radiotherapy is of limited use. Interferon-alpha may increase survival in patients with tumours more than 1.5 mm thick.

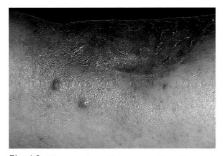

Fig. 10 **Hypomelanotic recurrent malignant melanoma.** Pink papules of recurrent tumour are evident at the edge of a previously excised and grafted site.

Prevention and public education

Early malignant melanoma is a curable disease, but thick lesions have a poor prognosis. Public health education should encourage early visits to the doctor for changing pigmented lesions and should discourage excessive sun exposure, especially in fair-skinned individuals or those with numerous melanocytic naevi. The best advice is:

- avoid burning in the sun
- report early any change in a mole.

> ### Malignant melanoma
>
> - The UK incidence is 15–20 per 100 000 per year.
> - The female to male ratio is 2:1.
> - The incidence has risen by 7% per year and doubled in the past two decades.
> - The incidence is proportional to the geographical latitude, suggesting an effect of ultraviolet radiation.
> - The prognosis is related to tumour thickness. Early lesions are curable by surgical excision.

Malignant epidermal tumours

Malignant skin tumours are among the most common of all cancers. They are more frequent in light-skinned races, and ultraviolet radiation seems to be involved in their aetiology. The incidence of *non-melanoma skin cancer* in caucasoids in the USA was recently estimated at 230 per 100 000 per year, compared with 3 per 100 000 for African Americans. The majority of malignant skin tumours (Table 1) are epidermal in origin and are either basal cell or squamous cell carcinomas or malignant melanomas (p. 96). Premalignant epidermal conditions are common (p. 100), but dermal malignancies are comparatively rare.

Basal cell carcinoma

Basal cell carcinomas (rodent ulcers) are the commonest form of skin cancer and are typically seen on the face in elderly or middle-aged subjects. They arise from the basal keratinocytes of the epidermis, are locally invasive, but very rarely metastasize.

Aetiopathogenesis

Malignant transformation of basal cells may be induced by:

- prolonged ultraviolet exposure (and acute sunburn)
- arsenic ingestion, e.g. in 'tonics' or in drinking water
- X-rays and other ionizing radiation
- chronic scarring, e.g. burns or vaccination scars
- genetic predisposition, e.g. basal cell naevus syndrome.

Basal cell carcinomas are most common in caucasoids with a fair 'celtic' skin who live near the equator, and are seen more in males than in females. In the UK, they mainly occur in those over the age of 40 years, although, in Australia, they may be seen in the third decade.

Pathology

The tumour is classically composed of uniform basophilic cells, in well-defined islands, that invade the dermis from the epidermis as buds, lobules or strands (Fig. 1).

Clinical presentation

Basal cell carcinomas occur mainly on light-exposed sites, commonly around the nose, the inner canthus of the eyelids and the temple. They grow slowly but relentlessly, are locally invasive and may destroy cartilage, bone and soft tissue structures. A lesion has often been present for 2 years or more before the patient seeks advice. Often more than one tumour is evident. There are four main types of basal cell carcinoma, all of which may occasionally be pigmented:

- *Nodular.* This is the commonest type of lesion and usually starts as a small, skin-coloured papule that shows fine telangiectasia and a glistening pearly

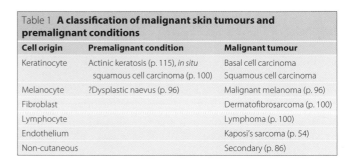

Table 1 **A classification of malignant skin tumours and premalignant conditions**

Cell origin	Premalignant condition	Malignant tumour
Keratinocyte	Actinic keratosis (p. 115), *in situ* squamous cell carcinoma (p. 100)	Basal cell carcinoma Squamous cell carcinoma
Melanocyte	?Dysplastic naevus (p. 96)	Malignant melanoma (p. 96)
Fibroblast		Dermatofibrosarcoma (p. 100)
Lymphocyte		Lymphoma (p. 100)
Endothelium		Kaposi's sarcoma (p. 54)
Non-cutaneous		Secondary (p. 86)

Lobules and islands of basal cell carcinoma

Invading strands of squamous cell carcinoma

Fig. 1 **The histological structure of a basal cell carcinoma and a squamous cell carcinoma.**

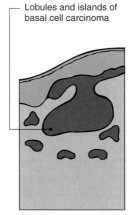

Fig. 2 **Basal cell carcinoma.** The lesion shows the typical pearly edge, telangiectasia and central crusting.

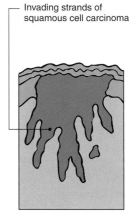

Fig. 3 **Basal cell carcinoma of the superficial multifocal type.** This was located on the trunk. A biopsy (scar visible) confirmed the diagnosis.

edge (Fig. 2). Central necrosis often occurs and leaves a small ulcer with an adherent crust. They are mostly less than 1 cm in diameter, but grow larger if present for several years.
- *Cystic.* These become tense and translucent and show cystic spaces on histology.
- *Multicentric.* Superficial tumours, often multiple, plaque-like and several centimetres in diameter, are sometimes seen especially on the trunk (Fig. 3). They have a rim-like edge and are frequently lightly pigmented.

- *Morphoeic.* This scarring (cicatricial) variant, most common on the face, often shows a white or yellow morphoea-like plaque that may be centrally depressed.

Differential diagnosis

The differential diagnosis depends on the type, pigmentation and location of the basal cell carcinoma:

- *Nodular/cystic*: intradermal naevus (p. 94), molluscum contagiosum (p. 50), keratoacanthoma (p. 100), squamous cell carcinoma, sebaceous hyperplasia (a benign proliferation of sebaceous glands).

- *Multicentric*: discoid eczema (p. 36), psoriatic plaque (p. 28), *in situ* squamous cell carcinoma (p. 100).
- *Morphoeic*: morphoea (p. 78), scar.
- *Pigmented*: malignant melanoma (p. 96), seborrhoeic wart (p. 92), compound naevus (p. 94).

Management

The most appropriate treatment for any one tumour depends on its size, site, type and the patient's age. If possible, complete *excision* is the best treatment, as this allows a histological check on the adequacy of removal. If excision is difficult or not possible, incisional biopsy (to confirm the diagnosis) and *radiotherapy* are suitable for those aged 60 years and over. Large tumours around the eye and the nasolabial fold, especially if of the morphoeic type, are best managed by surgical excision. *Mohs' micrographic surgery* (p. 108) may be employed, as the margins of these tumours are often difficult to determine and may be extensive. *Curettage and cautery* is sometimes used for lesions on the trunk or upper extremities. *Cryosurgery* or topical *imiquimod* (p. 111) are acceptable modalities for multiple, superficial lesions, e.g. on the trunk.

The recurrence rate is about 5% at 5 years for most methods of treatment. Follow-up is particularly important if there is concern about the adequacy of treatment.

Squamous cell carcinoma

Squamous cell carcinoma is a malignant tumour, derived from keratinocytes, which usually arises in an area of sun-damaged skin. It mainly occurs in white-skinned people over 55 years of age, is three times more common in males than in females and may metastasize.

Aetiopathogenesis

Squamous cell carcinoma is derived from moderately well-differentiated keratinocytes. Predisposing factors include:

- chronic actinic damage, accumulating over a lifetime of sun exposure (p. 102); psoralen with ultraviolet A (PUVA) treatment can predispose
- X-rays or other ionizing radiation; radiant heat (e.g. from a fire; see erythema ab igne, p. 68)
- chronic ulceration and scarring (e.g. a burn, lupus vulgaris or discoid lupus erythematosus)
- smoking pipes and cigars (relevant for lip lesions)
- industrial carcinogens (e.g. coal tars, oils)
- human papilloma (wart) virus and immunosuppression, e.g. in renal transplant patients (p. 55)
- genetic (e.g. albinos, xeroderma pigmentosum, p. 90).

Pathology

The malignant keratinocytes, which retain the ability to produce keratin, destroy the dermoepidermal junction and invade the dermis in an irregular manner (Fig. 1).

Clinical presentation

Squamous cell carcinomas usually develop in sun-exposed sites such as the face, neck, forearm or hand. The tumour may start within an actinic keratosis as a small papule that, if left, progresses to ulcerate and form a crust. This type of squamous cell carcinoma does not commonly metastasize. The nodular type of squamous cell carcinoma develops as a dome-shaped nodule sometimes, but not invariably, in sun-damaged skin (Fig. 4). Its shape

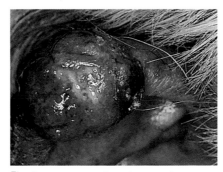

Fig. 4 **Squamous cell carcinoma.** The cancer is seen here on the upper pinna in a patient with actinically damaged skin.

differentiates it from the keratosis-derived variety. More aggressive ulcerating forms of squamous cell carcinoma are seen developing at the edge of ulcers (Fig. 5), in scars and at sites of radiation damage. Metastasis is found in 10% or more of these cancers.

Differential diagnosis

A squamous cell carcinoma needs to be distinguished from keratoacanthoma, actinic keratosis, basal cell carcinoma, *in situ* squamous cell carcinoma, amelanotic malignant melanoma and seborrhoeic keratosis. Excisional or incisional biopsy is needed in every case to confirm the diagnosis or adequacy of excision.

Management

Surgical excision is the treatment of choice. Large lesions may require a skin graft. In the elderly, squamous cell carcinomas of the face or scalp can be treated by *radiotherapy* (after an incisional biopsy for histological diagnosis). Patients are examined for lymph node metastasis at presentation; suspicious nodes are biopsied. Prognosis relates to tumour thickness.

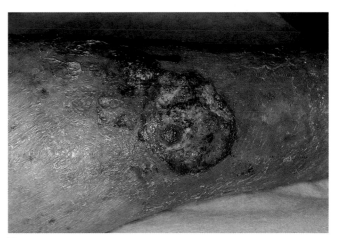

Fig. 5 **Squamous cell carcinoma on the lower leg.** The tumour occurred at the site of a longstanding ulcer.

Malignant epidermal tumours

- **Basal cell carcinoma** (rodent ulcer) is a common tumour often seen on the face in elderly or middle-aged patients who may have had excessive sun exposure. It:
  – is locally invasive but almost never metastasizes
  – is best removed by surgical excision with an adequate margin
  – can be treated by radiotherapy, by curettage and cautery, using cryosurgery or with topical imiquimod in certain biopsy-proven tumours.
- **Squamous cell carcinoma** is often seen in the sun-exposed skin of white people in association with signs of actinic damage. A more aggressive form of the tumour is found with chronic scarring. All types are treated by surgical excision. Prognosis relates to tumour thickness.

Premalignant epidermal disorders and malignant dermal tumours

Most premalignant epidermal conditions occur in sun-exposed sites, and ultraviolet radiation seems to play a role in their aetiology. Malignant tumours of the dermis are infrequent. The commonest causes are *secondary deposits* (p. 86), *Kaposi's sarcoma* (p. 54), a malignant tumour of dermal fibroblasts (*dermatofibrosarcoma*) and *cutaneous T-cell lymphoma*.

In situ squamous cell carcinoma (Bowen's disease)

In situ squamous cell carcinoma is common and typically occurs on the lower leg in elderly women. The lesions are solitary or multiple. Previous exposure to arsenicals predisposes to the condition.

Pink or lightly pigmented scaly plaques, up to several centimetres in size, are found on the lower leg or trunk (Fig. 1). Transformation into invasive squamous cell carcinoma is infrequent. Bowen's disease may resemble discoid eczema, psoriasis or superficial basal cell carcinoma. Histologically, the epidermis is thickened and the keratinocytes are atypical, but not invasive.

After histological confirmation, the area is treated by cryotherapy, curettage, excision, topical 5-fluorouracil, diclofenac or imiquimod, or photodynamic therapy (p. 109).

Keratoacanthoma

A keratoacanthoma is a rapidly growing tumour usually arising in the sun-exposed skin of the face or arms (Fig. 2); it is not normally regarded as malignant. The tumour grows rapidly over a few weeks into a dome-shaped nodule up to 2 cm in diameter. There is often a keratin plug, which may fall out to leave a crater. Spontaneous resolution will occur but takes several months and leaves an unpleasant scar.

Histologically, a keratoacanthoma may resemble a squamous cell carcinoma, although it shows more symmetry and shouldering. Excision is the preferred treatment, but thorough curettage and cautery will usually be satisfactory. If recurrence occurs after curettage, excision is recommended.

Cutaneous T-cell lymphoma (CTCL: mycosis fungoides)

CTCL describes a lymphoma that evolves in the skin, although extracutaneous T-cell tumours often produce secondary skin deposits. CTCL is a slowly progressive tumour of CD3+, CD 4+ T lymphocytes that becomes systemic only in its terminal stage.

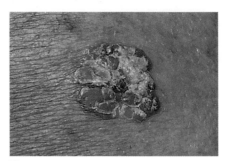

Fig. 1 *In situ* **squamous cell carcinoma on the lower leg.**

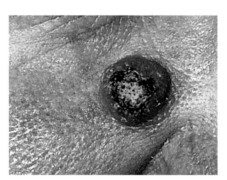

Fig. 2 **Keratoacanthoma on the face.**

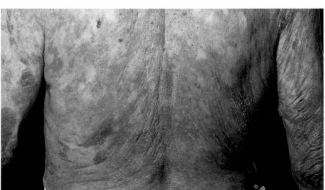

Fig. 3 **Cutaneous T-cell lymphoma showing infiltrated plaques on the back and arms.**

The course is usually protracted, although it is occasionally more rapidly progressive. The diagnosis may be secured only after repeated skin biopsy. CTCL can be regarded as having four stages, namely:

- *Patch stage.* In this phase, there are small scaly erythematosus patches, typically on the trunk (p. 40), that can resemble eczema. It may persist for 10 years or more. Occasionally, the skin becomes atrophic, pigmented and telangiectatic (poikiloderma).
- *Infiltrated plaques.* Fixed plaques develop, usually on the trunk but sometimes more widely distributed (Fig. 3). This stage may last for years.
- *Tumour stage.* This later phase, characterized by tumorous nodules or ulcers within the plaques, has a 5-year survival of 40–65%.
- *Systemic disease.* Involvement of lymph nodes or internal organs is a late finding. The Sézary syndrome (p. 42) is a variant of this phase.

Current treatment is not curative but aimed at controlling the lymphoma. The patch-stage lesions often improve with moderately potent topical steroids and ultraviolet B therapy. More infiltrated plaques require psoralen with UVA (PUVA), topical nitrogen mustard, photopheresis (p. 110) or electron beam therapy. Localized nodules or tumours respond to conventional radiotherapy. Oral bexarotene (p. 110) helps 50% of cases.

Premalignant epidermal disorders and malignant dermal tumours

- *In situ* **squamous cell carcinoma** is a common premalignant condition seen as a scaly plaque often on the lower leg or trunk. Treatment is by cryotherapy, excision or topical 5-fluorouracil, diclofenac or imiquimod.

- **Keratoacanthoma** is a rapidly growing dome-shaped tumour on the face or arm, which often shows a central keratin plug. Treatment is by excision or curettage.

- **Cutaneous T-cell lymphoma** is an uncommon condition resulting from malignant T lymphocytes. It progresses through patch stage to indurated plaques, and then to tumours and systemic involvement. Treatment involves several modalities and requires a specialized team approach.

Special Topics in Dermatology

Ultraviolet radiation and the skin

An interaction between skin and sunlight is inescapable. The potential for harm depends on the type and length of exposure. Photoageing is a growing problem, because of an increasingly aged population and a rise in the average individual exposure to ultraviolet (UV) radiation.

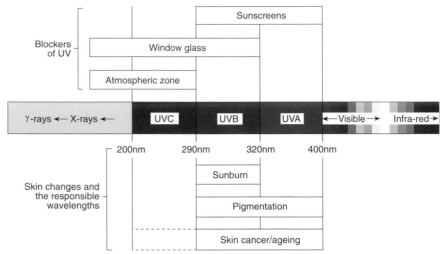

Fig. 1 **The sun's emission spectrum.**

The electromagnetic radiation spectrum

The sun's emission of electromagnetic radiation ranges from low-wavelength ionizing cosmic, gamma and X-rays to the non-ionizing UV, visible and infrared higher wavelengths (Fig. 1). The ozone layer absorbs UVC, but UVA and smaller amounts of UVB reach ground level. UV radiation is maximal in the middle of the day (11.00 to 15.00 h) and is increased by reflection from snow, water and sand. UVA penetrates the epidermis to reach the dermis. UVB is mostly absorbed by the stratum corneum – only 10% reaches the dermis. Most window glass absorbs UV less than 320 nm in wavelength. Artificial UV sources emit in the UVB or UVA spectrum. Sunbeds largely emit UVA.

Effects of light on normal skin

Physiological
UVB promotes the synthesis of vitamin D3 from its precursors in the skin, and UVA and UVB stimulate immediate pigmentation (due to photo-oxidation of melanin precursors), melanogenesis and epidermal thickening as a protective measure against UV damage (p. 7).

Sunburn
If enough UVB is given, erythema always results. The threshold dose of UVB – the *minimal erythema dose* (MED) – is a guide to an individual's susceptibility. Excessive UVB exposure results in tingling of the skin, followed 2–12 h later by erythema. The redness is maximal at 24 h and fades over the next 2 or 3 days to leave desquamation and pigmentation. Severe sunburn causes oedema, pain, blistering and systemic upset. The early use of topical steroids may help sunburn; otherwise, a soothing shake lotion (e.g. calamine lotion) is applied. Individuals may be skin typed by their likelihood of burning in the sun (Table 1). Prevention is better than cure, and 'celts' with a fair 'type 1' skin should not sunbathe and must use a high

Table 1 Skin type according to sunburn and suntan histories	
Skin type	**Reaction to sun exposure**
Type 1	Always burns, never tans
Type 2	Always burns, sometimes tans
Type 3	Sometimes burns, always tans
Type 4	Never burns, always tans
Type 5	Brown skin (e.g. Asian caucasoid)
Type 6	Black skin (e.g. black African)

protection factor sunblock cream on exposed sites (p. 104).

Sunbeds
Sunbeds emit UVA radiation and have been used by 10–20% of adults in the UK. They will produce a tan in people with skin types 3 and over, but those with type 1 and 2 skin will not tan so well, if at all. Side-effects, particularly redness, itching and dry skin, are seen in half of all users. More serious effects can occur in patients taking drugs or applying preparations with a photosensitizing potential. An acute photosensitive eruption may develop, and intense pigmentation sometimes follows. Sunbeds can exacerbate polymorphic light eruption and systemic lupus erythematosus, and may induce porphyria-like skin fragility and blistering. They are a weak risk factor for malignant melanoma, and animal studies suggest that they can cause premature skin ageing.

Dermatologists discourage the use of sunbeds, particularly in the fair-skinned, those with several melanocytic naevi and in anyone with a history of skin cancer. Patients who, despite these

warnings, wish to use a sunbed should not do so more than twice a year and should limit each course to 10 sessions. Sunbeds are not recommended for the treatment of skin disease.

Phototherapy and photochemotherapy
Natural sunlight helps certain skin diseases (p. 44), and both UVB and UVA are extensively used therapeutically. UVA alone has little effect and is combined with photosensitizing psoralens given systemically or topically.

Ultraviolet B
UVB (290–320 nm) is given three times a week. The starting dose is decided from the patient's MED or skin type. The dosage is increased on each visit according to a schedule. A course of 10–30 treatments is usual. Narrow-band (311 ± 2 nm: TL01) UV lamps are superior to broadband and allow a lower dose of UV to be used.

UVB is used to treat psoriasis and mycosis fungoides and, occasionally, atopic eczema and pityriasis rosea. It can be given to children and women during pregnancy. Its main side-effects are acute sunburn and an increased long-term risk of skin cancer.

When used to treat psoriasis, UVB may be combined with a topical preparation such as a vitamin D analogue (p. 30), tar or dithranol, or with oral acitretin.

Photochemotherapy (PUVA)
In psoralen plus UVA (PUVA) therapy, 8-methoxypsoralen, taken orally 2 h

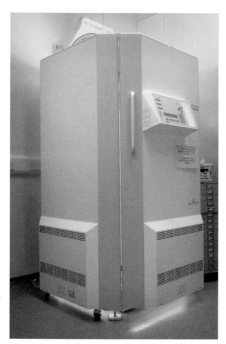

Fig. 2 **Photochemotherapy using UVA-emitting tubes.**

before UVA (320–400 nm) exposure (Fig. 2), is photoactivated. This causes cross-linkage in DNA, inhibits cell division and suppresses cell-mediated immunity. PUVA is usually given for psoriasis or mycosis fungoides, and

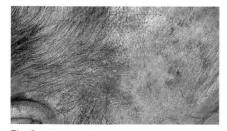

Fig. 3 **Photoageing of the skin.** Keratoses and pigmentation are evident.

sometimes for atopic eczema, polymorphic light eruption (p. 44) or vitiligo (p. 72). The initial dose of UVA is determined by the minimum toxic dose (the MED for PUVA) or skin type, and is increased according to a schedule. PUVA is given two or three times a week and leads to clearance of psoriasis (with tanning) in 15–25 treatments. Maintenance PUVA is not recommended. PUVA can be combined with acitretin ('Re-PUVA') but not methotrexate.

The immediate side-effects of pruritus, nausea and erythema are usually mild. The long-term risks of skin cancer and premature skin ageing are related to the number of treatments or total UVA dose. Careful records must be kept. Cataracts are theoretically possible, and UVA-opaque sunglasses must be worn for 24 h after taking the psoralen.

Bath PUVA, in which the patient soaks in a bath containing a psoralen, is an alternative, especially if systemic side-effects make the oral route impractical. A lower dose of UVA is needed. *Local PUVA* using topical psoralen is useful for psoriasis or dermatitis of the hands or feet.

Photoageing

Photoageing describes the skin changes resulting from chronic sun exposure. Photoaged skin is coarse, wrinkled, pale-yellow in colour, telangiectatic, irregularly pigmented, prone to purpura and subject to benign and malignant neoplasms (Fig. 3). Some of these changes resemble those of intrinsic ageing, but the two are not identical, as may be judged by comparing, in an elderly patient, the sun-exposed face with the sun-protected buttock. The features of photoageing are usually more striking, particularly the development of premalignant and malignant tumours. Some rare conditions, e.g. xeroderma pigmentosum (p. 90), predispose to photoageing.

Histologically, the photoaged dermis shows tangled clumps of elastin with proliferation of glycosaminoglycans (Fig. 4). The epidermis is variable in thickness, with areas of atrophy and hypertrophy and a variation in the degree of pigmentation. *In vitro,* keratinocytes and fibroblasts from sun-exposed sites have a reduced proliferative ability compared with cells from sun-protected sites. The specific clinical changes of photoageing are discussed on page 114.

Management of photoageing

Prevention is the most effective treatment and is particularly important for those with a fair (type 1 or 2) skin. Avoidance of prolonged, direct sun exposure by wearing long-sleeved shirts and a wide-brimmed hat is useful, and sunscreens (p. 104) are applied to sites that are likely to receive some sun, such as the face or hands. The use of tretinoin or alpha hydroxy acids, in cream formulations, has been shown partially to reverse the clinical and histological changes of photoageing. Chemical peels and laser resurfacing are also used.

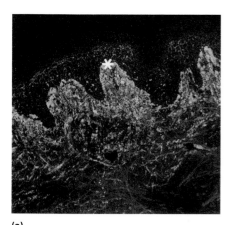

(a)

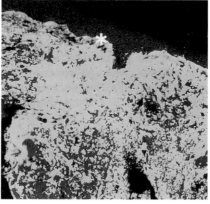

(b)

Fig. 4 **(a) Sun-protected skin.** Preservation of the normal pattern of glycosaminoglycan (GAG: green, hyaluronan) and fibriform elastin (red) is shown. Asterisk (*) shows the dermoepidermal junction: DEJ).
(b) Sun-exposed elastotic skin. Tangled clumps of elastin (red) are shown, with proliferations of GAG (chondroitin sulphate) co-localized to elastin (yellow) throughout the dermis. Asterisk (*) shows DEJ.

Cosmetics

A cosmetic may be defined as any substance that is applied to the body for cleansing, beautifying, promoting attractiveness or altering the appearance. Cosmetics in some form are used by almost everyone. The market for cosmetic sales is vast and far exceeds that of dermatological products. Over recent years, the fields of cosmetology and dermatology have converged so that patients often present having had a reaction to a cosmetic or asking for advice about cosmetic usage. Some cosmetics are now being marketed with the claim that they have an 'active' ingredient, for example one that can 'reverse ageing'.

The range of cosmetics and their usage

Cosmetics are normally used to enhance the appearance of the body, to clean it, to impart a pleasing smell or to mask an unpleasant one, or as a fashion accessory. Table 1 shows the range of common types of cosmetics.

Constituents of cosmetics

The exact contents of a cosmetic depend on its proposed function. However, commonly used ingredients, some of which will be found in most cosmetics, are detailed in Table 2. Many cosmetics contain perfumes, preservatives and, quite often, a sunblock agent. Cosmetics are often emulsions (e.g. oil-in-water or water-in-oil). Full labelling of contents is required in the European Union, a measure strongly supported by dermatologists. This is a useful development for patients allergic to cosmetic ingredients because they are now able to avoid products that would be problematic. Certain preparations deserve special mention. They are discussed below.

Table 1	The range of cosmetics
Site	Product
Skin	Moisturiser, cleanser, soap, make-up remover, powder, rouge, foundation, 'tonic', perfume, aftershave, bath additive, sunscreen
Hair	Shampoo, conditioner, bleach, colorant, permanent waving, straightening, lacquer, gel, hair-removing agents
Eyelids	Mascara, eyeshadow, eyeliner, pencil
Nails	Nail varnish, false nails
Lips	Lipstick, lipgloss, sunscreen

Paraphenylenediamine (PPD) hair dye

Hair dyes, principally PPD, are widely used. Adverse reactions occur in 5%, usually as a scalp or facial eczema. 'Henna' tattoos often contain 15–30% PPD and can induce allergy to PPD.

Nail preparations

Nail varnish is composed of a tosylamide–formaldehyde resin and colorants. Artificial nails are made of methacrylate acid esters and stuck on with acrylic glues.

Sunscreens

A sunscreen absorbs or reflects ultraviolet (UV) radiation. Absorbent agents are shown in Table 2. Titanium dioxide and zinc oxide are reflectant pigments. The sun protection factor (SPF) indicates the ratio of the reaction time to erythema when exposed to UV radiation for treated compared with untreated skin. Thus, using a factor 10 cream means that it should take 10 times longer for erythema to develop when in the sun. Some sunscreen creams are waterproof. Most need to be applied several times a day. Preparations available on prescription in the UK for patients with photodermatoses include Delph Lotion, E45 Sun, RoC Sante Soleil 25, SpectraBan 25, Sunsense Ultra and Uvistat Ultrablock.

Camouflage cosmetics

These pigmented camouflage creams can be mixed to match the colour of the patient's skin and are useful for individuals who have vitiligo, disfiguring birthmarks or scars. Prescribable examples include Covermark, Dermacolor, Keromask and Veil.

Skin-lightening creams

These may contain mercury or hydroquinone, both of which can cause contact allergy or, paradoxically, pigmentation.

Hypoallergenic formulations

These cosmetics are made of highly purified ingredients, selected with the knowledge of their allergenic and irritant potential. However, they still contain compounds that are potential irritants and allergens.

Reactions to cosmetics

Side-effects are comparatively rare when the vast usage of cosmetics is considered but, nonetheless, 12% or more of adults have had a reaction to a cosmetic. Some responses, e.g. stinging with aftershave due to the alcohol base, are expected and do not constitute a reaction. Some patients undoubtedly have a 'sensitive' skin and experience abreactions to a number of products. The preparations most likely to cause a problem are eye and facial cosmetics, antiperspirants and deodorants, hair colorants and soaps (Table 3). Reactions can be categorized as follows.

Irritant contact dermatitis

This is particularly seen in atopics and those with a 'sensitive' skin. Soaps, which are drying and alkaline (the normal pH of facial skin is about 5.5), and deodorants cause mostly irritant dermatitis (Fig. 1). Lanolins, detergents and preservatives may also be irritant.

Table 2	Some ingredients of cosmetics	
Ingredient	Action	Examples
Antioxidant	Prevent degradation	Butylhydroxyanisole, gallates, tocopherol
Colorant, dye	Colour	Cochineal, azo compounds, iron dioxides, paraphenylenediamine, titanium dioxide, dihydroxyacetone in fake tan
Perfume	Smell or for masking smell	Myroxylon pereirae, eugenol, oak moss absolute, lyral
Preservative	Antimicrobial	Parabens, formaldehyde, methyl dibromoglutaronitrile, methyl isothiazolin-one/chloro methyl isothiazolin-one, Dowicil 200, Bronopol, Germall 115
Polyol	Humectant (retains water), emollient	Glycerol, propylene glycol, sorbitol
Oil, fat, wax	Emollient, lustre	Vaseline, almond oil, lanolin
Sun filter	Absorb or reflect UV	Titanium dioxide, Eusolex 4360, Parsol 1789
Tensioactive agent	Emulsifier, surfactant, detergent	Soaps, stearic and oleic acids
Water	Hydration	Purified water

Table 3 **Frequent adverse reactions to cosmetics**

Cosmetic	Reaction
Soap, detergent	Mostly irritant
Deodorant, antiperspirant	Irritant, sometimes allergic
Moisturizer	Irritant and allergic
Eyeshadow	Mostly irritant
Mascara	Mostly irritant
Permanent wave agent	Irritant and allergic
Hair dye (mostly paraphenylenediamine)	Allergic
Shampoo	Mostly irritant

Allergic contact dermatitis

Allergic contact dermatitis most commonly develops to fragrances, preservatives, dyes (e.g. PPD), lanolins and the permanent wave agent glyceryl mono-thioglycolate (Figs 2 and 3). The eruption usually develops at the place of application of the product (usually the face), but this is not always so, as substances can be transferred to another site where they cause symptoms. For example, contact allergy to tosylamide–formaldehyde resin (Fig. 4) in nail varnish most often manifests as an eruption around the eyelids or on the neck.

Contact urticaria and other adverse reactions

Contact urticaria presents as a wheal and flare response within a few minutes of the application of a substance. It may occur with compounds in perfumes, shampoos and hair dyes.

Other adverse reactions include nail dystrophies caused by nail cosmetic use, hair breakage and weathering due to improper use of permanent waving, hair straighteners or dyes, pigmentation and acne.

Management of cosmetic reactions

A patient intolerant of a cosmetic should stop the use of all cosmetics. If necessary, a topical steroid is prescribed until the reaction subsides. All the cosmetics and preparations that have been used must be examined for ingredients, and patch testing (p. 122) performed if appropriate. Alternative cosmetics can then be introduced, but kept to a minimum.

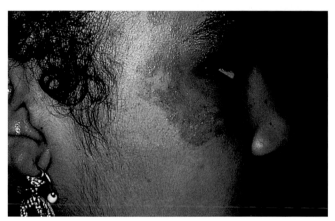
Fig. 1 **Irritant contact dermatitis to a component of a hair-removing cream.**

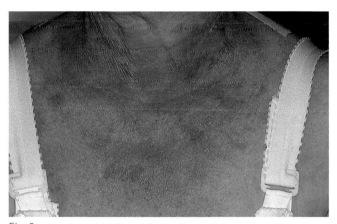
Fig. 2 **Allergic contact dermatitis on the neck due to fragrances.**

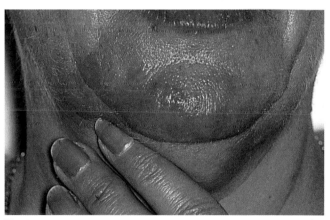
Fig. 4 **Contact sensitivity to tosylamide–formaldehyde resin in nail varnish, causing a facial dermatitis.**

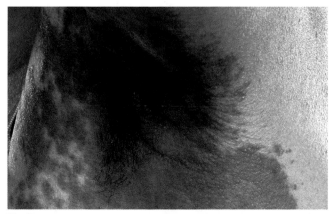
Fig. 3 **Allergic contact dermatitis at the axilla due to a component of a roll-on deodorant.**

Cosmetics

- *A cosmetic* is a substance applied to the body for cleansing, to promote attractiveness or to alter the appearance. Now used by both sexes.

- *A cosmetic cream* typically contains emollients, emulsifiers, colorants, perfumes and preservatives to prevent oxidation and the growth of microorganisms. Sun filters may also be included to prolong shelf-life and for their 'anti-photoageing' effect.

- *Reactions to cosmetics* may take the form of irritant or allergic contact dermatitis, contact urticaria or pigmentary change.

- The commonest causes of *irritant reactions* are soaps, shampoos and deodorants, often because of detergents or preservatives.

- The substances that most frequently cause *allergic contact dermatitis* are fragrances or preservatives (found in most cosmetics, e.g. moisturizers) and dyes (e.g. paraphenylenediamine (PPD) found in hair colorants).

Basic dermatological surgery

The demand for the removal of benign and malignant skin lesions has increased considerably, such that skin surgery is now practised by many general practitioners as well as by dermatologists. Knowledge of basic surgical techniques is mandatory for all those who treat skin disease.

Instruments and methods

No-one should attempt a procedure if unsure about it. Those with limited experience should remove only benign lesions. All procedures are ideally performed in an *operating theatre* with trained nurses and adequate lighting. Sterile instruments, an aseptic technique and sterile gloves are essential. The operator plans the procedure, explains it to the patient, discusses the scar and obtains written consent. The direction of crease marks is assessed: any excision is usually made parallel to these lines.

The *basic instruments* (Fig. 1) include a #3 scalpel handle and #15 blade, a toothed Adson's forceps, a small smooth-jawed needle-holder, a pair of fine scissors, artery forceps and a Gillies skin hook. Curettes and skin punches come in various sizes. A solution of 1% lidocaine (Xylocaine) with 1/200 000 adrenaline (epinephrine) is usually satisfactory as the *local anaesthetic*, but plain lidocaine must be used on the fingers, toes and penis. The skin is prepared (but not sterilized) using, e.g. 0.05% aqueous chlorhexidine (Unisept). Alcohol-based preparations are avoided as, if cautery is used, the solution may ignite. Sterile towels, placed around the operation site, reduce the chance of infection.

The commonest *suture materials* are braided nylon (e.g. Ethilon) and polypropylene (e.g. Prolene), and these are now preferred to silk as they give less of a tissue reaction and a lower rate of wound infection. Use 5/0 sutures on the face, 3/0 on the back and legs, and

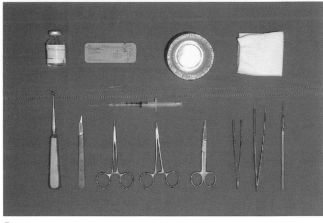

Fig. 1 **A typical surgical set for skin surgery.** A curette is included.

4/0 elsewhere. Stitches are preferably removed at 5 days on the face, 10–14 days on the legs or trunk, and 7–8 days at other sites. Steristrips give extra support to a wound either in addition to sutures or when applied after their removal. A non-adherent dressing is used if necessary.

Every biopsied lesion is sent for histology. If more than one specimen is taken from a patient, separate pots are used and each labelled before the biopsy is placed in it. The usual fixative is 10% formalin.

Basic surgical techniques

Excisional biopsy

An excisional biopsy is planned after considering the local anatomy. The excision's axis depends on the skin creases (Fig. 2) and its margin on the nature of the lesion. The ellipse to be excised is drawn on the skin using a marker pen. An ellipse has an apical angle of about 30° and is usually three times as long as it is wide. If any shorter, 'dog-ears' appear at either end, although these can easily be corrected. After cleaning, local anaesthetic is infiltrated, using a fine needle, into the area of the lesion. Once numbed, the skin is incised vertically down to fat with the scalpel, in a smooth continuous manner to complete both arcs of the ellipse. The ellipse is freed from surrounding skin, secured at one end with a skin hook and removed from the underlying fat, usually using the scalpel blade (Fig. 3). In most cases, the wound can now be repaired, although first any bleeding vessels will need to be tied off.

In a simple *interrupted skin suture*, the needle is inserted vertically through the skin surface down through the dermis and up the other side of the incision to trace a flask-shaped profile (Fig. 3). The wound is apposed and slightly everted. Stitches should not be tied too tightly. Nylon or polypropylene

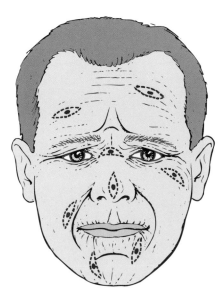

Fig. 2 **Facial crease lines, with some examples of excision ellipses.**

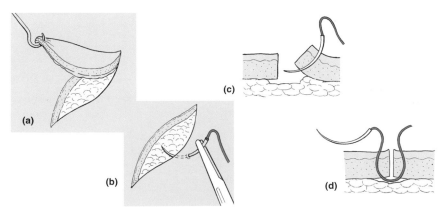

Fig. 3 **Ellipse removal and suture insertion. (a)** The ellipse is removed, one end being secured with a skin hook. **(b)** The suture needle is inserted vertically through the skin surface. **(c)** The suture needle pierces the full thickness of the epidermis and dermis. **(d)** The tied suture is 'flask' shaped and slightly everts the skin surface.

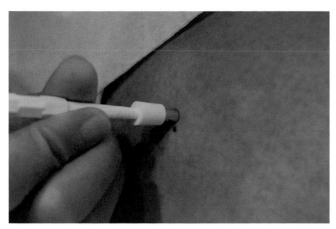

Fig. 4 **Punch biopsy.** After anaesthetizing, the skin is stretched at right angles to the tension lines, the punch blade is placed on the skin over the area to be biopsied and rotated under gentle pressure by rolling it between the thumb and the forefinger until it penetrates down to subcutaneous fat. The full-thickness cylinder of skin floats up and can be snipped off at the base. The defect is repaired with a single suture, cauterized or left to heal by secondary intention.

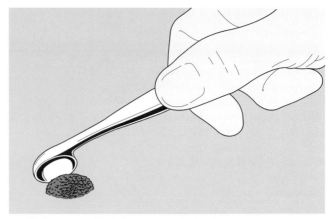

Fig. 5 **Curettage.** The lesion is removed using the curette spoon in a gentle scooping fashion. Most of the curettes now employed are disposable (use only once) ring curettes.

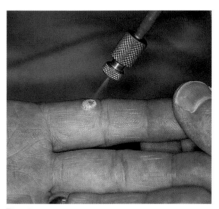

Fig. 6 **Liquid nitrogen treatment using a cryotherapy apparatus.**

sutures are tied with two knots on each of three throws, which are done in alternating directions to produce a square knot. Care is exercised at sites where keloids may form (e.g. the upper back, chest or jawline), where scars may be obvious (e.g. the face of a young woman) and when healing may be poor (e.g. the lower leg). Absorbable subcutaneous sutures (e.g. polyglactin; Vicryl) are used for excisions where the wound may be deep or under tension.

Incisional, punch and shave biopsies

An *incisional biopsy* is done for diagnostic purposes. The technique is similar to an excision except that less tissue is taken. A *punch biopsy* employs a punch (normally about 4 mm in diameter) for removing small lesions or for diagnostic biopsies (Fig. 4).

Shave biopsy is employed for benign lesions, usually intradermal naevi or seborrhoeic warts. The lesion is shaved off parallel to, but slightly above, the skin surface. Haemostasis is achieved with cautery. Not all the lesion is removed, and shaving is not used if malignancy is a possibility. Skin tags can be removed by simply snipping them off with scissors and cauterizing any bleeding points.

Curettage

Curettage is performed for seborrhoeic warts, pyogenic granulomas, keratoacanthomas or single viral warts (e.g. on the face), but not for naevi. After being anaesthetized, the lesion is removed by a gentle scooping motion with the curette spoon or ring (Fig. 5), and then the base is cauterized.

Other surgical techniques

Cautery

Cautery secures haemostasis and destroys tissue. The conventional cautery machine has an electrically heated wire and is self-sterilizing. The *Birtcher hyfrecator*, a unipolar diathermy, gives better controlled electrocautery. It is used to treat spider naevi and telangiectasia, and to give haemostasis, but needs to be employed with care in patients with cardiac pacemakers. Aluminium chloride 20% in an alcohol base (Driclor; Anhydrol Forte) or silver nitrate sticks provide chemical cautery.

Cryotherapy

Cryotherapy using liquid nitrogen is effective for viral warts, molluscum contagiosum, seborrhoeic warts, actinic keratoses, *in situ* squamous cell carcinoma and, in some instances, biopsy-proven basal cell carcinoma. The liquid nitrogen (at −196°C) is delivered by spray gun (e.g. Cry-Ac) or cotton wool bud and injures cells by ice formation. After immersion in a flask containing liquid nitrogen, a cotton wool bud on a stick is applied to the lesion for about 10 s until a thin frozen halo appears at the base. The spray gun is used from a distance of about 10 mm for a similar length of freeze (Fig. 6). Longer freeze times are given for suitable malignant lesions. Blisters may develop within 24 h. They are punctured and a dry dressing applied. Side-effects include hypopigmentation of pigmented skin and ulceration of lower leg lesions, particularly in the elderly. Treatment is repeated after 4 weeks if necessary.

Dermatological surgery

- **Skin surgery** is best performed in an operating theatre with aseptic technique, adequate lighting and trained nurses.
- **Local anaesthetic:** 1% lidocaine with 1/200 000 adrenaline is an adequate local anaesthetic for most sites.
- **Nylon or polypropylene sutures** are preferred to silk as they give a better scar with less wound infection.
- **Histopathology** is performed on all biopsy material, which needs to be labelled carefully.
- **Excisions** are done as an ellipse, parallel to the crease marks, and are about three times as long as wide, with 30° angles at the ends.
- **Shave biopsy** is a technique suitable for the removal of benign naevi.
- **Punch biopsy** is a useful technique for removing small lesions or for full-thickness diagnostic biopsy.
- **Curettage** is a good treatment for seborrhoeic warts, single viral warts and pyogenic granulomas.
- **Cautery,** e.g. hyfrecation, secures haemostasis and destroys tissue.
- **Cryotherapy** is used for viral and seborrhoeic warts, premalignant conditions and some tumours.

http://www.aafp.org/afp/20020315/1155.html ■ http://www.npcentral.net/talks/sharpen.your.bx.tech.pdf

Advanced dermatological surgery

Some dermatologists specialize in the field of skin surgery. All registrars and residents in dermatology are trained in these techniques. An outline of the subject is given here, including the use of flaps, grafts and Mohs' surgery, along with mention of lasers and photodynamic therapy, and of some basic cosmetic procedures.

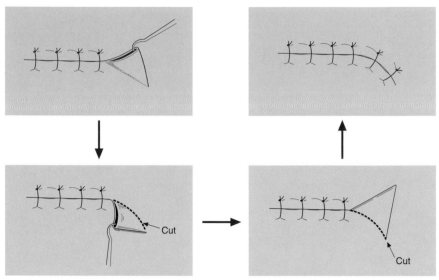

Fig. 1 **Dog-ear repair.**

Simple plastic repairs

Simple plastic repairs are carried out by:

- *Dog-ear excision*: Dog-ears are redundant tissue at the end of an excision line. They occur when the sides of an excision are unequal or when the excision defect is nearly circular. The redundant skin is lifted like a tent using a skin hook then excised each side, and the extended wound is sutured (Fig. 1).
- *M-plasty*: The M-plasty is an excision that reduces the length of an ellipse where space is limited, e.g. on the face. The 'M' end of the ellipse is formed by imagining one tip of the ellipse is folded in.

Skin flaps

Side-to-side closure of a surgical defect is often possible by undermining the edges of the wound using scissors to free the tissue but, when this is not possible, a skin graft or flap is considered. The simplest types of flap are advancement and rotational.

- *Advancement flap*: In this, the skin flap is advanced in one direction over the defect. The flap of skin is created by making excision lines away from the defect to be covered, undermining to free the pedicle, advancing it into the defect and then suturing it in place (Fig. 2).
- *Rotation flap*: A defect may be covered by rotating in skin from one side. One side of the excision wound is extended as an arc that is up to three times the length of the primary defect, depending on the elasticity of the skin at that body site (the scalp and dorsal hand are the least elastic). The pedicle is undermined, rotated in to the defect and sutured in place (Fig. 3).

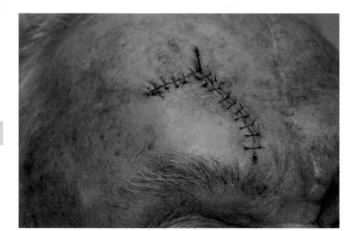

Fig. 2 **Advancement flap of the O to L type.**

- *Full thickness*: Full-thickness skin is excised completely from the donor site, e.g. behind the ear or upper inner arm, which is then sutured. This is the usual method for repairing an excision defect.
- *Split thickness*: In a spilt-thickness graft, the donor site skin is cut through the dermis leaving re-epithialization to occur from the epidermal cells of the hair follicles left behind. This method is usually used by plastic surgeons for covering large defects.

Skin grafts

When a defect cannot be closed directly or by a flap, healing by secondary intention is often considered. This can produce excellent results on concave aspects of the nose, eye, ear and temple, but less satisfactory appearances on convex surfaces of the nose, lips, cheeks and chin. If it is essential to cover a defect and other techniques cannot be employed, a skin graft may be used. Skin grafts are relatively simple to perform, but give relatively poor cosmetic results. A graft is either full or split thickness.

Mohs' micrographic surgery

Mohs' surgery describes the serial removal of a cancer that is mapped and examined microscopically during the procedure to define the extent of the tumour and the adequacy of the excision. It is indicated mostly for basal cell carcinomas that:

- are of the morphoeic type
- have recurred
- have developed in embryonic folds, e.g. nasolabial site
- require tissue conservation as a priority.

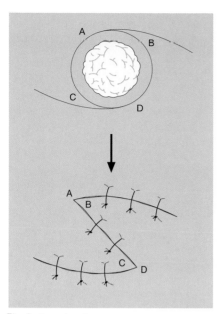

Fig. 3 **Rotation flap.**

The bulk of the tumour is removed by curettage and then a saucer-like piece of skin is excised. This specimen is marked and flattened, and frozen sections are taken and read immediately by microscope, giving a 'map' that shows the extent of the tumour and the areas from which further excision is needed (Fig. 4). The defect is repaired conventionally, sometimes in collaboration with plastic surgeons. The cure rate is 98% for basal cell carcinoma.

Lasers

The technology of *lasers* (*l*ight *a*mplification by *s*timulated *e*mission of *r*adiation) has advanced rapidly, and lasers can be used to treat vascular or pigmented lesions, tumours and tattoos and for hair removal. The variation in absorption of different wavelengths of light means that a range of different lasers is needed (Table 1). Treatment is carried out in specialized centres. Several visits are usually required.

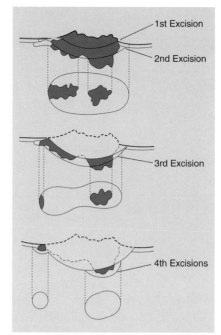

Fig. 4 **Mohs' micrographic surgery.** Microscopic examination of the removed saucer of skin shows where tumour is still present and indicates the sites at which further excision is required.

Photodynamic therapy

Photodynamic therapy (PDT), in which the porphyrin precursor 5-amino-laevulinic acid is applied to a lesion that is then irradiated with visible or laser light, is very effective for extensive *in situ* squamous cell carcinoma, actinic keratoses and superficial basal cell carcinoma.

Cosmetic procedures

Cosmetic procedures are part of the day-to-day practice of the average dermatologist in many countries, although not yet in the UK. Lasers are used extensively for telangiectasia or areas of pigmentation. Other procedures include botulinum toxins for wrinkles, dermabrasion, chemical peels, resurfacing and the use of fillers.

- *Botulinum toxins*: Injection of botulinum toxins into facial muscle paralyses the action of the muscle, thus reducing the prominence of frown lines. It is also used for axillary and sometimes palmar hyperhidrosis.
- *Dermabrasion*: The technique of dermabrasion is used for the removal of pitted or depressed scars on the face. It involves abrasive planing in a sedated and prepared patient of the epidermis and superficial dermis using a high-speed rotary brush. Regeneration of the epidermis occurs rapidly due to abundant pilosebaceous structures.
- *Laser resurfacing*: An erbium:YAG laser is used to remove the epidermis with minimal dermal damage, allowing regeneration of epidermis and the elimination of scars or photodamage.
- *Chemical peels*: Chemical peel is an alternative to dermabrasion to improve the appearance of photodamaged or wrinkled facial skin. Alpha-hydroxy acids or weak trichloroacetic acid solutions are used.
- *Fillers*: Soft tissue defects, e.g. depressed scars or wrinkles, often on the face, may be corrected by the injection of biocompatible materials such as bovine collagen or hyaluronic acid derivatives.
- *Liposuction*: In liposuction, a small cannula and suction equipment are used to remove subcutaneous fat and produce a slimmer body shape.
- *Hair transplant*: Punch biopsies are taken from areas of normal hair density on the scalp. The hair follicles are dissected out one by one and inserted individually into areas of alopecia.

http://www.mohscollege.org/ ■ http://www.surgical-tutor.org.uk/default-home.htm?core/trauma/skin_grafts.htm~right

Table 1 **The application of commonly used lasers**		
Laser	**Wavelength**	**Application**
Q-switched Nd:YAG	532 nm and 1064 nm	Pigmented lesions; adult port wine stains, black/blue tattoos; hair removal (1064 nm)
Pulsed dye rhodamine	585–600 nm	Port wine stains in children, warts, telangiectasia, hypertrophic scars
Ruby normal mode	694 nm	Hair removal, lentigines, freckles
Q-switched alexandrite	755 nm	Multicoloured tattoos, naevus of Ota, viral warts, hair removal
Diode	800 nm	Hair removal
Erbium:YAG	2940 nm	Resurfacing
Carbon dioxide pulsed	10 600 nm	Resurfacing, epidermal naevi, warts, tumours, rhinophyma

Advanced dermatological surgery

- **Dog-ear excision** removes redundant tissue at the ends of an excision to give a better quality scar.
- **Skin flaps** are used to repair a defect by the mobilization and advancement or rotation of skin.
- **Skin grafts** are used to close a defect, but secondary intention healing may give a better cosmetic result.
- **Mohs' surgery** describes the microscopically controlled serial excision of difficult-to-treat skin cancers, giving a high cure rate.
- **Lasers** are used to treat vascular or pigmented skin lesions, tattoos, some skin cancers and for hair removal.
- **Photodynamic therapy** is a very effective method of treating widespread *in situ* squamous cell carcinomas.
- **Cosmetic procedures** are increasingly seen as part of dermatological practice in many countries.

New trends in dermatological treatment

Therapeutic advances have revolutionized the treatment of skin disease over the last 40 years. The 1960s saw the introduction of topical steroids, the 1970s the development of psoralen with ultraviolet A (PUVA), the 1980s retinoids, and the 1990s lasers and ciclosporin. The major advance of the 'noughties' is the biologics.

There have been changes in the delivery of care. Over the last two decades, the number of inpatient dermatology beds has fallen dramatically, and patients who would have been admitted are now managed as outpatients with potent drugs. Nurse practitioners have a higher profile and run their own clinics, e.g. for patients with leg ulcers, eczema or psoriasis, prescribe treatments and perform surgical procedures.

Androgenetic alopecia

The enzyme 5-alpha reductase converts testosterone to the more potent dihydrotestosterone (DHT), which plays a part in the miniaturization of hair follicles seen in androgenetic alopecia. *Finasteride*, a 5-alpha reductase inhibitor, reduces DHT levels and is beneficial in male balding (p. 64).

Atopic eczema

The topical calcineurin inhibitors *tacrolimus* (Protopic) and *pimecrolimus* (Elidel) are alternatives to topical steroids and do not cause skin atrophy (Fig. 1). The systemic immunosuppressors *mycophenolate mofetil* and *methotrexate* (the latter often used in psoriasis) may be beneficial in severe atopic eczema.

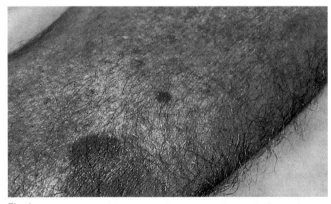

Fig. 1   **Skin atrophy with purpura due to excessive topical use of a potent steroid.**

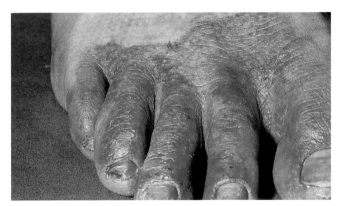

Fig. 2   **Tinea pedis.**

Bullous diseases

Intravenous *immunoglobulin* is used for severe pemphigus or mucous membrane pemphigoid. The biologic *rituximab* has been used in resistant cases.

Cutaneous T-cell lymphoma

The retinoid receptor agonist *bexarotene* (Targretin) seems to be effective in some patients with cutaneous T-cell lymphoma. *Photophoresis*, in which a lymphocyte-enriched blood fraction from the patient, who has taken a psoralen, is exposed to UVA outside the body and then re-infused, is sometimes effective, especially for the Sézary syndrome (p. 42).

Fungal infections

Terbinafine (Lamisil) cream, applied once or twice daily for 1 week, cures tinea pedis (Fig. 2). Pulse treatment with oral *itraconazole* (Sporanox) or *terbinafine* (Lamisil) has given cure rates of 80% for fungal infection of the toenails. The pulse consists of itraconazole 200 mg twice daily or terbinafine 500 mg daily for 7 days followed by a 3-week drug-free interval. This course is taken twice for fingernail infections and three times for infected toenails. *Fluconazole* (Diflucan) 450 mg once weekly for 9 months is also effective. Three-weekly pulses of *terbinafine* (Lamisil) given over 8 weeks produces a 90% cure rate for childhood tinea capitis (Fig. 3).

Hidradenitis suppurativa

Hidradenitis suppurativa (p. 63) is characterized by abscesses, sinuses and scars in the axillae and groin (Fig. 4) and is very difficult to treat. *Acitretin* is helpful in suitable patients, as can be the combination of the antibiotics *clindamycin* and *rifampicin*.

Hirsutism

Eflornithine (Vaniqa) cream is a topical treatment for hirsutism, and may reduce hair density by about 20%. The diode or ruby laser can be used for hair removal.

Hyperhidrosis

The injection of *botulinum toxin A* (Botox, Dysport) into the axillary or palmar skin will control excessive sweating in these areas (p. 63) but needs to be repeated every 9 months.

Leg ulcers

Larval therapy with sterile maggots (LarvE) can be used for managing sloughy leg ulcers (p. 70). *Recombinant platelet-derived growth factor* (becaplermin) is licensed for use in neuropathic ulcers, e.g. in diabetes. *Tissue-engineered skin equivalents*, e.g. Apligraf, can be effective in therapy-resistant wounds.

Psoriasis

The receptor-selective retinoid *tazarotene* (Zorac) modulates keratinocyte proliferation and inflammatory markers and is of proven benefit for plaque psoriasis. Fumaric acid esters and the combination of methotrexate and ciclosporin are useful for patients with 'difficult' psoriasis.

The biological response modifiers are a breakthrough in the treatment of psoriasis. The 'biologics' work by having a blocking effect on tumour necrosis factor (TNF) and

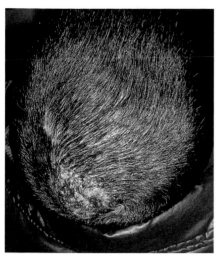

Fig. 3 **Kerion with associated alopecia.** The boggy pustular lesion results from a zoophilic fungal infection (p. 64).

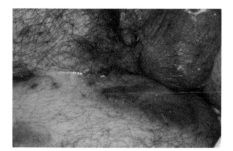

Fig. 4 **Hidradenitis suppurativa.** Multiple inflammatory nodules are evident. Scarring is common.

T lymphocytes, which are involved in causing the disease. Biologics are based on recombinant cytokines, fusion proteins or monoclonal antibodies (mouse or human) that bind to TNF or block T-cell receptors to have their effect. They are given by intravenous infusion or subcutaneous injection, at intervals that vary from twice weekly to once monthly.

The most commonly used biologics for psoriasis at present are the anti-TNF agents *infliximab, etanercept* and *adalimumab*, and the anti-T-cell agents *alefacept* and *efalizumab*. The biologics are very effective drugs, producing up to 88% improvement over a 10-week period. The main problems with biologics are related to reactivation of latent tuberculosis, exacerbation of heart failure, demyelination and expense. The National Institute for Health and Clinical Excellence (NICE) has approved *etanercept* and *efalizumab* for use in patients whose psoriasis is severe and has failed to respond to other systemic drugs. It is anticipated that the use and efficacy of biologics will increase in psoriasis and other skin diseases over the next few years.

Scabies

Ivermectin, a drug used to treat onchocerciasis (p. 59), may be effective for scabies, especially of the crusted (Norwegian) type (p. 114) and for use in institutional outbreaks.

Scleroderma

Topical *calcipotriene* (0.005%) has been shown to improve lesions of localized scleroderma (morphoea). Oral *methotrexate* is beneficial in certain types of morphoea, e.g. en coup de sabre. Systemic sclerosis (Fig. 5) can respond to *photophoresis* (see above) and *PUVA*.

Skin cancer

Topical use of the immunomodulator *imiquimod* (Aldara) is effective for actinic

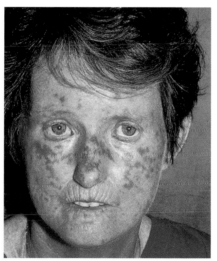

Fig. 5 **Systemic sclerosis of the face.** Telangiectasia and furrowing around the mouth are prominent changes.

keratosis, *in situ* squamous cell carcinoma and superficial basal cell carcinoma. *Dacarbazine* and *interferon-α* are used in the chemotherapy of metastatic malignant melanoma. Some centres use 'sentinel' lymph node biopsy in the management of malignant melanoma.

Vitiligo

The *Excimer 308-nm laser* (Fig. 6) is effective in the treatment of localized areas of vitiligo affecting the cosmetically sensitive sites, e. g. the face.

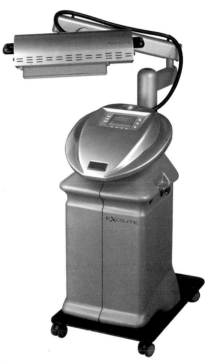

Fig. 6 **The Excimer 308-nm laser.** It can be used for treating localized areas of vitiligo, psoriasis or cutaneous T-cell lymphoma.

New trends in dermatological treatment

Disease	Topical therapy	Systemic therapy
Androgenetic alopecia	–	Finasteride
Atopic eczema	Pimecrolimus, tacrolimus	Mycophenolate, methotrexate
Bullous disease	–	Immunoglobulin, rituximab
Cutaneous T-cell lymphoma	–	Bexarotene, photophoresis
Fungal infection	Terbinafine	Pulse itraconazole, terbinafine, fluconazole
Hidradenitis suppurativa	–	Acitretin, clindamycin/rifampicin
Hirsutism	Eflornithine	Diode or ruby laser
Hyperhidrosis	Botulinum toxin (intralesional)	–
Leg ulcer	Sterile larvae, skin equivalent	–
Psoriasis	Tazarotene	Biologics, e.g. etanercept, infliximab
Scabies	–	Ivermectin
Scleroderma	Calcipotriene	Methotrexate, photophoresis
Skin cancer	Imiquimod (superficial basal cell carcinoma)	Dacarbazine/ interferon-α (malignant melanoma)
Vitiligo	–	Excimer laser

http://www.nice.org.uk/page.aspx?o=appraisals.inprogress.psoriasis ■ http://www.besttreatments.co.uk/btuk/home.jsp

Paediatric dermatology

Some conditions are almost exclusive to childhood (e.g. napkin dermatitis and juvenile plantar dermatosis), and others are more common in children (e.g. atopic eczema or viral exanthems). The common childhood dermatoses not mentioned elsewhere are detailed here along with some rare but important disorders.

Childhood eczemas and related disorders

Forms of eczema found in childhood include:

- napkin (diaper) dermatitis
- infantile seborrhoeic dermatitis
- candidiasis
- juvenile plantar dermatosis
- napkin psoriasis (p. 29)
- atopic eczema (p. 34)
- pityriasis alba (p. 41).

Napkin (diaper) dermatitis
Napkin dermatitis is the commonest type of napkin eruption. It is usually seen in infants who are only a few weeks old, and is rare after the age of 12 months. It is an irritant dermatitis due to the macerating effect of prolonged contact of the skin with faeces and urine. A glazed erythema is seen in the napkin area, sparing the skin folds. Erosions or ulceration may follow (Fig. 1), and hypopigmentation is a complication in pigmented skin. Secondary bacterial or *Candida albicans* infection is frequent, and the latter may account for the development of erythematous papules or pustules.

The *differential diagnosis* is from infantile seborrhoeic eczema and candidiasis, both of which tend to affect the flexures. The treatment of napkin

dermatitis is aimed at keeping the area dry. The use of disposable superabsorbent nappies helps, as may more frequent changes. A bland preparation such as aqueous cream is used as an emollient and soap substitute, and a silicone-based cream (e.g. Drapolene) may have a protective action. Topical 1% hydrocortisone, with an antifungal (e.g. Daktacort or Canesten-HC creams), is also effective.

Infantile seborrhoeic eczema
Infantile seborrhoeic eczema starts in the first few weeks of life and tends to affect the body folds, including the axillae, groin and neck, but it also may involve the face and scalp. Flexural lesions present as moist, shiny well-demarcated scaly erythema (Fig. 2), but a yellowish crust is often found on the scalp. The condition can usually be differentiated from *napkin dermatitis* (which spares the flexures), *candidiasis* (which is usually pustular) and *atopic eczema* (which is more pruritic, although differentiation can be difficult in some cases). Infantile seborrhoeic eczema is treated by emollients and 1% hydrocortisone ointment, or with a hydrocortisone–antifungal combination. Scalp lesions respond to 2% ketoconazole shampoo. Olive oil or arachis oil will help to soften the scalp scales of cradle cap.

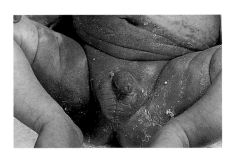

Fig. 2 **Infantile seborrhoeic eczema.** The condition involves the flexures.

Candidiasis
Infection with *C. albicans* is relatively common in the neonatal period. The organism can also secondarily complicate infantile seborrhoeic eczema or napkin dermatitis. Erythema, scaling and pustules are seen, often involving the flexures, and there may be satellite lesions. Treatment is with a topical

anticandidal agent, e.g. 2% ketoconazole cream, and 2% miconazole gel orally.

Juvenile plantar dermatosis
Juvenile plantar dermatosis, first recognized in 1968, presents with red, dry, fissured and glazed skin, principally over the forefeet but sometimes involving the whole sole (Fig. 3). It usually starts in the primary school years and resolves spontaneously in the early to mid-teens. The condition is thought to be linked to the wearing of socks and shoes made from synthetic materials, although it may be a manifestation of atopy in some children. It is usual to advise cotton socks and less occlusive footwear, preferably made of leather. Topical steroids are ineffective but emollients help.

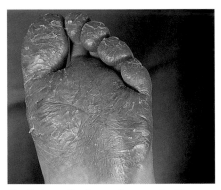

Fig. 3 **Juvenile plantar dermatosis.** The forefoot is mainly affected.

Other childhood dermatoses

Some uncommon but characteristic eruptions are found in childhood. These include:

- urticaria pigmentosa
- Langerhans cell histiocytosis
- Kawasaki disease and other viral infections (p. 51)
- ichthyosis (p. 88)
- epidermolysis bullosa (p. 89).

Urticaria pigmentosa
Urticaria pigmentosa is characterized by multiple reddish-brown macules or papules on the trunk and limbs of an infant. The lesions may become red, swollen and itchy after a bath or when rubbed, and blistering may occur. Histologically, there are accumulations of mast cells in the dermis. The disorder

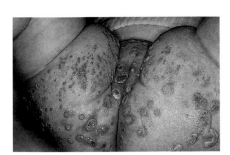

Fig. 1 **Napkin dermatitis.** A severe erosive variant is seen here.

normally resolves spontaneously before adolescence. There is a form with a later onset, usually beginning in adolescence or adult life, which rarely resolves and may involve internal organs – something that is rare in the childhood variety.

Langerhans cell histiocytosis (histiocytosis X)

Langerhans cell histiocytosis is a rare and serious condition that normally involves internal organs. The skin signs are common, variable and include a seborrhoeic-like dermatitis, papules or pustules on the trunk and ulceration, particularly of the flexures. The skin, abdominal organs, lungs and bones are infiltrated by clonal Langerhans cells, which may behave in a malignant fashion, although the condition is believed to be reactive and not a true malignancy. Skin biopsy is usually diagnostic. The prognosis is poorer when the onset is before 2 years of age.

Vascular naevi

Vascular naevi are common and are present at birth or develop soon after. Superficial lesions are due to capillary networks in the upper or mid-dermis, but larger angiomas show multiple vascular channels in the lower dermis and subcutis.

Clinical presentation

There are four main clinical pictures, which are described below.

Salmon patch

This is the commonest vascular naevus, seen in 20–60% of neonates. Patches at the upper eyelid fade quickly, but the 'stork mark' at the posterior neck persists in 20–30% of cases. Parents should be reassured: no investigation or treatment is required.

Port wine stain naevus

Present at birth, the port wine stain (or *naevus flammeus*) is an irregular red or purple macule that often affects one side of the face (Fig. 4), although other sites can be affected. Lesions vary from millimetres to centimetres in diameter. In middle age, it can darken and become lumpy. A port wine stain involving the ophthalmic division of the trigeminal nerve may have an associated intracranial vascular malformation (the *Sturge–Weber syndrome*). Port wine stains near the eye can be associated with glaucoma.

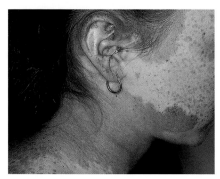

Fig. 4 **Port wine stain naevus.** These are often present at birth. Neurological and ophthalmological assessments may be needed. Early treatment with a flashlamp–pulsed dye laser is often recommended.

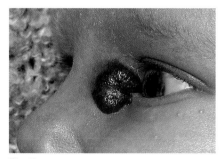

Fig. 5 **Strawberry naevus in an infant.** These haemangiomas develop during the first few weeks of life but often involute by the age of 4–7 years. Treatment is needed if they compromise vital structures such as the eye.

Strawberry naevus

Also known as a capillary cavernous haemangioma, this lesion usually develops during the first few weeks of life and grows to reach its maximum in the first 12 months (Fig. 5). It remains static for the next 6–12 months and then involutes; most cases will have regressed by the age of 5–7 years, leaving an area of atrophy. They occur anywhere on the skin surface.

Cavernous haemangioma

Similar to a strawberry naevus, this is composed of larger and deeper vascular channels and presents as a nodular swelling. The overlying skin may be normal or show a superficial vascular component. Regression is not as complete as in a strawberry naevus. Ulceration with bleeding and secondary infection can develop. Large haemangiomas may trap platelets and cause thrombocytopenia (the *Kasabach–Merritt syndrome*).

Arteriovenous malformation (AVM)

Aberrant vascular channels may occur in the skin, subcutis or deeper structures. Arteriovenous fistulae can be found, e.g. in a limb, and hypertrophy of the involved part sometimes is seen.

Management

Port wine stains may be covered with camouflage cosmetics (p. 104), but treatment is now available with the flashlamp-pulsed dye laser (p. 108), which obliterates the abnormal dermal vessels and improves the appearance. A child with a facial port wine stain needs neurological and ophthalmic assessment. Strawberry naevi should be allowed to involute unless they compromise vital structures such as the eye or airway. In this case, a short course of prednisolone or even emergency surgery is needed. The Kasabach–Merritt syndrome is treated in a similar fashion. Cavernous haemangiomas at the lower back may have associated tethering of the spinal cord: a neurological assessment and imaging are indicated. An AVM requires the opinion of a vascular surgeon.

Paediatric dermatology		
Disorder	**Age at onset**	**Clinical features**
Napkin dermatitis	First few weeks to 12 months	Glazed erythema that spares body folds. Erosions may occur
Infantile seborrhoeic eczema	First few weeks	Moist scaly erythema Flexures and scalp affected
Candidiasis	Infancy	Erythema, with scaling and pustules. Flexures affected Secondary infection found
Juvenile plantar dermatosis	School age to mid-teens	Glazed red fissured skin on the forefeet and soles
Urticaria pigmentosa	Mostly at 3–9 months	Reddish-brown macules or papules on trunk, which urticate when rubbed
Langerhans cell histiocytosis	All ages (different types)	Seborrhoeic-like dermatitis, papules/pustules, ulceration
Vascular naevi	At birth, in first few weeks	Salmon patch on neck, port wine naevus (e.g. on face), strawberry naevus

http://www.pharmj.com/Editorial/20000729/education/childhood_skin.html

The skin in old age

In westernized societies, the proportion of people aged over 65 is high and continues to rise. Poor nutrition, lack of self-care and general illness contribute to skin disease in the elderly. Few people die from old skin, but many suffer from it.

Intrinsic ageing of the skin

The changes in aged, sun-protected skin are more subtle than those of photoageing (p. 103) and consist of laxity, fine wrinkling and benign neoplasms. In addition, androgenetic alopecia (p. 64) and greying of the hair are age related.

Histologically, the epidermis is thinned with the loss of the rete ridge pattern and a reduction in the numbers of melanocytes and Langerhans cells. Individual epidermal cells are smaller. The dermis is thinned due, mainly, to loss of proteoglycans. Functionally, the skin is less elastic and has a reduced tensile strength. Resistance to injury, irritants and infection is reduced, and wound healing is slower.

Some inherited disorders, e.g. pseudoxanthoma elasticum (p. 91), show features of aged skin. The misuse of potent topical steroids induces atrophy and purpura (p. 110), signs also seen in old skin.

Dermatoses in the elderly

Few skin conditions are exclusive to old age, but some are seen more frequently (Table 1).

Dry skin and asteatotic eczema

Dryness with itching is common in elderly skin. It may be a mild roughness and scaling, or more severe, with fissuring and inflammation (asteatotic eczema, p. 36). The changes often occur on the legs and are aggravated by low humidity, central heating and excessive washing. Emollients, sometimes with a mild or moderate potency topical steroid ointment, usually help.

Seborrhoeic dermatitis (p. 36) in the elderly (Fig. 1) may be flexural and resemble psoriasis, candidiasis or erythrasma. In old people, *allergic contact dermatitis* (p. 32) to allergens in topical medicaments or toiletries, e.g. lanolin, neomycin, fragrances and

local anaesthetics, particularly needs to be considered.

Pruritus

Itch in old age can be severe and unrelenting. Examination will usually show asteatotic eczema, scabies, urticaria or the prebullous phase of pemphigoid (p. 76), or investigations may reveal renal or liver disease or underlying malignancy (p. 86). The small group of patients in whom no cause is found have '*senile pruritus*'. Topical treatments and sedating antihistamines are often ineffective.

Psoriasis

Psoriasis has its peak onset in the teens with a second peak in the sixth decade. In the elderly patient, it is frequently flexural (p. 28), but all patterns, except guttate, are seen. Management can be difficult due to inability to apply topical therapy, attend hospital or stand for ultraviolet treatment. Methotrexate is used quite often and is mostly well tolerated.

Infections and infestations

Herpes zoster (p. 52) at some time affects 25% of people over 65. Post-herpetic neuralgia increases with age, occurring in 75% of shingles victims over 70. Early treatment with aciclovir, famciclovir or prednisolone makes neuralgia less likely.

Infection with *Candida albicans* (p. 56) is common in the flexures of obese elderly women. *Onychomycosis* (p. 66) is a frequent incidental finding in old people, especially men. Treatment is not always needed unless the nail produces pain.

Scabies epidemics are a problem in old people's homes and are difficult to control (p. 60). Any itchy old person should be examined carefully, as burrows are easily missed. Elderly patients who are debilitated, paralysed, immunosuppressed or who cannot scratch may develop crusted 'Norwegian' scabies (Fig. 2), which is highly contagious due to the thousands of mites present.

Photodamage and skin tumours

Most benign and malignant skin tumours are more common in the elderly (Table 1). Many are related to sun exposure (p. 103). Specific disorders of photodamage include:

Table 1 **Skin disorders common in the elderly**			
The eczemas	Asteatotic/dry skin (p. 36)	Benign tumours	Seborrhoeic wart (p. 92)
	Seborrhoeic (p. 36)		Cherry angioma (p. 92)
	Contact (p. 32)		Skin tag (p. 92)
	Venous (p. 36)		Chondrodermatitis nodularis
Other eruptions	Psoriasis (p. 28)	Photodamage	Photoageing (p. 103)
	Drug eruption (p. 84)		Actinic elastosis
	Erythema ab igne (p. 68)	Premalignant	Actinic keratosis
Infections	Herpes zoster (p. 52)		*In situ* squamous cell carcinoma (p. 100)
	Candidiasis (p. 56)	Cancers	Basal cell carcinoma (p. 98)
	Onychomycosis (p. 66)		Squamous cell carcinoma (p. 98)
	Scabies (p. 60)		Lentigo malignant melanoma (p. 96)
Ulceration	Leg ulcer (p. 70)		Cutaneous T-cell lymphoma (p. 100)
	Pressure ulcer	Other	Senile pruritus
Autoimmune	Pemphigoid (p. 76)		

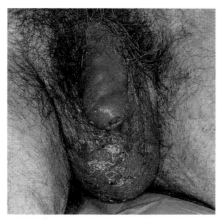

Fig. 1 **Flexural seborrhoeic dermatitis affecting the scrotum and penis.**

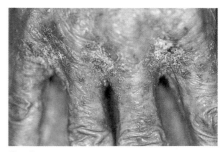

Fig. 2 **Crusted 'Norwegian' scabies.**

- *Actinic (solar) keratoses*: These are single or multiple discrete scaly hyperkeratotic rough-surfaced areas, usually less than 1 cm in diameter. They are seen on sun-exposed sites, especially the dorsal aspects of the hands, face and neck (Fig. 3). They are most common in those with a fair skin.

Histologically, they show hyperkeratosis, abnormal keratinocytes with loss of maturation and dermal elastosis. Actinic keratoses may regress spontaneously. However, they can progress to squamous cell carcinoma, although this is relatively uncommon. Treatment is normally by cryosurgery, but certain lesions may be best treated with curettage, excision or by applying 5% fluorouracil cream (Efudix) once or twice daily for 3–4 weeks, 3% diclofenac gel (Solaraze) twice daily for 60–90 days or imiquimod (Aldara).

A *cutaneous horn* may occasionally develop in an actinic keratosis (Fig. 4). It is best treated by excision.

- *Actinic (solar) elastosis*: In solar elastosis, the sun-exposed skin is yellowed, thickened and wrinkled. On the neck, furrowed rhomboidal patterns are sometimes seen (Fig. 5), particularly in those with outside occupations such as farmers. 'Senile' comedones or thickened yellowish

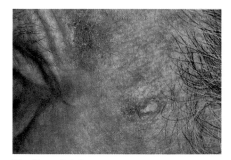

Fig. 3 **Actinic keratoses.**

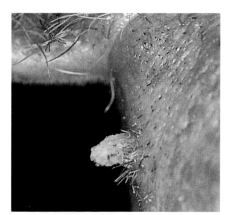

Fig. 4 **A cutaneous horn.**

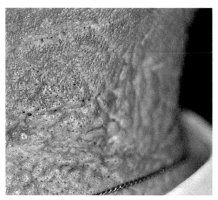

Fig. 5 **Actinic elastosis.** The characteristic rhomboid pattern is seen on the neck, associated with senile comedones. A history of chronic sun exposure, often occupational, is invariably obtained.

plaques may develop. Photodamage is worse in smokers.
- Damaged dermal collagen with inflammation in the dermis and cartilage is a feature of *chondrodermatitis nodularis* (p. 93, Fig. 6). Treatment is by excision.
- *Actinic cheilitis*: Excessive exposure to sun, often occupational, can induce inflammation and scaling of the lower lip. Treatment is by cryosurgery or excision.

Ulceration

- *Leg ulcers*: Venous ulcers often start in middle age but, because of their chronicity, are a problem in the elderly. Ischaemic ulcers become more common with advancing years (p. 71).
- *Pressure ulcers*: A pressure ulcer starts as an area of erythema and progresses to widespread necrosis of tissue with ulceration. Deep ulcers develop over the sacrum (Fig. 7), heels, ischia and greater trochanters. Secondary infection with *Pseudomonas aeruginosa* is common.

Pressure ulcers mainly occur in the elderly who are recumbent and

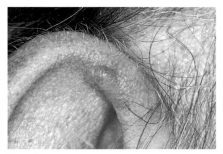

Fig. 6 **Chrondrodermatitis nodularis.**

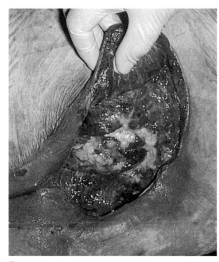

Fig. 7 **Pressure ulcer over the sacrum.**

immobile, e.g. due to a fractured femur, arthritis, unconsciousness or paraplegia. Malnutrition, reduced cutaneous sensation and arterial disease predispose to tissue breakdown.

Prevention is possible if at-risk patients are identified. Regular repositioning, the use of an antipressure mattress and attention to diet and to the patient's general condition help in prevention and treatment. A necrotic eschar separates by itself in 2–4 weeks. The resulting ulcer can be covered by a semipermeable dressing, e.g. Opsite. Proteolytic enzymes (Varidase) may be used to debride heel lesions. Pain relief is vital. Surgical excision and flap repair are often possible provided the patient's general condition is satisfactory.

> ### The skin in old age
>
> - **Asteatotic eczema** (also known as eczéma craquelé) is a dry, scaly, fissured eruption that commonly affects the elderly. Treatment is with emollients and mild topical steroids.
> - **Pruritus** in old people nearly always has a cause. Scabies, urticaria or prebullous pemphigoid are easily missed. Investigation for underlying systemic disease may be indicated.
> - **Herpes zoster** is common in old age. Aciclovir or famciclovir may make neuralgia less likely.
> - **Actinic keratoses** are roughened hyperkeratotic areas in sun-exposed sites. They are often treated by cryosurgery or the application of fluorouracil cream or diclofenac gel.
> - **Actinic elastosis** is a yellowed, thickened, wrinkled change in sun-exposed skin, e.g. on the neck, often seen in men who have had outdoor occupations.
> - **Pressure ulcers** result from reduced sensation, immobility, malnutrition and ischaemia. It is vital to identify at-risk patients and institute means to prevent these ulcers from developing.

Genitourinary medicine

In the UK and Ireland, genitourinary medicine has traditionally been a separate specialty from dermatology, but the two are combined as 'dermatovenereology' in many countries. It has become increasingly important for those treating skin disease to know more about genitourinary disorders. Genitourinary diseases range as follows (see also Table 1):

- syphilis
- gonorrhoea
- human immunodeficiency virus (HIV) infection (p. 54)
- chlamydial infection
- pelvic inflammatory disease
- vaginitis
- chancroid
- viral warts (p. 50)
- genital herpes simplex (p. 52)
- hepatitis B and hepatitis C
- vulval/perianal dermatoses
- penile/scrotal dermatoses.

Syphilis (lues)

Syphilis is a chronic infectious disease due to *Treponema pallidum*. Skin signs are seen in all three stages.

Clinical presentation

T. pallidum may rarely be acquired congenitally or from a contaminated blood transfusion, but the normal mode of transmission is through sexual intercourse.

- *Primary chancre.* About 3 weeks after sexual contact, a primary chancre, a painless ulcerated button-like papule, develops at the site of inoculation. This is usually genital (Fig. 1), but oral and anal chancres are seen in men who have sex with men. Regional lymphadenopathy is common. Without treatment, the chancre clears spontaneously in 3–8 weeks. Serology is not positive until 4 weeks after infection, but spirochaetes can be isolated from the chancre.
- *Secondary stage.* This phase starts 4–12 weeks after the onset of the chancre. It is characterized by a non-itchy pink or copper-coloured papular eruption on the trunk, limbs, palms and soles (p. 40). Untreated, the eruption resolves in 1–3 months. Serology is positive.
- *Tertiary stage.* About 40% of patients with untreated syphilis will develop late lesions, usually after a latent period of years. Painless nodules, sometimes with scaling, develop in annular or arcuate patterns on the face or back. Subcutaneous granulomatous gumma – usually on the face, neck or calf – ulcerate, scar and never heal completely (Fig. 2). Cardiovascular syphilis or neurosyphilis may coexist.

Table 1	**Other genitourinary infections**		
Condition	**Organisms**	**Clinical features**	**Therapy**
Non-gonococcal urethritis	*Chlamydia trachomatis, Ureaplasma urealyticum*	Males: dysuria, frequency, urethral discharge	Doxycycline or erythromycin for 7 days or 1-dose azithromycin
Mucopurulent cervicitis	*Chlamydia trachomatis,* (*Neisseria gonorrhoeae*)	Females: asymptomatic or yellow cervical exudate	Doxycycline or erythromycin for 7 days or 1-dose azithromycin
Pelvic inflammatory disease	*Chlamydia trachomatis, Neisseria gonorrhoeae*	Acute abdominal pain and tenderness, fever, raised WBC	Ofloxacin and metronidazole for 14 days
Vaginitis	*Trichomonas vaginalis, Gardnerella vaginalis,* Bacteroides, *C. albicans*	Asymptomatic or erythema, itch and discharge: male partners get urethritis and balanitis	Trichomonal/bacterial – oral metronidazole for 7 days; anticandidal topicals
Chancroid	*Haemophilus ducreyi*	Single or multiple tender, necrotic, erosive ulcers	Oral erythromycin for 7 days
Hepatitis B	Hepatitis B virus	Only one third to one half show symptoms of acute hepatitis	Vaccinate at-risk groups; interferon-α, lamivudine

WBC, white blood count.

Management

Primary or secondary syphilis is treated with procaine penicillin 600 mg intramuscularly daily for 14 days as first-line therapy. Doxycycline (200 mg daily for 14 days) and erythromycin are alternatives. Patients need contact tracing and assessment for other venereal diseases, and should be managed in a genitourinary medicine department.

Gonorrhoea

Gonorrhoea is caused by the Gram-negative diplococcus *Neisseria gonorrhoeae*. Infection may be symptomatic or asymptomatic.

Clinical presentation

Symptomatic males usually present with dysuria, frequency of micturition and a purulent urethral discharge. Females, when symptomatic, can have an abnormal vaginal discharge, dysuria, menstrual irregularity or abdominal pain. Pharyngeal and anorectal infection may produce symptoms, or may be asymptomatic. The diagnosis relies on the microscopic

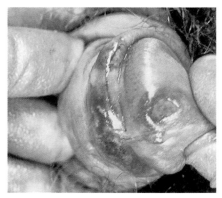

Fig. 1 **Primary chancre of syphilis.**

identification of Gram-negative intracellular diplococci from urethral (males and females) or endocervical (females) smears, and culture for *N. gonorrhoeae*. Serological tests are unreliable. Women with untreated gonorrhoea are at risk of developing pelvic inflammatory disease and infertility. In men, complications include urethral stricture, infertility and epididymitis.

Gonococcaemia is rare but, when observed, results in fever, arthritis and

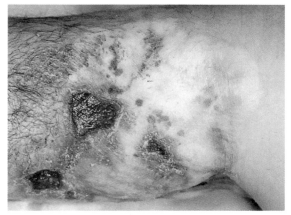

Fig. 2 **Gumma of tertiary syphilis.**

pustules that are few in number and generally distributed on the hands, feet or near the large joints. This is a type of septic vasculitis which, like some other systemic infections (e.g. *Neisseria meningitidis*), may be purpuric.

Management

Uncomplicated acute gonorrhoea should be treated with ciprofloxacin 500 mg, or ofloxacin 400 mg, as a single oral dose. Amoxicillin, 3 g as a single oral dose with probenecid 1 g orally, is an alternative. Infection acquired abroad should be presumed to be multiantibiotic resistant. Pharyngeal and rectal infection may be particularly difficult to eliminate. A repeated culture to test for a cure is made 4–7 days after treatment. Patients with gonorrhoea should be screened for coexisting sexually transmitted diseases, e.g. chlamydia. Management is most appropriate in a department of genitourinary medicine where contact tracing can be organized.

Vulval disorders

The vulva can be involved in many conditions, and itching (pruritus vulvae), often followed by secondary lichenification, is frequent. Commonly seen dermatoses include:

- lichen sclerosus (p. 39)
- eczemas including allergic contact dermatitis (Fig. 3) and seborrhoeic dermatitis (p. 36)
- psoriasis (p. 28)
- lichen planus (p. 38).

Herpes simplex (p. 52), viral warts (p. 50), candidiasis (p. 56), venereal infections (see above) and extramammary Paget's disease (p. 86) also occur. Other specific disorders include:

- *Vulval intraepithelial neoplasia* (VIN) includes *in situ* squamous cell carcinoma and Bowenoid papulosis

(Fig. 4). Cervical intraepithelial neoplasia can coexist and screening is required. Human papillomavirus infection may predispose to the precancerous change. There is a small risk of progression to invasive squamous cell carcinoma. Treatment is by cryosurgery or excision (for small areas), topical fluorouracil and laser therapy. Follow-up is needed.
- *Vulvodynia* is chronic vulval discomfort, often with burning and soreness. It is sometimes due to erosive vulvitis, e.g. from lichen planus or VIN. Some patients have underlying psychological problems.
- *Genital ulceration* may occur with pemphigoid or pemphigus (p. 76), or acutely with erythema multiforme. It is also seen with Behçet's syndrome, a multisystem disorder in which recurrent oral aphthous ulceration and iridocyclitis also occur.

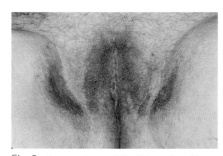

Fig. 3 **Contact dermatitis of the vulva.** This was caused by allergy to neomycin in a cream.

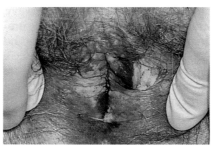

Fig. 4 **A hyperkeratotic variant of vulval intraepithelial neoplasia (VIN).**

Penile and scrotal eruptions

Balanitis (inflammation of the penile skin; Fig. 5) and scrotal eruptions can be caused by a similar list of conditions to those outlined above for vulval dermatoses. Specific disorders include:

- *Circinate balanitis*, an eroded or crusted penile eruption seen in Reiter's syndrome (p. 40)
- *Scrotal gangrene*, a necrotizing cellulitis of rapid onset, seen in diabetics. It has a mortality of 45%.

Pruritus ani

The perianal skin is frequently involved in infective, inflammatory and occasionally neoplastic conditions, as for the genitalia. Pruritus ani is common in middle-aged men. Whatever the underlying dermatosis, faecal contamination of the perianal skin with bacteria, enzymes and allergens causes inflammation and itch. Persistent rubbing induces lichen simplex (p. 37) or maceration, and secondary infection with bacteria or fungi. A compounding contact dermatitis due to allergy to 'over-the-counter' creams is common. Anal carcinoma, fissure or haemorrhoids, and threadworm infestation in children, should be excluded.

Treatment requires attention to personal hygiene (daily baths are helpful but avoid the use of soap) and the topical application of an emollient, antiseptic or steroid preparation.

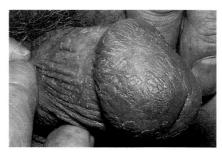

Fig. 5 **Eczema of the glans penis.**

Genitourinary medicine

Syphilis
- The primary chancre appears 3 weeks after sexual contact.
- The papular non-pruritic eruption of the secondary stage is seen 4–12 weeks following the chancre.
- Tertiary syphilis may be delayed several years.
- Treatment is with procaine penicillin or doxycycline.
- Patients need contact tracing and should be screened for other venereal diseases.

Gonorrhoea
- Men present with dysuria, frequency and a urethral discharge.
- Women complain of a vaginal discharge, dysuria and abdominal pain.
- Infection may be asymptomatic.
- Late sequelae include pelvic inflammatory disease and infertility.
- Treatment is with a single oral dose of ciprofloxacin or ofloxacin (or amoxicillin with probenecid).

Vulval disorders
- Common vulval disorders include lichen sclerosus, eczemas, psoriasis and vulvodynia.
- Vulval intraepithelial neoplasia requires long-term follow-up and cervical screening.
- Chronic ulceration may indicate a blistering disorder or Behçet's syndrome.
- Secondary contact dermatitis, e.g. due to medicament allergy, is common.

Pruritus ani
- Is common in middle-aged men.
- May be due to the irritant effects of faecal contamination on perianal skin.
- Anal carcinoma, anal fissure and haemorrhoids must be excluded.
- Local hygiene measures and a topical antiseptic or steroid are prescribed.
- Secondary allergic contact dermatitis is common.

Racially pigmented skin

Common dermatoses may show variable manifestations in different races due to differences in pigmentation, hair or the response of skin to external stimuli. In addition, some conditions have a distinct racial predisposition. The response of darkly pigmented skin to injury and to certain therapeutic modalities needs to be taken into account when planning a programme of management.

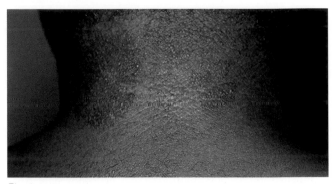

Fig. 1 **Lichen simplex chronicus showing hyperpigmentation and lichenification.**

Definition of race

The characteristics of our species, *Homo sapiens*, are continuously variable, and hence the division into 'races' is – to some extent – artificial. However, there are obvious differences between groups of humans, and these differences have an influence on the appearance of and susceptibility to disease. Most definitions of a '*race*' are unsatisfactory, but perhaps the best is 'a population which differs significantly from other populations in regard to the frequency of one or more of the genes that it possesses'. Obviously, this definition allows even rather small groups to be classified as a race!

It is generally assumed that changes in gene frequency result from mutation, natural selection and 'accidental' loss. Some changes are thought to be the result of adaptation to environmental conditions, although it is not always obvious what advantage is conferred. Racial classification has relied on physical characteristics, often skeletal, although hair form and skin colour are taken into account. The main divisions are:

- *Australoid*: e.g. Australian aborigines
- *Capoid*: e.g. bushmen, hottentots
- *Caucasoid*: Europeans, people of the Mediterranean, Middle East and most of the Indian subcontinent
- *Mongoloid*: peoples of East Asia, Eskimos, American Indians
- *Negroid*: e.g. black Africans.

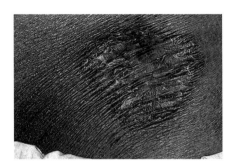

Fig. 2 **Lichen planus with hyperpigmentation.**

Table 1 Causes of hypopigmentation in a pigmented skin

Division	Disorder
Infections	Leprosy, onchocerciasis, pinta, pityriasis versicolor
Papulosquamous disorders	Pityriasis rosea/alba, psoriasis (occasionally), seborrhoeic dermatitis
Physical/chemical agents	Burns, cryotherapy, hydroquinone, topical potent steroids
Post-inflammatory	Discoid lupus erythematosus, systemic sclerosis, sarcoidosis
Other	Albinism, vitiligo

caucasoids. Body hair is most profuse in caucasoids. The black African stratum corneum differs from the caucasoid by showing greater intercellular adhesion and a higher lipid content.

Diseases that show racially dependent variations

In pigmented skin, eruptions that appear red or brown in white caucasoid skin may be black, grey or purple, and pigmentation can mask an erythematous reaction. Inflammation in pigmented skin often provokes a hyperpigmentary (Figs 1 and 2) or hypopigmentary reaction (Table 1). Follicular, papular and annular patterns are more common in pigmented skin than in caucasoid. In addition, some skin disorders show an inter-racial variation in prevalence (Table 2).

Racial differences in normal skin

The most obvious difference is in pigmentation (p. 72), but hair forms and colour also vary. Mongoloid hair is straight and has the largest diameter; black African hair is short, spiralled, drier and more brittle than that of other races; and caucasoid hair may be wavy, straight or helical. Hair colour is predominantly black in mongoloids and Africans, and black, blond or red in

Table 2 Diseases with racially dependent variations

Skin disorder	Caucasoid	Mongoloid	Black African
Acne	Most severe	Least common	Hyperpigmented lesions
Atopic eczema	Most common with western lifestyle	Lichenification is seen	Follicular and hyperpigmented lesions are found
Keloid	May occur	More frequent	More frequent
Lichen planus	Can show some pigmentation	Often hyperpigmented	Often hyperpigmented
Melanocytic naevi	Very common	A few may be present	Uncommon
Psoriasis	Common (2% prevalence)	Rare (0.3% prevalence but increasing)	East > West Africans: plaques bluish, leave hyper- or hypopigmentation
Sarcoidosis	Less common	Less common	In US, 10 times more common than in caucasoids
Skin cancer	Most common in northern Europeans	Intermediate prevalence	Uncommon
Vitiligo	Same prevalence, least obvious	Same prevalence, more obvious	Same prevalence, most obvious

Diseases with a distinct racial or ethnic predisposition

Hair disorders

Racially dependent hair conditions are most common in black Africans and include the following:

- *Folliculitis keloidalis* describes discrete follicular papules, often keloids, at the back of the neck in African males (Fig. 3). Intralesional steroids may help.
- *Pseudofolliculitis barbae* is a common disorder in black African men and is characterized by inflammatory papules and pustules in the beard area. It is thought to result from hairs growing back into the skin (Fig. 4). Treatment is difficult but includes attention to shaving technique and the topical use of antibiotics and steroids.
- *Traction alopecia* is mainly seen in black Africans because of the practice of plaiting or tightly braiding the hair (Fig. 5). Hairs are loosened from their follicles. The temples are often affected.
- *Hot-comb alopecia* is a traction alopecia caused by applying a hot comb to oiled hair in order to straighten it (curly black African hair is usually straightened by chemical methods).

Pigmentary changes

Pigmentary abnormalities, as both a variation of 'normal' and otherwise, are also common. These include the following:

- *Dermatosis papulosa nigra* describes small, seborrhoeic wart-like papules often seen on the face in black Africans.
- *Lines of hypo- or hyperpigmentation*, often on the upper arms, are not infrequently found in black Africans.
- *Longitudinal nail pigmentation* and macular pigmentation of palms and soles occur mainly in black Africans.
- *Mongolian spot* is a slate-brown pigmentation at the sacral area in a baby and is found in 100% of mongoloids, 70% or more of Africans and 10% of caucasoids. It usually fades by the age of 6 years.

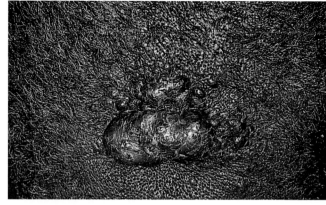

Fig. 3 **Folliculitis keloidalis.**

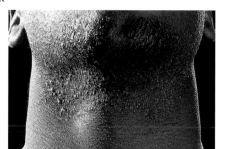

Fig. 4 **Pseudofolliculitis barbae.**

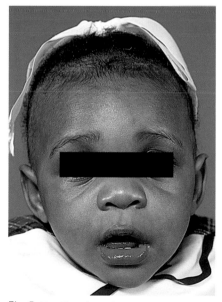

Fig. 5 **Traction alopecia.**

- *Naevus of Ota* is a macular, slate-grey pigmentation in the upper trigeminal area, which may involve the sclera (Fig. 6). It is seen most frequently in mongoloids.

Other conditions

A racial preponderance is also seen with the following conditions.

- *Sickle cell disease* occurs in black Africans. The main cutaneous findings are painful oedema of the hands and feet, caused by infarction in the small bones, and leg ulceration.
- *Vascular naevi*, such as the port wine stain naevus, are more common in caucasoids than in other races.

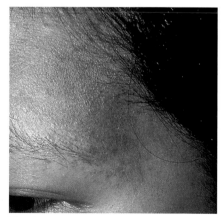

Fig. 6 **Naevus of Ota**

Racially pigmented skin

- **A race** is a genetically defined group, although the characteristics of *Homo sapiens* are continuously variable.
- **The most numerous races** are mongoloids, black Africans and caucasoids (the last include Middle East and Indian subcontinent peoples).
- **Eruptions that are red or brown** in caucasoid skin may appear *black, grey or purple* in subjects with pigmented skin.
- **Lichenification**: inflammatory dermatoses tend to become lichenified in mongoloids and may be *follicular* in black Africans.
- **Hypopigmentation** may follow from skin trauma, e.g. burns or from cryotherapy, topical steroids and some dermatoses, in pigmented skin.
- **Hair disorders**, e.g. pseudofolliculitis, keloidal change or traction alopecia, are common in black Africans.
- **Pigmentary lines** are frequently found on the limbs (e.g. the outer upper arm) or nails in black Africans and other races.
- **Sacral mongolian spots** are found in most mongoloid and black African babies, but in only a few caucasoid infants.
- **Vascular and melanocytic naevi** (e.g. port wine stain) are more common in caucasoids than in other races.

Occupation and the skin

Skin disorders, after stress and musculoskeletal problems, are the commonest reported cause of occupational disease and are responsible for much lost productivity. An occupational dermatosis is defined as a skin condition that is primarily due to components of the work environment that would not have occurred unless the individual were doing that job.

Diagnosis

Proving a work association can be difficult. The following give clues:

- contact with a known noxious agent
- similar skin disease in other workers
- consistent exposure-to-onset time course
- attacks appear with exposure, improve on withdrawal
- site and type of eruption consistent with exposure
- corroboration by patch testing.

Contact dermatitis is the most common work-related skin disease and is more often irritant than allergic. Contact urticaria, particularly to latex, is now well recognized. Other occupational dermatoses are listed in Table 1. Certain infections, e.g. anthrax (p. 48), orf (p. 50) and tinea corporis (p. 56) may be occupational. Heat, cold, ultraviolet radiation, vibration and X-rays can cause industrial disease.

Contact dermatitis

It is often difficult to differentiate between allergic and irritant causes.

Aetiopathogenesis

Many industrial substances are irritants and some are allergens as well (p. 32). Water, detergents, alkalis, coolant oils and solvents are important irritants. Common allergens include chromate, rubber chemicals, preservatives, nickel, fragrances, epoxy resins and phenol-formaldehyde resins (Table 2).

Irritant dermatitis frequently results from cumulative exposure to multiple types of irritant. An irritant dermatitis increases epidermal penetration by allergens and, because of this, it predisposes to superimposed contact sensitization. Similarly, allergic contact dermatitis renders skin vulnerable to attack by irritants.

Constitutional factors, especially atopic eczema, predispose to contact dermatitis. Environmental factors such as physical friction, occlusion, heat, cold, dry air from air conditioning or sudden swings in air temperature or humidity also have an effect.

Clinical presentation

The hands are affected, alone or with other sites, in 80–90% of occupational cases. The arms can be involved if not covered, and the face and neck are affected if there is exposure to dust or fumes. Cement workers often have lower leg and foot dermatitis in addition to hand changes. Allergy to rubber chemicals can cause dermatitis from rubber gloves or boots. Some workers develop 'hardening', an adaptive tolerance to irritants or allergies.

Occupational dermatitis appears at any age, but peaks at each end of working life. In bakers and hairdressers, dermatitis appears early. In cement workers, chromate dermatitis requires a few years to develop. Cumulative irritant dermatitis appears after several years' exposure.

Table 1 **Rarer occupational skin disorders**		
Condition	**Presentation**	**Occupational exposure**
Argyria (Fig. 4)	Slate-grey pigmentation on face, hands, sclerae	Industrial processes, e.g. silver smelters
Chloracne (Fig. 5)	Multiple open and closed comedones on cheeks and behind ears	Halogenated aromatic hydrocarbons, e.g. contamination during manufacture
Occupational vitiligo (p. 72)	Symmetrical pigment loss on face and hands	Substituted phenols or catechols in oils, at coking plant
Tar keratoses (Fig. 6)	Small keratotic warts on face/hand, premalignant	Tar and pitch, e.g. road work or coking plant: UV is co-carcinogen
Vibration white finger	Blanching and pain in digits, later swelling and impaired fine movement	Handheld vibrating tools, as used by rock drillers or chainsaw operators

Table 2 **Contact dermatitis hazards in selected occupations**		
Occupation	**Irritants**	**Allergens**
Bakers	Flour, detergent, sugar, enzymes	Flavouring, oil, antioxidant
Building trade workers	Cement, glass wool, acid, preservatives	Cement (Cr, Co), rubber, resin, wood
Caterers, cooks	Meat, fish, fruit, veg, detergent, water	Veg/fruit, cutlery (Ni), rubber gloves, spice
Cleaners	Detergent, solvent, water	Rubber gloves, nickel, fragrance
Dental personnel	Detergent, soap, acrylate, flux	Rubber, acrylate, fragrance, mercury
Electronics assemblers	Solder, solvent, fibreglass, acid	Cr, Co, Ni, acrylate, epoxy resin
Hairdressers	Shampoo, bleach, perm lotion, soap	Paraphenylenediamine dye, rubber, fragrance, thioglycolate
Metal workers	Cutting fluid, cleanser, solvent	Preservative, Ni, Cr, Co, antioxidant
Office workers	Paper, fibreglass, dry atmosphere	Rubber, Ni, dye, glue, copying paper
Textile workers	Solvent, bleach, fibre, formaldehyde	Formaldehyde resin, dye, Ni
Veterinarians, farmers	Disinfectant, animal secretion	Rubber, antibiotics, plants, preservative

Case history 1

Hand dermatitis

A 17-year-old girl who had had childhood atopic eczema started as a hairdressing apprentice. Within 8 weeks, she developed hand dermatitis (Fig. 1) unresponsive to emollients and topical steroids. Patch testing was positive for ammonium thioglycolate (a permanent wave agent) and nickel. A diagnosis was made of contact dermatitis with irritant and allergic components, in an individual with underlying endogenous eczema. Her dermatitis cleared within weeks when she left hairdressing to work in an office.

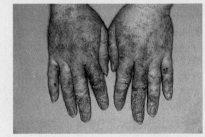

Fig. 1 **Hand dermatitis in a hairdresser.**

Differential diagnosis

Contact dermatitis due to non-occupational exposure and endogenous eczemas need considering. Often, occupational dermatitis is multifactorial, with irritants, allergens, endogenous factors and secondary bacterial infection all causally involved.

Management

Patch testing (p. 122) is required if there is exposure to known allergens. A factory visit helps to ascertain the exact nature of irritant or allergen exposure.

Once recognized, occupational exposure to a causative agent can be minimized, but this does not always produce an improvement. Chromate allergy is particularly intransigent. Any dermatitis is treated along standard lines with special attention to hand care. Barrier creams are of dubious value.

Contact urticaria

Some proteins and chemicals provoke immediate urticaria (p. 104). The release of mast cell histamine or other mediators may or may not be immunoglobulin (Ig)E mediated. Pruritus, erythema and whealing appear within minutes and last a few hours.

Occupational contacts include latex in rubber gloves, foods (e.g. fish, potato, eggs, flour, spices, meats and numerous fruits), *Myroxylon pereirae* (a perfume and flavouring agent) and animal saliva. Contact dermatitis may coexist.

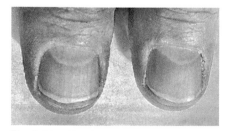

Fig. 4 **Blue discoloration of the nails due to argyria in a silver smelter.**

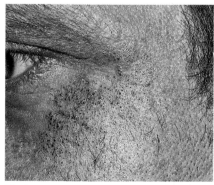

Fig. 5 **Chloracne showing comedones in a man exposed to dioxin contaminants.**

Case history 2

Chromate dermatitis

A 30-year-old man had been employed for 3 years making pipes out of cement. This involved exposure to wet cement. Despite him wearing gloves and overalls, he developed dermatitis on the hands (Fig. 2), arms and lower legs. Patch testing showed chromate allergy. He received compensation for having an industrial disease but, despite changing his occupation to driving, he continued to have hand dermatitis.

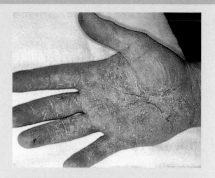

Fig. 2 **Hand dermatitis in a cement worker.**

Case history 3

Contact urticaria

A 40-year-old female nurse gave a 12-month history of itching, swelling and redness on her hands (Fig. 3), which developed within minutes of wearing disposable latex gloves. Patch testing was negative, but a prick test was positive for latex (confirmed by specific IgE test). Her symptoms resolved when she changed to polyvinyl chloride gloves. Provision of non-powdered latex or nitrile gloves to healthcare workers may reduce the development of latex allergy.

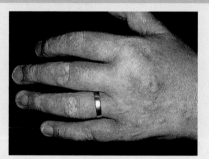

Fig. 3 **Contact urticaria to latex.**

Latex contact urticaria is a problem in healthcare workers and other occupations. Anaphylaxis may occur if there is a massive latex exposure, e.g. in a patient exposed to surgeon's gloves during abdominal surgery.

Prevention

Reducing the contact time between the skin and noxious substances is the aim. It is achieved by:

- improved work practices, e.g. increased automation

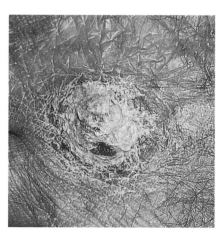

Fig. 6 **A tar keratosis in a coking plant worker.**

- substituting an alternative, e.g. nitrile gloves instead of rubber
- provision of protective clothing
- taking better care of the skin.

Recognizing an occupational disease may highlight faulty work practices that can be corrected. Compensation may be due.

Occupation and the skin

- **Occurrence:** industrial skin disease is common, especially contact dermatitis.

- **Causation:** occupational contact dermatitis is caused more by irritants than allergens but is often multifactorial, with endogenous factors frequently being engaged in addition.

- **Predisposition:** previous atopic eczema predisposes to occupational contact dermatitis.

- **Patch testing:** can help identify an allergen, e.g. chromate or rubber chemicals.

- **Contact urticaria** to latex is a risk in healthcare workers and other occupations.

- **Prevention:** occupational skin disease is minimized by reducing the contact time of noxious agents with the skin and by increasing awareness of the problem.

http://www.nsc.gov.sg/cgi-bin/WB_ContentGen.pl?id=169 ■ http://hse.gov.uk/pubns/ms24.pdf

Immunological tests

Clinical and laboratory tests of an immunological nature are valuable in the diagnosis and management of certain skin diseases. Patch tests are helpful in the investigation of *contact dermatitis*, serum immunoglobulin (Ig)E tests or prick tests are sometimes of use in *atopic disease*, and immunofluorescent studies on biopsied skin (or on serum) are essential in the diagnosis of *bullous disorders* and in some other conditions such as connective tissue diseases (e.g. lupus erythematosus) or vasculitis.

Prick tests

Prick testing detects *immediate (type I) hypersensitivity*. The reaction is mediated by the antigen-triggered IgE-mediated release of vasoactive substances from skin mast cells (p. 11). Small drops of commercially prepared antigen solutions are placed on marked areas on the forearm and lightly pricked into the skin using separate blunt lancets. The epidermis is punctured by gently pressing the blunt lancet in a horizontal manner onto the skin surface through the test solution. The sites are inspected at 15 min, and a positive result is regarded, by convention, as one showing a wheal of 4 mm or greater (Fig. 1). Patients should have stopped antihistamines 48 h before the test. Prick tests are used, in atopic subjects, to demonstrate allergy to inhalants (e.g. house dust mite) or to foods (e.g. hen's egg or peanuts), and are positive in patients with contact urticaria to latex (p. 116). A positive test correlates well with a positive allergen-specific IgE test (usually an

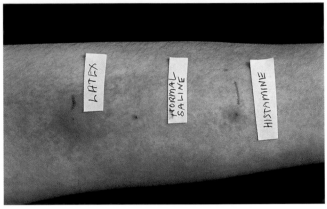

Fig. 1 **A positive prick test to latex is seen in a latex-allergic subject.** The wheal to histamine is shown as a positive control.

enzyme-linked immunosorbent assay (ELISA); the RAST (radioallergosorbent test) is no longer used). The risk of anaphylaxis is small, but resuscitation facilities, including adrenaline (epinephrine) for intramuscular injection and oxygen, are mandatory.

Patch testing

The epicutaneous patch test detects *cell-mediated (type IV) hypersensitivity* (p. 11). It is very helpful in the investigation of contact dermatitis. Commercially prepared allergens are available in the correct concentration for testing, usually in petrolatum (or sometimes water) as a diluent. Details of the procedure are shown in Figure 2.

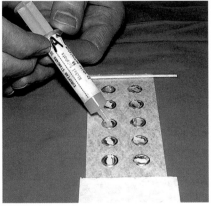

(a)

Fig. 2 **Patch testing methodology.**

(a) *Patch tests are prepared.*
Small amounts of the test substances are applied to the 8-mm-diameter aluminium discs on adhesive tape (Finn chambers) that are used for patch testing. The exact selection of test substances depends on the clinical problem, the site of the dermatitis, the environmental contacts and the patient's occupation.

(b) *Patch tests are applied.*
A 'standard series' of 35 substances is applied to every patient, with additional allergens as

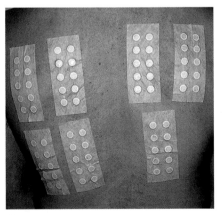

(b)

necessary. A record sheet is kept. The patches are fixed to the upper back, left on for 2 days and then removed after marking the top margin of each text strip with adhesive tape or with a marker pen.

(c) *Patch tests are read.*
Numerous *allergic-positive patch test sites* are shown. A positive allergic response is manifest by a localized eczema reaction, which is scored according to the following convention:

?+   doubtful: faint erythema only
+   weak: erythema, maybe papules

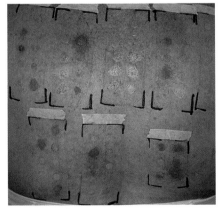

(c)

++   strong: vesicles, infiltration
+++   extreme: bullous
IR   irritant (of various types, but often showing a glazed circumscribed area, frequently with increased skin markings).

The test sites are read for a second time at 4 days, as positive reactions commonly do not appear until this time. The results are interpreted in the light of the clinical situation: a positive reaction is not always relevant to the current skin problem. Common allergens and their sources are shown on page 32.

Immunofluorescence

Immunofluorescence, either direct (on the patient's skin) or indirect (using the patient's serum reacted with an animal substrate) (Fig. 3), is helpful in making a diagnosis in the *autoimmune blistering diseases* (Table 1). Bullous disorders such as pemphigoid (Fig. 4) and pemphigus (Fig. 5) (p. 76) are characterized by the deposition of organ-specific autoantibodies (usually IgG) in the skin and, less easily demonstrated, by the presence of these autoantibodies in the serum. Dermatitis herpetiformis (Fig. 6) and other conditions such as leucocytoclastic vasculitis or lupus erythematosus often show the deposition of immunoglobulin or complement components in the patient's skin.

Table 1 Immunofluorescence in bullous disease		
Bullous disorder	Direct immuno-fluorescence (skin)	Indirect immuno-fluorescence (serum)
Bullous pemphigoid	Linear IgG/C3 at BMZ in 80%	Linear IgG at BMZ in 75% (IgA/IgM in 25%)
Pemphigus vulgaris	Intercellular epidermal IgG/C3 in 100% (IgA/IgM in 20%)	Intercellular IgG in 80% (the antibody titre reflects disease activity)
Dermatitis herpetiformis	Granular IgA deposition at dermal papilla (100%)	Absent
Linear IgA disease	Linear IgA at BMZ in 80% (IgG/IgM/C3 in 10%)	Linear IgA at BMZ found in some cases

BMZ, basement membrane zone.

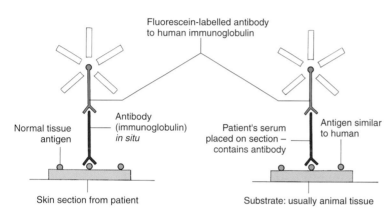

Direct immunofluorescence

Indirect immunofluorescence

Fluorescein-labelled antibody to human immunoglobulin

Normal tissue antigen

Antibody (immunoglobulin) *in situ*

Skin section from patient

Patient's serum placed on section – contains antibody

Antigen similar to human

Substrate: usually animal tissue

Fig. 3 **Immunofluorescence.** In *direct immunofluorescence*, usually done on perilesional skin, the antibodies or complement components are detected by reacting the freshly cut skin sections with an antibody directed against the specific immunoglobulin or complement fraction and labelled with a marker (usually fluorescein), which shows up when the section is examined under ultraviolet radiation. The *indirect method* is a two-step procedure that involves the use of cut sections of an animal substrate (e.g. monkey oesophagus) or human skin. The patient's diluted serum (containing the putative antibody) is placed on this section, incubated for an hour or so and then revealed using a fluorescein-tagged antihuman immunoglobulin antibody that is demonstrated by examining with ultraviolet radiation. Human skin, split at the dermoepidermal junction by saline incubation, may be used as a substrate to distinguish variants of pemphigoid, when deposition of the antibody on the epidermal or dermal side of the split can be diagnostic.

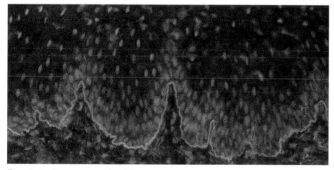

Fig. 4 **Bullous pemphigoid.** Indirect immunofluorescence demonstrates a linear band of IgG antibodies along the basement membrane zone (BMZ) using monkey oesophagus as substrate. These antibodies are directed against bullous pemphigoid antigens (MW 230 and 180 kDa), proteins located within the adhesion complex of the hemidesmosomes and synthesized by basal keratinocytes.

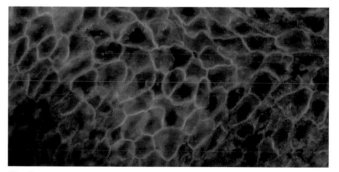

Fig. 5 **Pemphigus vulgaris.** Direct immunofluorescence demonstrates IgG antibodies, directed against desmoglein 3 (MW 130 kDa), a desmosomal cadherin involved in mediating epidermal intercellular adhesion, showing up in a chicken-wire pattern throughout the epidermis.

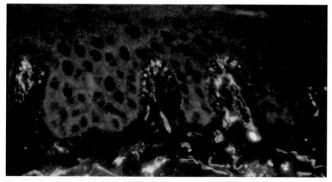

Fig. 6 **Dermatitis herpetiformis.** Direct immunofluorescence reveals the deposition of IgA in a granular pattern at the dermal papillae. This is diagnostic for dermatitis herpetiformis (p. 76), although it is unlikely that the eruption is solely due to the presence of this IgA.

Immunological tests

- **Prick tests** reveal type I (IgE-mediated) hypersensitivity and can demonstrate inhalant (e.g. house dust mite), food and latex allergies.

- **Patch tests** detect type IV (cell-mediated) hypersensitivity and are helpful in investigating contact dermatitis, e.g. in hand eczema.

- **Direct immunofluorescence** demonstrates immunoglobulin and complement deposition in the skin and is very useful in the diagnosis of bullous disorders, e.g. pemphigoid or pemphigus.

- **Indirect immunofluorescence** uses an animal substrate to detect antibodies in a patient's serum. It is often positive in pemphigus and pemphigoid, and sometimes in linear IgA disease, but is negative in dermatitis herpetiformis.

- **Autoantibodies in bullous pemphigoid (BP)** are against BP antigens of molecular weight (MW) 230 and 180 kDa and, in pemphigus vulgaris, against desmoglein 3 antigen (MW 130 kDa). The autoantigen, if any, in dermatitis herpetiformis is not currently known.

Dermatology and the Internet

The widespread availability of access to the Internet has had profound effects on dermatology. Doctors and students now have unlimited access to medical information, patients have readily available facts or opinions about their conditions, and both clinicians and patients have the possibility for remote consultation by 'teledermatology'.

The Internet as a library

Doctors in many countries have access to the Internet, which gives them an unrivalled and rapid entrée to the world's medical literature.

Databases. Searches can be made through databases such as PubMed (http://www.ncbi.nlm.nih.gov/entrez/query.fcgi) (Fig. 1) and online written information obtained through search engines such as Google (http://www.google.com/). Other useful resources are McKusick's catalogue of inherited diseases (http://www.ncbi.nlm.nih.gov/entrez/query.fcgi?db= OMIM) and a site concerned with cutaneous drug reactions (http://www.geocities.com/HotSprings/4809/Drugerup.htm).

Organizations. All the major dermatological organizations have their own websites that give practical details for clinicians and patients, e.g. the British Association of Dermatologists (http://www.bad.org.uk/), the European Academy of Dermatology and Venereology (http://www.eadv. org/) (Fig. 2) and the American Academy of Dermatology (http://www.aad.org/). Most large international institutions have their own websites, e.g. the World Health Organization (http://www.who.int/).

Education. There are websites specifically dedicated to education, such as emedicine (http://www.emedicine.com/ derm/contents.htm), MedlinePlus (http://www.nlm.nih.gov/ medlineplus/skindiseasesgeneral.html) (Fig. 3) and the New Zealand Dermatological Society (http://www.dermnet. org.nz/index.html). Other useful sites are an online atlas, e.g. the Dermatology Image Atlas (http://dermatlas.med.jhmi. edu/derm/) or a histopathology collection, e.g. the Bristol Biomedical Image Archive (http://www.brisbio.ac.uk/).

Evidence-based medicine. In an age when the clinician is called upon to defend his or her practice, it is useful to know that there are web pages dedicated to providing details and analysis on the true benefit or otherwise of many evaluable therapies. The Cochrane Skin Group's website (http://www. nottingham.ac.uk/~muzd/) and the National Library for Health (http://www.library.nhs.uk/skin) are invaluable resources.

Journals. Many journals are available online, often through a publisher's website, e.g. Synergy (http://www. blackwell-synergy.com/) provides the *British Journal of Dermatology*, and Nature (http://www.nature.com/jid/index. html) provides the *Journal of Investigative Dermatology*. *Archives of Dermatology* can be obtained at http://archderm. ama-assn.org/, *Dermatology in Practice* at http://www. dermatologyinpractice. co.uk/dip/current.asp and Elsevier journals at http://www.elsevier.com/wps/find/homepage.cws_ home. Often, only abstracts of articles are provided, although, for subscribers, a password will permit full access.

Guidelines. Clinicians in search of guidelines will find useful the web pages from the British Association of Dermatologists (http://www.bad.org.uk/healthcare/

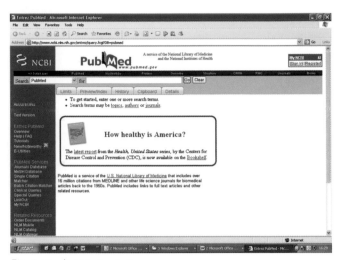

Fig. 1 **The PubMed website.**

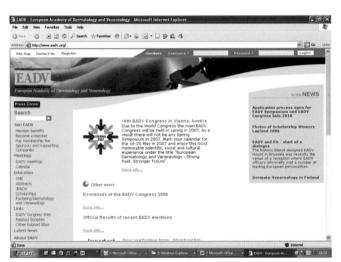

Fig. 2 **The website of the European Academy of Dermatology and Venereology.**

guidelines/) and from the National Institute for Health and Clinical Excellence (NICE; http://www.nice.org.uk/).

Links. Some web pages specialize in providing links to other resources, e.g. one hosted by Michigan State University (http://www.com.msu.edu/omi/greenejo/index2.html# Dermatology), the Hardin Library (http://www.lib.uiowa.edu/ hardin/md/derm.html.the) and the British Association of Dermatologists (http://www.bad.org.uk/links/rslinks.asp).

Resources for patients

Many patients are familiar with searching the Internet, and some find this useful, especially if they find material specifically written for the lay public. Unfortunately, the Internet is not regulated, and some of the information posted is unreliable. Nonetheless, a better informed clientele means that physicians have to be well briefed and able to discuss the pros and cons of suggested treatments.

Patient websites. Web pages designed for use by patients can be very informative. Good examples include DermIS (http://www.dermis.net/index_e.html) and ones from the

New Zealand Dermatological Society (http://www.dermnetnz.org/) and the American Academy of Dermatology (http://www.skincarephysicians.com/). MedlinePlus (see above) also has an excellent medical encyclopaedia for patients, and reliable information can be obtained at Yahoo Health (http://health.yahoo.com/).

Patient support groups. Many excellent web pages are available (p. 128). The Iowa University web page (http://tray.dermatology.uiowa.edu/SuprtGrps.html) contains a comprehensive list including groups for rare conditions. Several sites give fact sheets about skin conditions and their treatment. Worth a particular mention are those from the Skin Care Campaign (http://www.skincarecampaign.org/), which gives a comprehensive list of patient support organizations, the National Eczema Association (http://www.nationaleczema.org/home.html) (Fig. 4) and the Psoriasis Association (http://www.psoriasis-association.org.uk/).

Handouts. Certain web pages specifically produce handouts for patients, e.g. RxMed (http://www.rxmed.com/).

Teledermatology

Telemedicine is the practice of medicine remote from the patient using some form of electronic transfer via the Internet or a more secure computer network of clinical data such as a photograph. It is particularly suited to dermatology because of the visual nature of the specialty. A specialist dermatologist may not serve subjects living in remote regions away from large urban centres regularly.

Electronic image. An accurate diagnosis and a suggested management plan obtained from the specialist examining an image on a computer is an attractive concept. Digitally captured still ('store and forward') or videoconference photographs can be transmitted electronically to a dermatologist hundreds or even thousands of miles away for an opinion. A good-quality image of high resolution is vital.

Accuracy. Teledermatology has been evaluated, mostly using the 'store and forward' method, for patients living in remote regions and has been found to be a useful adjunct to clinical medicine. It can be an accurate method for differentiating between benign and

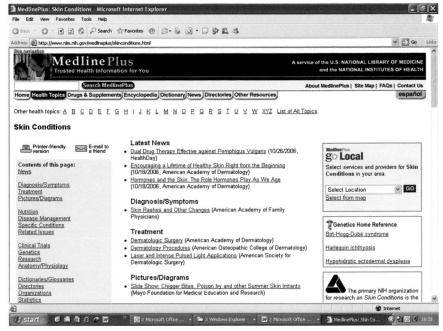

Fig. 3 **The MedlinePlus web page.**

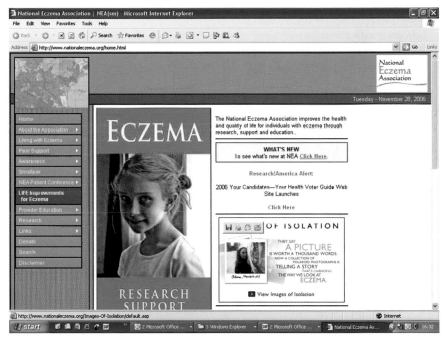

Fig. 4 **The website of the National Eczema Association.**

malignant skin lesions, but is not a substitute for face-to-face consultation, which should be available when indicated.

Dermatology and the Internet

- **Databases,** e.g. PubMed, are used to search for medical information.
- **Professional organizations,** e.g. the European Academy of Dermatology and Venereology, have web pages for use by clinicians and patients.
- **Educational resources** for students include MedlinePlus and the Dermatology Image Atlas.
- **Evidence-based dermatology** is accessed via the Cochrane Skin Group's web page.
- **Online journals** are obtained via the publishers' websites.
- **Guidelines** can be viewed, e.g. from NICE or the British Association of Dermatologists.
- **Patient support groups** have numerous web pages, e.g. Skin Care Campaign.
- **Teledermatology** may be of value for skin problems that occur in people who live in remote areas.

Bibliography

Many medical students and qualified health professionals like to have suggestions for further reading. Recommended references are given mainly in the form of recently published books. Journal papers are offered where appropriate, mostly in widely available periodicals.

Microanatomy, derivatives, physiology and biochemistry of the skin

Archer C B 2004 *Functions of the Skin* (ch. 4). In: Burns T, Breathnach S, Cox B, Griffiths C (eds) *Textbook of Dermatology*, 7th edn. Blackwell Publishing, Oxford.

Forslind B, Lindberg M (eds) 2004 *Skin, Hair, and Nails: Structure and Function*. Marcel Dekker, New York.

Hori Y, Hearing V J, Nakayama J 1996 *Melanogenesis and Malignant Melanoma: Biochemistry, Cell Biology, Molecular Biology, Pathophysiology, Diagnosis and Treatment*. Elsevier Science, Amsterdam.

Immunology of the skin

Roitt I, Brostoff J, Male D 2002 *Immunology*, 6th edn. Mosby, London.

Molecular genetics and the skin

Mueller R F, Young I D 2001 *Emery's Elements of Medical Genetics*, 11th edn. Churchill Livingstone, Edinburgh.

Terminology of skin lesions, taking a history and examining the skin

Cox NH, White GM 2006 *Diseases of the Skin: a Color Atlas and Text*, 2nd edn. Mosby, London.

Stolz W, Landthaler M, Braun Falco O, Cognetta AB, Bilek P (eds) 2002 *Color Atlas of Dermatoscopy*, 2nd edn. Blackwell, Oxford.

White GM 2004 *Color Atlas of Dermatology*, 3rd edn. Mosby, Edinburgh.

Basics of medical therapy

Lebwohl M G, Heymann W R, Berth-Jones J, Coulson I 2006 *Treatment of Skin Disease*, 2nd edn. Mosby, London.

Shelley W B, Shelley B 2001 *Advanced Dermatologic Therapy*, 2nd edn. WB Saunders, Philadelphia.

Williams H, Bigby M, Diepgen T, Herxheimer A, Naldi L, Rzany B 2003 *Evidence Based Dermatology*. BMJ Books, London.

Epidemiology of skin disease

Parish L C, Millikan L E (eds) 1994 *Global Dermatology: Diagnosis and Management According to Geography, Climate and Culture*. Springer, Berlin.

William H C 1997 *Dermatology: Health Care Needs Assessment*. Radcliffe Medical Press, Oxford.

Body image, the psyche and the skin

Thiers BH, Gupta MA 2005 *Psychocutaneous Disease*. Dermatologic Clinics. WB Saunders, Philadelphia.

Psoriasis

Davison S, Barker J, Poyner T 2000 *Pocket Guide to Psoriasis*. Blackwell, Oxford.

Camisa C 2005 *Handbook of Psoriasis*, 2nd edn. Blackwell Publishing, Oxford.

The eczemas

Frosch P J, Menné T, Lepoittevin J P 2006 *Contact Dermatitis*, 4th edn. Springer, Berlin.

Holden C, Ostlere L 2000 *Pocket Guide to Eczema and Contact Dermatitis*. Blackwell, Oxford.

Reitamo S, Luger TA 2006 *Textbook of Atopic Dermatitis*. Taylor & Francis, Abingdon.

Lichenoid eruptions

Boyd A S, Neldner K H 1991 Lichen planus. *J Am Acad Dermatol* 25: 593–619.

Papulosquamous eruptions

Kempf W, Burg G 2000 Pityriasis rosea – a virus-induced skin disease? An update. *Arch Virol* 145: 1509–1520.

Erythroderma

Rothe M J, Bialy T L, Grant-Kels J M 2000 Erythroderma. *Dermatol Clin* 18: 405–415.

Photodermatology

Elder G H, Hift R J, Meissner P N 1997 The acute porphyrias. *Lancet* 349: 1613–1617.

Ferguson J, Dover JS 2006 *Photodermatology*. Manson, London.

Bacterial, viral and fungal infections

Anaissie E, McGinnis M R, Pfaller M A 2000 *Clinical Mycology*. Churchill Livingstone, Edinburgh.

Bisno A L, Stevens D L 1996 Streptococcal infections of skin and soft tissue. *N Engl J Med* 334: 240–245.

Richardson M, Johnson E 2006 *Pocket Guide to Fungal Infection*, 2nd edn. Blackwell, Oxford.

Syrjanen K J, Syrjanen S M 2000. *Papillomavirus Infection in Human Pathology*. John Wiley, New York.

HIV disease and immunodeficiency syndromes

Alcamo E 2001 *A Primer on AIDS*. Blackwell, Boston.

Tropical infections and infestations

Tyring S, Lupi O, Hengge U 2005 *Tropical Dermatology*. Churchill Livingstone, Edinburgh.

Infestations

Chosidow O 2000 Scabies and pediculosis. *Lancet* 355: 819–826.

Sebaceous and sweat gland disorders

Darvey A, Chu A 2000 *Pocket Guide to Acne*. Blackwell, Oxford.

Marks R 2006 *Facial Skin Disorders*. Taylor & Francis, Abingdon.

Mortimer P S, Lunniss P J 1999 Hidradenitis suppurativa. *J Roy Soc Med* 93: 420–422.

Disorders of hair

Dawber R, van Neste D 2004 *Hair and Scalp Disorders*. Taylor & Francis, Abingdon.

Disorders of nails

Scher R K, Daniel C R 2005 *Nails: Diagnosis, Therapy, Surgery*. WB Saunders, Philadelphia.

Vascular and lymphatic diseases and leg ulcers

Grey J, Harding K (eds) 2005 *ABC of Wound Healing*. BMJ Books, London.

Wasser M, Suen J V 1999 *Hemangiomas and Vascular Malformations of the Head and Neck.* John Wiley, New York.

Pigmentation

Nordlund J, Boissy R, Hearing V, King R, Oetting W, Ortonne JP (eds) 2006 *The Pigmentary System,* 2nd edn. Blackwell Publishing, Oxford.

Urticaria and angioedema

Greaves M W, Kaplan A P (eds) 2004 *Urticaria and Angioedema.* Marcel Dekker, New York.

Blistering disorders

Chan L 2006 *Blistering Skin Disease.* Manson, London.

Connective tissue diseases

Morrow J, Nelson J L, Watts R, Isenberg D 1999 *Autoimmune Rheumatic Diseases.* Oxford University Press, Oxford.

Vasculitis and the reactive erythemas

Ball E, Bridges S L (eds) 2001 *Vasculitis.* Oxford University Press, Oxford.

Skin changes in internal medicine

Callen J P, Jorizzo J L, Bologna J L, Piette W, Zone J J 2003 *Dermatological Signs of Internal Disease.* WB Saunders, Philadelphia.

Drug eruptions

Gruchalla G, Gruchalla R 2006 *Drug-Induced Skin Disease.* Marcel Dekker, New York.

Association with malignancy

Provost T T, Flynn J A 2000 *Cutaneous Medicine.* BC Decker, London.

Inherited keratinization, blistering, neurocutaneous and other syndromes

Spritz J L 2005 *Genodermatoses,* 2nd edn. Lippincott Williams & Wilkins, Philadelphia.

Benign tumours and naevi

Schaffer J V, Bolognia J L 2000 The clinical spectrum of pigmented lesions. *Clin Plast Surg* 27: 391–408.

Malignant melanoma

National Collaborative Centre for Cancer 2006 *Improving Outcomes for People with Skin Tumours Including Melanoma.* National Institute for Health and Clinical Excellence, London.

Thompson J F, Morton D L, Kroon B B R 2004 *Textbook of Melanoma.* Martin Dunitz, London.

Malignant epidermal and dermal tumours and premalignant epidermal disorders

Rigel P S, Friedman R, Dzubow L M, Reintgen D S, Bystryn J C, Marks R 2005 *Cancer of the Skin.* WB Saunders, Philadelphia.

Ultraviolet radiation and the skin

Gilchrest B (ed) 1995 *Photodamage.* Blackwell, Boston.

Zanolli M D, Feldman S 2004 *Phototherapy Treatment Protocols for Psoriasis and Other Skin Diseases.* Parthenon Publishing, New York.

Cosmetics

Baran R, Maibach HI 2004 *Textbook of Cosmetic Dermatology,* 3rd edn. Taylor & Francis, New York.

Basic dermatological surgery

Burge S, Colver G, Lester R 1996 *Simple Skin Surgery,* 2nd edn. Blackwell, Oxford.

Dawber R, Colver G, Jackson A 1998 *Cutaneous Cryosurgery: Principles and Clinical Practice,* 2nd edn. Martin Dunitz, London.

Lanigan S W 2000 *Lasers in Dermatology.* Springer, Berlin.

Thiers B H, Brown M D 2005 *Advanced Surgical Techniques.* Dermatologic Clinics. WB Saunders, Philadelphia.

New trends in dermatological treatment

James W D, Cockerell C J, Maloney M, Paller A S 2005 *Advances in Dermatology.* Mosby, St Louis.

Malignant melanoma
Smith C H, Anstey A V, Barker J N et al. 2005 British Association of Dermatologists' guidelines for use of biological interventions in psoriasis 2005. *Br J Dermatol* 153(3): 486–497.

Wakelin S H 2002 *A Handbook of Systemic Drug Treatment in Dermatology.* Manson, London.

Paediatric dermatology

Harper J, Oranje A, Prose N (eds) 2005 *Textbook of Pediatric Dermatology,* 2nd edn. Blackwell Publishing, Oxford.

Eichenfield L F, Frieden I J, Esterly N B 2001 *Textbook of Neonatal Dermatology.* WB Saunders, Philadelphia.

The skin in old age

Zylicz Z, Twycross R, Jones E A 2004 *Pruritus in Advanced Disease.* Oxford University Press, Oxford.

Genitourinary medicine

Black M M, McKay M, Braude P R, Vaughn-Jones S 2002 *Obstetric and Gynecologic Dermatology,* 2nd edn. Mosby, St Louis.

Bunker C B 2004 *Male Genital Skin Disease.* WB Saunders, Philadelphia.

Racially pigmented skin

Johnson B L, Moy R L, White G M 1998 *Ethnic Skin Medical Surgical.* Mosby, St Louis.

Occupation and the skin

English J S C (ed) 1999 *A Colour Handbook of Occupational Dermatology.* Manson, London.

Kanerva L, Elsner P, Wahlberg J E, Maibach H I (eds) 2000 *Handbook of Occupational Dermatology.* Springer, Berlin.

Immunological tests

Kalaaji A N, Nicolas M E O 2006 *Mayo Clinic Atlas of Immunofluorescence in Dermatology.* Taylor & Francis, New York.

Dermatology and the Internet

Rigel D 2003 *Dermatology – an Internet Resource Guide.* Medical Economics Co., New Jersey.

Self-help groups

Patients with skin disease, especially those with a chronic condition, often find it helpful to meet and speak to others with the same problem. *Patient help groups (known as patient advocate groups in the USA) fulfil a particular need by helping the patient to come to terms with his or her condition, by informing the patient through meetings and publications of advances in treatments and benefits that may be available to them, and by providing support through difficult times. Several of them are also actively engaged in fundraising to support research and are involved in advancing their cause, and that of dermatology generally, in the local and national media. The addresses of some of the patient help groups, and of other organizations that are of service to those with skin problems, are given here. In the UK, details of support groups can be obtained through the Skin Care Campaign (details below); in the USA, through the Coalition of Skin Diseases, PO Box 418, Mt. Freedom, NJ 07970-0418 (email: kball@ sturge-weber.com).

Acne

Acne Support Group
PO Box 9
Newquay TR9 6WG
Web: www.stopspots.org

All skin disorders

Skin Care Campaign
163 Eversholt Street
London NW1 1BU
Web: www.skincarecampaign.
org

Inflammatory Skin Disease Institute
PO Box 1074
Newport News, VA 23601,
USA
Web: www.isdionline.org

Allergy

Allergy UK
3 White Oak Square
London Road
Swanley BR8 7AG
Web: www.allergyuk.org

Alopecia

Alopecia UK
5 Titchwell Road
London SW18 3LW
Web: www.alopeciaonline.
org.uk

National Alopecia Areata Foundation
14 Mitchell Boulevard
San Rafael, CA 94903, USA
Web: www.naaf.org

Camouflage

British Red Cross
4 Nasmith Place
Glasgow G52 4PR
Web: www.redcross.org.uk

Cutaneous lymphoma

Lymphoma Association
PO Box 386
Aylesbury HP20 2GA
Web: www.lymphoma.org.uk

Cutaneous Lymphoma Foundation
PO Box 374
Birmingham, MI 48102, USA
Web: www.clfoundation.org

Darier's disease

Darier's Disease Support Group
29 St Annes Road
Hakin
Milford Haven SA73 3LQ
Web: www.dariers.co.nr

Dermatitis herpetiformis

Gluten Intolerance Group
15110 10th Avenue SW,
Suite A
Seattle, WA 98166, USA
Web: www.gluten.net

Dermatomyositis

Dermatomyositis and Polymyositis Support Group
146 Newtown Road
Southampton SO19 9HR
Web: www.myositis.org.uk

Ectodermal dysplasia

Ectodermal Dysplasia Society
108 Charlton Lane
Cheltenham GL53 9EA
Web: www.
ectodermaldysplasia.org

National Foundation for Ectodermal Dysplasias
410 E. Main Street
Mascoutah, IL 62258, USA
Web: www.nfed.org

Eczema

National Eczema Society
Hill House
Highgate Hill
London N19 5NA
Web: www.eczema.org

National Eczema Association for Science and Education
4460 Redwood Hwy, Suite 16D
San Rafael, CA 94903, USA
Web: www.nationaleczema.
org

Ehlers–Danlos syndrome

Ehlers–Danlos Support Group
PO Box 337
Aldershot GU12 6WZ
Web: www.ehlers-danlos.org

Ehlers–Danlos National Foundation
3200 Wilshire Blvd, Ste 1601
Los Angeles, CA 90010, USA
Web: www.ednf.org

Epidermolysis bullosa

Dystrophic Epidermolysis Bullosa Research Association
13 Wellington Business Park
Crowthorne RG45 6LS
Web: www.debra.org.uk

DebRA of America, Inc.
5 West 36th Street, Suite 404
New York, NY 10018, USA
Web: www.debra.org

Facial disfigurement

Changing Faces
33–37 University Street
London WC1E 6JN
Web: www.changingfaces.org.
uk

Herpes virus

Herpes Viruses Association
41 North Road
London N7 9DP
Web: www.herpes.org.uk

HIV infection

Terrence Higgins Trust
314–320 Gray's Inn Road
London WC1X 8DP
Web: www.tht.org.uk

Ichthyosis

Ichthyosis Support Group
PO Box 9213
Reading RG6 4ZQ
Web: www.ichthyosis.org.uk

Foundation for Ichthyosis and Related Skin Types
1601 S. Valley Forge Road
Lansdale, PA 19446, USA
Web: www.scalyskin.org

Latex allergy

The Latex Allergy Support Group
PO Box 27
Filey YO14 9YH
Web: www.lasg.co.uk

Leprosy

LEPRA – The British Leprosy Relief Association
Fairfax House
Causton Road
Colchester CO1 1PU
Web: www.lepra.org.uk

Lichen sclerosus

National Lichen Sclerosus Support Group
PO Box 5830
Lyme Regis DT7 3ZU
Web: www.lichensclerosus.org

Lupus erythematosus

LUPUS UK
St James House
Eastern Road
Romford RM1 3NH
Web: www.lupusuk.org.uk

Lupus Foundation of America, Inc.
1300 Piccard Drive, Suite 200
Rockville, MD 20850-4303, USA
Web: www.lupus.org

Melanocytic naevi

Congenital Melanocytic Naevus Support Group
Bridge Chapel Centre
Heath Road
Liverpool L19 4XR
Web: www.caringmattersnow.co.uk

Nevus Outreach, Inc.
616 Alpha Street
Lansing, MI 48910, USA
Web: www.nevus.org

Neurofibromatosis

Neurofibromatosis Association
Quayside House
8 High Street
Kingston upon Thames
Surrey KT1 1HL
Web: www.nfauk.org

Pemphigus

Pemphigus Vulgaris Network
26 St Germans Road
London SE23 1RJ
Web: www.pemphigus.org.uk

International Pemphigus Foundation
1540 River Park Drive, Suite 208
Sacramento, CA 95818, USA
Web: www.pcmphigus.org

Porphyria

American Porphyria Foundation
PO Box 22712
Houston, TX 77227, USA
Web: www.porphyriafoundation.com

Pseudoxanthoma elasticum

Pseudoxanthoma Elasticum (PXE) Support Group
15 Mead Close
Marlow SL7 1HR
Web: www.pxe.org.uk

National Association for Pseudoxanthoma Elasticum
4301 Connecticut Avenue
Washington, DC 20008, USA
Web: www.pxe.org

Psoriasis

Psoriasis Association
7 Milton Street
Northampton NN2 7JG
Web: www.psoriasis-association.org.uk

Psoriatic Arthropathy Alliance
PO Box 111
St Albans AL2 3JQ
Web: www.thepaa.org

National Psoriasis Foundation
6600 SW 92nd, Suite 300
Portland, OR 97223, USA
Web: www.psoriasis.org

Raynaud's disease and scleroderma

Raynaud's and Scleroderma Association Trust
112 Crewe Road
Alsager ST7 2JA
Web: www.raynauds.org.uk

Scleroderma Foundation
89 Newbury Street, Suite 201
Danvers, MA 01923-1075, USA
Web: www.scleroderma.org

Skin cancer

British Association of Cancer United Patients (Cancerbackup)
3 Bath Place
London EC2A 3JR
Web: www.cancerbackup.org.uk

Skin Cancer Information Network MARC'S LINE (Melanoma and Related Cancers of the Skin)
Dermatology Treatment Centre
Salisbury District Hospital
Salisbury SP2 8BJ
Web: www.wessexcancer.org

Basal Cell Carcinoma Nevus Syndrome/Gorlin Syndrome
BCCNS Life Support Network
PO Box 321
Burton, OH 44021, USA
Web: www.bccns.org

Tuberous sclerosis

Tuberous Sclerosis Association
PO Box 12979
Barnt Green
Birmingham B45 5AN
Web: www.tuberous-sclerosis.org

Tuberose Sclerosis Alliance
801 Roeder Road, Suite 750,
Silver Spring, MD 20910, USA
Web: www.tsalliance.org

Vitiligo

Vitiligo Society
125 Kennington Road
London SE11 6SF
Web: www.vitiligosociety.org.uk

Vitiligo Support International, Inc.
PO Box 4008
Valley Village, CA 91617, USA
Web: www.VitiligoSupport.org

Vulval disorders

National Vulvodynia Association
PO Box 4491
Silver Spring, MD 20914, USA
Web: www.nva.org

Xeroderma pigmentosum

Xeroderma Pigmentosum Society
437 Snydertown Road
Craryville, NY 12521, USA
Web: www.xps.org

Index